RADIOLOGY

CASE REVIEW SERIES | Brain Imaging

RADIOLOGY

CASE REVIEW SERIES | Brain Imaging

Chang Yueh Ho, MD

Assistant Professor of Clinical Radiology
Director of Pediatric Neuroimaging
Riley Hospital for Children at IU Health
Indiana University School of Medicine
Indianapolis, Indiana

Rocky Saenz, DO, FAOCR

Vice-Chairman, Botsford Department of Radiology
Director of MRI, Botsford Hospital
Clinical Faculty, Michigan State University
Farmington Hills, Michigan

SERIES EDITOR

Roland Talanow, MD, PhD

President
Department of Radiology Education
Radiopolis, a subdivision of InnoMed, LLC
Stateline, Nevada

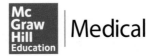

New York   Chicago   San Francisco   Athens   London
Madrid   Mexico City   Milan   New Delhi   Singapore
Sydney   Toronto

Radiology Case Review Series: Brain Imaging

1 2 3 4 5 6 7 8 9 0   CTP/CTP   19 18 17 16 15

ISBN 978-0-07-182691-4
MHID 0-07-182691-2

This book was set in Times LT Std. by Thomson Digital.
The editors were Michael Weitz and Brian Kearns.
The production supervisor was Richard Ruzycka.
Project management was provided by Sarita Yadav, Thomson Digital.
China Translation & Printing Services, Ltd., was printer and binder.

This book is printed on acid-free paper.

Library of Congress Cataloging-in-Publication Data
Brain imaging / editors, Chang Yueh Ho, Rocky Saenz.
    p. ; cm. — (Radiology case review series)
  Includes bibliographical references and index.
  ISBN 978-0-07-182691-4 (pbk.) — ISBN 0-07-182691-2 (pbk.)
  I. Ho, Chang Yueh, editor. II. Saenz, Rocky, 1973- , editor. III. Series: Radiology case review series.
  [DNLM: 1. Neuroimaging—Case Reports. 2. Neuroimaging—Problems and Exercises.
3. Central Nervous System Diseases—diagnosis—Case Reports. 4. Central Nervous System Diseases—diagnosis—Problems and Exercises. WL 18.2]
  RC386.6.M34
  616.8'047548—dc23
                                                                            2015009958

To my family, especially my wife Angel and my daughters,
as well as good friends in the work and church communities:
You keep me grounded, supported,
and focused on the most important relationships in life.
— Chang Yueh Ho, MD

First, I would like to thank Roland Talanow, as the mastermind
behind this case review series and its larger online component.
I would also like to give special thanks to my coauthor Chang Ho
for his dedication and brilliance in making this book
the quality project that it is. Next, I would like to thank my
residents Sharon Kreuer and Deeshali Patel-Shah for contributing cases.
Lastly and most importantly, I thank my mother Angelita, wife Blanca,
and sons Rocky, Russell, Ronin, and Rex. Without my strong family support,
I would not be able to complete this academic project or any
of my other creative works.
— Rocky Saenz, DO

Contents

Series Preface

Maybe I have an obsession for cases, but when I was a radiology resident I loved to learn especially from cases, not only because they are short, exciting, and fun—similar to a detective story in which the aim is to get to "the bottom" of the case—but also because, in the end, that's what radiologists are faced with during their daily work. Since medical school, I have been fascinated with learning, not only for my own benefit but also for the sake of teaching others, and I have enjoyed combining my IT skills with my growing knowledge to develop programs that help others in their learning process. Later, during my radiology residency, my passion for case-based learning grew to a level where the idea was born to create a case-based journal: integrating new concepts and technologies that aid in the traditional learning process. Only a few years later, the *Journal of Radiology Case Reports* became an internationally popular and PubMed indexed radiology journal—popular not only because of the interactive features but also because of the case-based approach. This led me to the next step: why not tackle something that I especially admired during my residency but that could be improved—creating a new interactive case-based review series. I imagined a book series that would take into account new developments in teaching and technology and changes in the examination process.

As did most other radiology residents, I loved the traditional case review books, especially for preparation for the boards. These books are quick and fun to read and focus in a condensed way on material that will be examined in the final boards. However, nothing is perfect and these traditional case review books had their own intrinsic flaws. The authors and I have tried to learn from our experience by putting the good things into this new book series but omitting the bad parts and exchanging them with innovative features.

What are the features that distinguish this series from traditional series of review books?

To save space, traditional review books provide two cases on one page. This requires the reader to turn the page to read the answer for the first case but could lead to unintentional "cheating" by seeing also the answer of the second case. Doesn't this defeat the purpose of a review book? From my own authoring experience on the *USMLE Help* book series, it was well appreciated that we avoided such accidental cheating by separating one case from the other. Taking the positive experience from that book series, we decided that each case in this series should consist of two pages: page 1 with images and questions and page 2 with the answers and explanations. This approach avoids unintentional peeking at the answers before deciding on the correct answers yourself. We keep it strict: one case per page! This way it remains up to your own knowledge to figure out the right answer.

Another example that residents (including me) did miss in traditional case review books is that these books did not highlight the pertinent findings on the images: sometimes, even looking at the images as a group of residents, we could not find the abnormality. This is not only frustrating but also time-consuming. When you prepare for the boards, you want to use your time as efficiently as possible. Why not show annotated images? We tackled that challenge by providing, on the second page of each case, the same images with annotations or additional images that highlight the findings.

When you are preparing for the boards and managing your clinical duties, time is a luxury that becomes even more precious. Does the resident preparing for the boards truly need lengthy discussions as in a typical textbook? Or does the resident rather want a "rapid fire" mode in which he or she can "fly" through as many cases as possible in the shortest possible time? This is the reality when you start your work after the boards! Part of our concept with the new series is providing short "pearls" instead of lengthy discussions. The reader can easily read and memorize these "pearls."

Another challenge in traditional books is that questions are asked on the first page and no direct answer is provided, only a lengthy block of discussion. Again, this might become time-consuming to find the right spot where the answer is located if you have doubts about one of several answer choices. Remember: time is money—and life! Therefore, we decided to provide explanations to *each* individual question, so that the reader knows exactly where to find the right answer to the right question. Questions are phrased in an intuitive way so that they fit not only the print version but also the multiple-choice questions for that particular case in our online version. This system enables you to move back and forth between the print version and the online version.

In addition, we have provided up to 3 references for each case. This case review is not intended to replace traditional textbooks. Instead, it is intended to reiterate and strengthen your already existing knowledge (from your training) and to fill potential gaps in your knowledge.

However, in a collaborative effort with the *Journal of Radiology Case Reports* and the international radiology community Radiolopolis, we have developed an online repository with more comprehensive information for each case, such as demographics, discussions, more image examples, interactive image stacks with scroll, a window/level feature, and other interactive features that almost resemble a workstation. In addition, we are planning ahead toward the new Radiology Boards format and are providing rapid fire online sessions and mock examinations that use the cases in the print version. Each case in the print version is crosslinked to the online version using a case ID. The case ID number appears to the right of the diagnosis heading at the top of the second page of each case. Each case can be accessed using the case ID number at the following web site: www.radiologycasereviews.com/case/ID, in which "ID" represents the case ID number. If you have any questions regarding this web site, please e-mail the series editor directly at roland@talanow.info.

I am particularly proud of such a symbiotic endeavor of print and interactive online education and I am grateful to McGraw-Hill for giving me and the authors the opportunity to provide such a unique and innovative method of radiology education, which, in my opinion, may be a trendsetter.

The primary audience of this book series is the radiology resident, particularly the resident in the final year who is preparing for the radiology boards. However, each book in

this series is structured on difficulty levels so that the series also becomes useful to an audience with limited experience in radiology (nonradiologist physicians or medical students) up to subspecialty-trained radiologists who are preparing for their CAQs or who just want to refresh their knowledge and use this series as a reference.

I am delighted to have such an excellent team of US and international educators as authors on this innovative book series. These authors have been thoroughly evaluated and selected based on their excellent contributions to the *Journal of Radiology Case Reports*, the Radiolopolis community, and other academic and scientific accomplishments.

It brings especially personal satisfaction to me that this project has enabled each author to be involved in the overall decision-making process and improvements regarding the print and online content. This makes each participant not only an author but also part of a great radiology product that will appeal to many readers.

Finally, I hope you will experience this case review book as it is intended to be: a quick, pertinent, "get to the point" radiology case review that provides essential information for the radiology boards in the shortest time available, which, in the end, is crucial for preparation for the boards.

Roland Talanow, MD, PhD

Preface

"Whatever good things we build end up building us."

—Jim Rohn

Countless hours upon hours were poured into the writing and image editing by my coauthor and me, which we hope ultimately benefits you, the reader. And yet the experience in the building of this book has already greatly benefited me as an educator in a field that I am passionate about: neuroradiology. Those of you familiar with teaching know that the teacher either gains or solidifies knowledge while preparing to teach. This has certainly been the case in writing this book for me.

We were ambitious for this book in that we did not want to only offer the usual format for a case review book. In addition to neuroradiology cases with probing questions and detailed but concise answers organized in easy, medium, and hard categories, we also wanted a practical reference book that showed a wide variety of cases organized by anatomy with practical pearls that help summarize the salient points. Most reference books are organized such that a radiologist must already have a relatively accurate differential diagnosis when considering abnormal imaging findings. The reference is then checked against the radiologist's best educated guess for the top pathologies in the differential, requiring significant preexisting knowledge and experience. In contrast, by using the index, and also because the cases are organized anatomically, it is our hope that this book can be a helpful, efficient tool at the workstation by comparing the real-time abnormal findings with the book cases that demonstrate a classic appearance of pathology, when possible. While the pure randomness and potpourri style of the prior board format is lost, we believe the systematic organization by anatomy will help solidify learning not by filling in holes from random chance, but by supporting anatomy-based learning which will in turn improve performance on the newer boards' format. It is our hope that this book is useful for both trainees just learning neuroradiology and more experienced practitioners.

Finally, I would like to thank Roland Talanow for the opportunity to author this book, and his creation of an efficient and easy-to-use authoring system; Rocky Saenz, my coauthor, for his shared dedication and input, who worked in the trenches with me despite being a whole state away; and Nucharin "Tanya" Supakul for her hard work and help in creating case material, particularly her desire to educate in pediatric neuroradiology. Most of all, I give much thanks and love to my wife, Angel, for her support and care of our young children while I was sequestered in front of a computer typing away like a madman. Without her this would not have been possible.

I hope you find this book useful and a treasure.

Chang Yueh Ho, MD

RADIOLOGY

CASE REVIEW SERIES | Brain Imaging

43-year-old male with progressive ataxia, and swallowing and balance difficulty

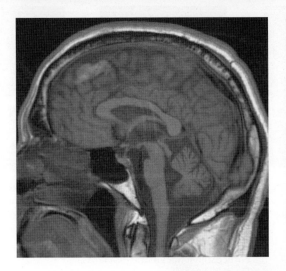 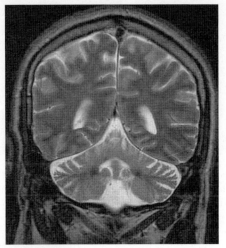

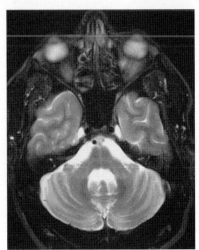

1. What are the described MRI findings for this disease?

2. What are the differential diagnoses for this finding?

3. What is the cause of hot cross bun sign?

4. What is a pathologic hallmark of multisystem atrophy?

5. What is the clinical presentation for this disease?

Case ranking/difficulty:

Category: Intra-axial infratentorial

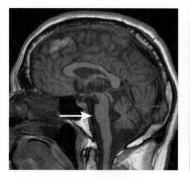

Sagittal T1 shows flattening of the pons *(white arrow)* and enlargement of the vermian folia *(red arrow)* from pontine and cerebellar atrophy.

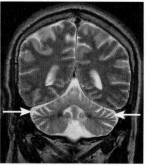

Coronal T2 shows prominence of the cerebellar folia from diffuse atrophy *(white arrows)*.

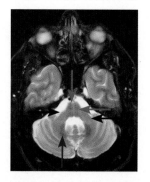

Axial T2 shows middle cerebellar peduncle atrophy *(black arrows)* and cruciate hyperintensity of the transverse pontocerebellar fibers *(red arrows)* with sparing of the corticospinal tract in the "hot cross bun" sign. There is decreased signal of the dentate nuclei *(blue arrow)* described with multisystem atrophy. Pontine atrophy with associated enlarged fourth ventricle is again noted.

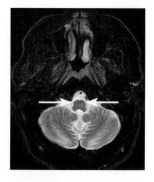

Axial T2 image through the medulla shows decreased prominence of the olivary nuclei *(white arrows)* from atrophy.

Answers

1. Cerebellar, pontine, and olivary atrophy, as well as putaminal atrophy and the "hot cross bun" sign, can be seen in some forms of olivopontocerebellar atrophy (OPCA). "Hot cross bun" sign is nonspecific and can be seen in other neurodegenerative diseases. Putaminal atrophy is seen in multisystem atrophy (MSA), which encompasses some sporadic forms of OPCA.

2. Spinocerebellar ataxias, alcohol abuse, congenital pontocerebellar hypoplasia, hyperthermia, and paraneoplastic syndromes can cause cerebellar atrophy with the addition of brainstem atrophy in neurodegenerative disorders such as spinocerebellar ataxias and congenital pontocerebellar hypoplasias.

3. The "hot cross bun" sign is T2 hyperintensity in a cruciate pattern within the atrophied pons and is thought to be from degeneration of transverse pontocerebellar fibers and pontine neurons as well as sparing of the corticospinal tract. This finding is nonspecific and can be seen in other neurodegenerative disorders including multisystem atrophy and spinocerebellar atrophy. Case reports have also described this finding in variant Creutzfeldt-Jakob disease and a patient with vasculitis presenting with parkinsonian symptoms.

4. Multisystem atrophy demonstrates cytoplasmic inclusions of alpha-synuclein within the cytoplasm of oligodendroglia, neurons, and axons.

5. Olivopontocerebellar atrophy, including the multisystem atrophy-C subtype, primarily presents with cerebellar symptoms. Furthermore, MSA-P subtype has more parkinsonian symptoms. Almost all MSA patients will eventually develop autonomic failure.

Pearls

- OPCA is a heterogeneous group of disorders that include sporadic forms primarily classified as multisystem atrophy and inherited familial forms.
- All OPCAs have similar findings of cerebellar and brainstem atrophy, including the pons and medullary olives.
- Sporadic OPCA classified in MSA can also have cerebral and putaminal atrophy.
- The "hot cross bun" sign of the pons is not specific but can be seen in many neurodegenerative disorders.
- No treatment is available: Most patients die of bronchopneumonia from central respiratory failure within a decade.

Suggested Readings

Naka H, Ohshita T, Murata Y, Imon Y, Mimori Y, Nakamura S. Characteristic MRI findings in multiple system atrophy: comparison of the three subtypes. *Neuroradiology.* 2002 Mar;44(3):204-209.

Ozawa T, Revesz T, Paviour D, et al. Difference in MSA phenotype distribution between populations: genetics or environment? *J Parkinsons Dis.* 2012 Jul;2(1):7-18.

Savoiardo M, Strada L, Girotti F, et al. Olivopontocerebellar atrophy: MR diagnosis and relationship to multisystem atrophy. *Radiology.* 1990 Mar;174(3, pt 1):693-696.

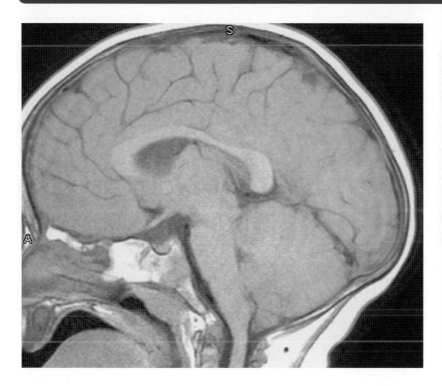
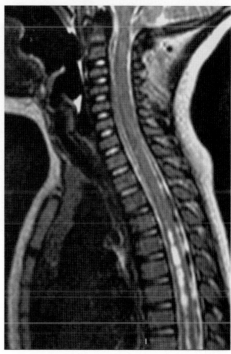

1. What is the diagnosis?

2. What are the classic imaging findings for this entity?

3. What are the symptoms seen with this entity?

4. What are the various causes of cerebellar ectopia/herniation?

5. What is the treatment for this entity when symptomatic?

Case ranking/difficulty:

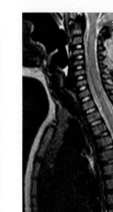

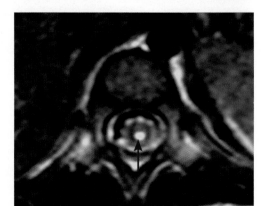

Sagittal T1 demonstrates herniation of cerebellar tonsil (*asterisk*) at foramen magnum. Cerebellar tonsils lie more than 5 mm below the line between basion (*blue arrow*) and opisthion (*green arrow*).

Sagittal T2 shows herniation of cerebellar tonsil (*green arrow*) at foramen magnum. Syringomyelia (*red arrow*) of the spinal cord.

Axial T2 image shows syringomyelia (*blue arrow*) of the spinal cord.

Answers

1. Chiari 1 malformation of hindbrain is more than 5 mm herniation of cerebellar tonsils below the foramen magnum.

2. CSF flow in Chiari 1 malformation shows decreased CSF flow at foramen magnum and through the vallecula cerebelli. Quantitative findings include prolonged CSF systole in the prepontine cistern, increased CSF velocity at the foramen magnum, reduced systolic velocities and duration of CSF systole just below foramen magnum, and increased duration of CSF systole at C-2 to C-3 level.

3. Occipital headache, swallowing dysfunction, nystagmus, lower cranial nerve palsies, vertigo, and tinnitus are some of the symptoms of Chiari 1 malformation.

4. Various causes of cerebellar ectopia/herniation include a small posterior fossa, chronic ventriculoperitoneal shunts, mass effect produced from tumors, chronic pseudotumor cerebri, larger hemorrhages, and intracranial hypotension.

5. The symptomatic Chiari I patient is usually treated with posterior fossa decompression surgery. Asymptomatic individuals are usually not treated.

Pearls

- Chiari 1 malformation is associated with an underdeveloped posterior cranial fossa.
- Adults may have cerebellar tonsil ectopia of 5 mm.
- Children less than 4 years can have tonsillar ectopia of up to 6 mm without any symptoms, if the subarachnoid space at foramen magnum remains patent.
- Pointed/compressed cerebellar tonsils with effacement of retrocerebellar cistern at foramen magnum are usually symptomatic.
- Posterior inclination of dens is associated with syringomyelia.
- MRI of the spine is needed given the approximate 20% incidence of syrinx.

Suggested Readings

Bunck AC, Kroeger JR, Juettner A, et al. Magnetic resonance 4D flow analysis of cerebrospinal fluid dynamics in Chiari I malformation with and without syringomyelia. *Eur Radiol.* 2012 Sep;22(9):1860-1870.

Heiss JD, Suffredini G, Smith R, et al. Pathophysiology of persistent syringomyelia after decompressive craniocervical surgery. Clinical article. *J Neurosurg Spine.* 2010 Dec;13(6):729-742.

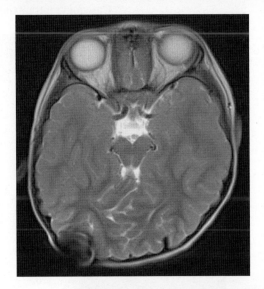 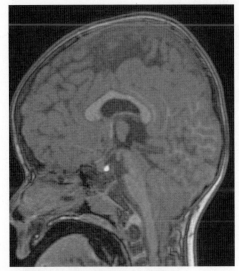

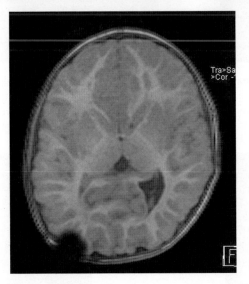 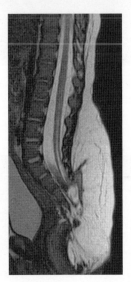

1. What are the typical brain MRI findings for this disease?

2. What differentiates the numbered subtypes of this entity?

3. What morphological changes involve the skeletal system in this disease?

4. What is the theoretic etiology of this disease?

5. What is the treatment for this disease?

Case ranking/difficulty:

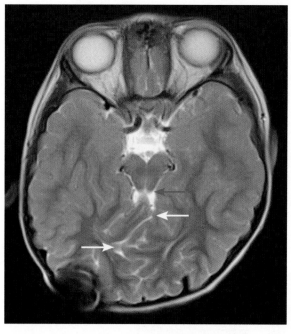

Axial T2 image at the midbrain level shows gyral interdigitation (*white arrows*) and beaked tectum (*red arrow*).

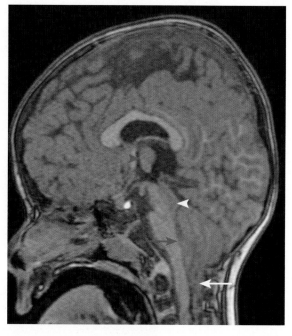

Sagittal T1 image of the brain at midline shows tonsillar herniation (*white arrow*), effacement of the fourth ventricle (*red arrow*), tectal beaking (*white arrowhead*), and enlarged massa intermedia (*red arrowhead*). These are typical findings of Chiari II malformation.

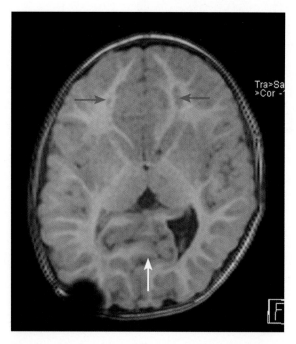

Axial T1 image though the ganglionic level shows falcine fenestration and gyral interdigitation (*white arrow*). Also note the bilateral frontal periventricular gray matter heterotopia (*red arrows*).

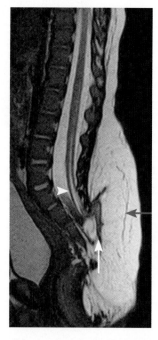

Sagittal T2 image of the lumbosacral spine shows dysraphic posterior elements in the sacral spinal canal with herniation of the cord (*white arrow*). The distal neural placode is attached to a lipoma distinguished from the subcutaneous fat by a fascial plane (*red arrow*). This is termed a lipomyelomenigocele. There is also a distal hydrosyringomyelia (*white arrowhead*).

Answers

1. Myelomeningocele, tonsillar herniation, beaked tectum, and fourth ventricular effacement are all hallmarks of Chiari II malformation.

   Additional findings include enlarged massa intermedia, corpus callosal dysgenesis, falcine fenestration and gyral interdigitation, stenogyria, and periventricular heterotopia.

2. Chiari I will usually only have cerebellar tonsillar herniation and fourth ventricular effacement. There may be a spinal cord syrinx without myelomeningocele.

   Chiari III has similar brain findings of Chiari II with a cranial cervical posterior encephalocele that involves dysraphism of the C1-C2 posterior elements.

3. Bony changes of Chiari II malformation include spinal dysraphism, clival notching, enlarged foramen magnum, and Lückenschädel.

   Lückenschädel (lacunar skull) describes craniolacunia involving both inner and outer tables due to a mesenchymal defect, not from increased intracranial pressure. This typically resolves by 6 months of age.

4. The favored theory includes CSF leakage through a myelomeningocele, leading to fourth ventricle collapse, and posterior fossa hypoplasia. This causes the cascade of tonsillar herniation, and towering cerebellum, inducing other brain abnormalities seen in Chiari II.

5. Folate supplementation prior to conception and for 6 weeks following helps prevent neural tube defects. Repair of the myelomeningocele and shunting of hydrocephalus are typically performed shortly after birth; however, in utero repair may help lessen brain malformations.

Pearls

- Chiari II malformation is nearly 100% associated with myelomeningocele.
- CSF loss theory through the neural tube defect is thought to give rise to small posterior fossa and resulting malformations.
- Abnormalities include (from most common to least common): myelomeningocele, hydrocephalus, small posterior fossa, tonsillar herniation, lacunar skull, brainstem descent, cervicomedullary kinking, towering cerebellum, beaked tectum, enlarged massa intermedia, dysgenesis of the corpus callosum, falcine fenestration/interdigitating gyri, syringohydromyelia, and nodular heterotopia.

Suggested Readings

Geerdink N, van der Vliet T, Rotteveel JJ, Feuth T, Roeleveld N, Mullaart RA. Essential features of Chiari II malformation in MR imaging: an interobserver reliability study—part 1. *Childs Nerv Syst.* 2012 Jul;28(7):977-985.

McLone DG, Naidich TP. Developmental morphology of the subarachnoid space, brain vasculature, and contiguous structures, and the cause of the Chiari II malformation. *AJNR Am J Neuroradiol.* 1999 Oct;13(2):463-482.

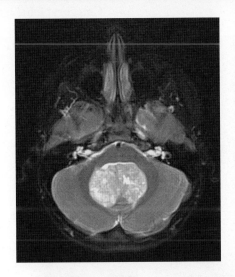
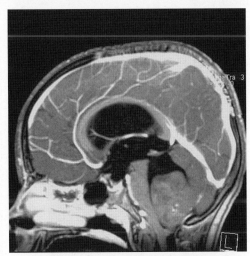
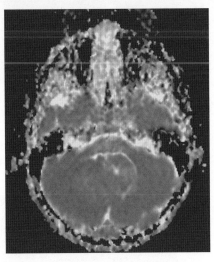
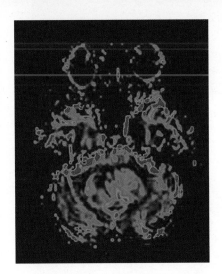

1. What is the differential diagnosis?

2. What imaging findings suggest high-grade neoplasm?

3. What morphological finding of the tumor can help differentiate this from other fourth ventricular tumors?

4. What is the typical mode of disease dissemination?

5. What are some molecular subtypes and prognosis associations?

Case ranking/difficulty: 🦫

Category: Intra-axial infratentorial

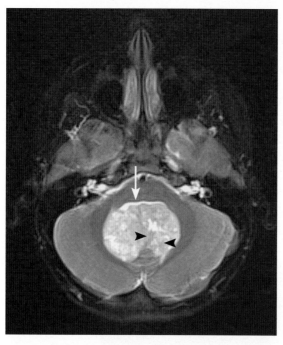

Axial T2 image of the posterior fossa shows a heterogeneous mass filling the fourth ventricle with areas of T2 hypointensity (*arrowheads*). Note the CSF cleft with the dorsal pons (*arrow*).

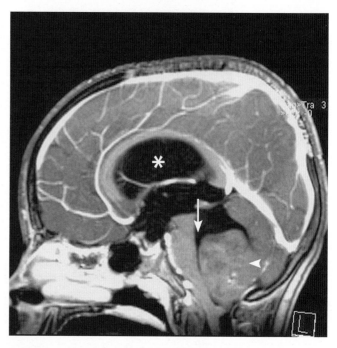

Sagittal post contrast T1 image shows the mildly enhancing and heterogeneous tumor, which causes hydrocephalus and ventricular dilatation (*asterisk*). Notice the CSF cleft separating the tumor from the dorsal brainstem (*arrow*) but with poor separation from the vermis, or roof of the fourth ventricle (*arrowhead*).

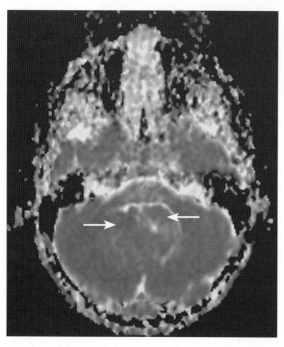

Axial DWI b = 1000 ADC map shows areas of decreased diffusion (*arrows*) consistent with a high-grade neoplasm.

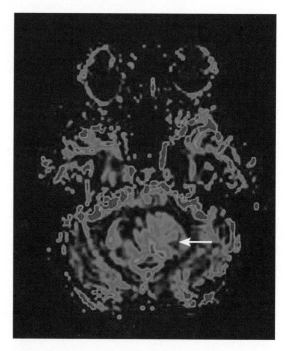

Axial relative cerebral blood volume map from dynamic susceptibility contrast technique shows significant hyperperfusion of the tumor (*arrow*).

Answers

1. Medulloblastoma and ependymoma are classic fourth ventricular tumors in the pediatric population. Pilocytic astrocytomas tend to be off midline and pedunculate into the fourth ventricle. Atypical teratoid rhabdoid tumors are difficult to separate from medulloblastoma by imaging as both are high-grade neoplasms but tend to be off midline compared to medulloblastoma. Brainstem gliomas with exophytic component into the fourth ventricle could be considered but is unlikely in this case due to a clean margin and a small CSF cleft between the mass and the dorsal surface of the brainstem.

2. Decreased diffusion and T2 signal can be seen in hypercellular components of tumors suggesting high grade. High-grade tumors also tend to cause neoangiogenesis, which will demonstrate increased cerebral blood volume on perfusion imaging.

3. Medulloblastomas classically arise from the roof of the fourth ventricle, and are difficult to separate from the cerebellar vermis on imaging. In contrast, ependymomas generally arise from the floor or dorsal brainstem ependymal surface of the fourth ventricle, and usually show some herniation of the tumor through the fourth ventricular foramina.

4. Up to 25% of medulloblastomas will demonstrate CSF/leptomeningeal dissemination at presentation. Careful evaluation of the leptomeninges along the entire neuraxis is indicated prior to surgery and treatment. Extraneural metastasis is rare, usually involving the bone, and can be seen in late stages of disease.

5. Molecular subgroups of medulloblastoma correlate with incidence of leptomeningeal dissemination and prognosis. A greater incidence of medulloblastomas is associated with familial cancer syndromes such as Li-Fraumeni, basal cell nevus, Turcot, Gardner, and Cowden. Amplification of the sonic the hedgehog (SHH) protein is seen with 30% of medulloblastomas and can involve different mutations. Mutations involving the SHH pathway is associated with a desmoplastic variant as in Gorlin syndrome as well as TP53 mutation in Li-Fraumeni syndrome, which carries a poorer prognosis. Subgroups with high amplification of the MYC proto-oncogene has the poorest prognosis with 5-year survival at 50% and is associated with the large cell anaplastic variant, with frequent leptomeningeal metastasis at diagnosis. In contrast, the wingless (WNT) protein pathway is the least common subgroup at 15% with 5-year survival of 95%, good prognosis, and less likely to metastasize. This subgroup is associated with Turcot syndrome.

Pearls

- Medulloblastomas are infratentorial primitive neuroectodermal tumors (PNET) and are the most common PNET of the brain, as well as the most common malignant brain tumor in children.
- As with all high-grade neoplasms, there are areas of T2 hypointensity, decreased diffusion, and increased perfusion from hypercellularity and increased neoangiogenesis.
- Tumor origin is from the medullary velum, or granular layer of the cerebellum, which explains the typical appearance of arising from the roof of the fourth ventricle, and causing obstructive hydrocephalus.
- Medulloblastomas uncommonly herniate out of the foramina Luschka and Magendie, which help distinguish it from ependymoma.
- Atypical teratoid rhabdoid tumor can appear very similar to medulloblastoma as both are high-grade tumors, but may present off midline in comparison.
- Spinal imaging for leptomeningeal metastasis is always indicated in medulloblastoma prior to surgery, as up to 25% of cases present with leptomeningeal disease.

Suggested Readings

Fruehwald-Pallamar J, Puchner SB, Rossi A, et al. Magnetic resonance imaging spectrum of medulloblastoma. *Neuroradiology*. 2011 Jun;53(6):387-396.

Yeom KW, Mobley BC, Lober RM, et al. Distinctive MRI features of pediatric medulloblastoma subtypes. *AJR Am J Roentgenol*. 2013 Apr;200(4):895-903.

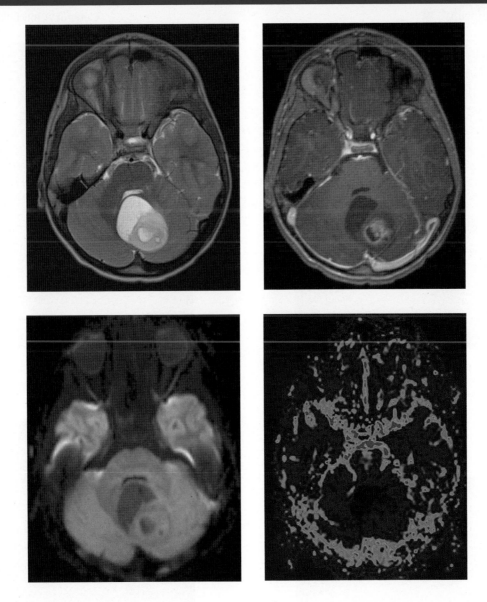

1. What is the differential diagnosis?

2. What imaging findings reflect a low-grade neoplasm?

3. What is the MR spectroscopic profile for this lesion?

4. Where are the common locations of occurrence for this tumor?

5. What is the prognosis of these lesions?

Case ranking/difficulty:

Category: Intra-axial infratentorial

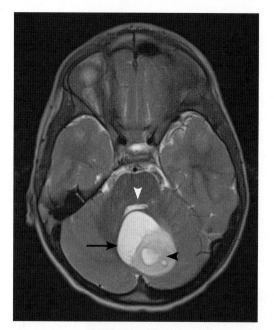

Axial T2 image of the posterior fossa shows a well-circumscribed mass arising from the vermis and left cerebellar hemisphere with little to no adjacent edema, and mass effect on the fourth ventricle (*white arrowhead*). There is a prominent cyst (*black arrow*) and relative T2 hyperintensity of the solid component (*black arrowhead*).

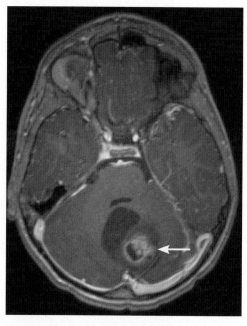

Axial T1 postcontrast image demonstrates heterogeneous enhancement of the solid component (*arrow*).

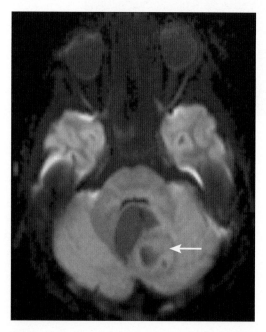

Axial DWI b = 1000 image shows no restricted diffusion of the tumor (*arrow*).

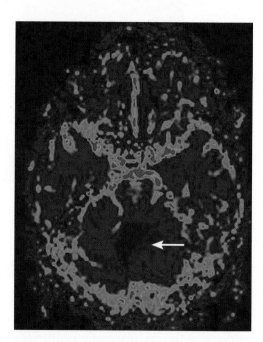

Axial relative cerebral blood volume map from dynamic susceptibility contrast perfusion shows no increased perfusion in the tumor (*arrow*).

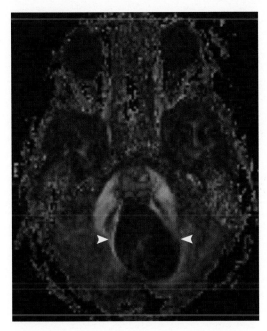

Axial fractional anisotropy map shows the mass displacing cerebellar white matter tracts (*arrowheads*) rather than invading the tracts suggestive of low-grade neoplasm.

Answers

1. Pilocytic astrocytoma and hemangioblastoma are classic differentials for the cyst with mural enhancing nodule in the posterior fossa, although hemangioblastomas are seen in adults associated with Von-Hippel Lindau disease. Medulloblastoma, ependymoma, and choroid plexus tumors should primarily arise from the fourth ventricle and do not typically have the cyst and nodule appearance. Furthermore, the tumor demonstrates low-grade characteristics, virtually excluding medulloblastoma from the differential.

2. Low-grade neoplasms generally have lower cellularity than high-grade neoplasms and demonstrate increased T2 signal and increased diffusion. Decreased perfusion can also suggest low-grade neoplasm. The presence of cysts can be seen in both high- and low-grade neoplasms.

3. MR spectroscopy for pilocytic astrocytomas can be paradoxical as a malignant tumor profile of decreased NAA, elevated choline, and the presence of lactate can be seen. However, when compared to ependymomas and medulloblastomas, the ratio of choline to NAA is increased for higher-grade tumors.

4. In decreasing order of frequency, pilocytic astrocytomas most commonly arise from the cerebellum, supratentorial structures around the third ventricle, and optic apparatus/hypothalamus. Rarely do they arise from peripheral lobar distributions.

5. The prognosis for pilocytic astrocytomas is excellent with greater than 95% survival in 10 years, regardless of complete surgical excision or chemoradiation.

Pearls

- Pilocytic astrocytomas are benign WHO grade I tumors with excellent prognosis with or without therapy.
- The classic cyst with an enhancing mural nodule appearance can be seen in half of cases.
- Solid portions of the tumor are usually T2 hyperintense and CT hypodense without decreased diffusion.
- Perfusion imaging is usually hypoperfused, although contrast leakage and areas of increased vascularity can cause some increase in CBV.
- MR spectroscopy is paradoxical in that there is elevated choline, decreased NAA, and the presence of lactate, although ratios of choline to NAA are lower than for malignant tumors.
- Most common locations include the cerebellum > around the third ventricle > optic pathway and hypothalamus > brainstem.

Suggested Readings

Arai K, Sato N, Aoki J, et al. MR signal of the solid portion of pilocytic astrocytoma on T2-weighted images: is it useful for differentiation from medulloblastoma? *Neuroradiology*. 2006 Apr;48(4):233-237.

Ho CY, Cardinal JS, Kamer AP, Kralik SF. Relative cerebral blood volume from dynamic susceptibility contrast perfusion in the grading of pediatric primary brain tumors. *Neuroradiology*. 2015 Mar;57(3):299-306.

Koeller KK, Rushing EJ. From the archives of the AFIP: pilocytic astrocytoma: radiologic-pathologic correlation. *Radiographics*. 2006 Apr;24(6):1693-1708.

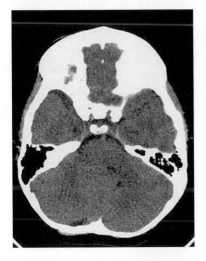
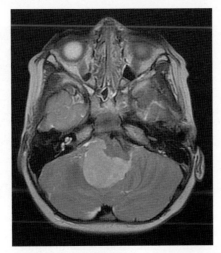
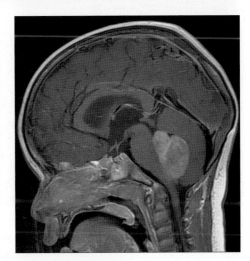

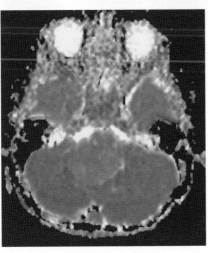
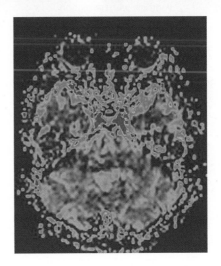

1. What is the differential diagnosis?

2. What is a morphologic finding of this tumor that can help distinguish it from other fourth ventricular tumors?

3. What syndrome has an increased incidence of this tumor?

4. What is the prognosis for this disease?

5. What is the most common location for this tumor in children?

Case ranking/difficulty:

Category: Intra-axial infratentorial

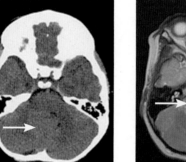

Axial CT image of the posterior fossa shows a hyperdense mass in the fourth ventricle (*arrow*).

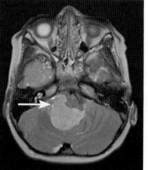

Axial T2 image of the posterior fossa shows a heterogenous mass centered in the fourth ventricle with herniation through the right foramen of Luschka (*arrow*). This is a typical finding for an ependymoma.

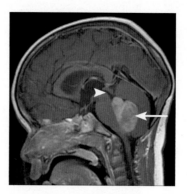

Sagittal T1 postcontrast shows a heterogeneous enhancing mass in the fourth ventricle (*arrow*) causing hydrocephalus with distention of the cerebral aqueduct (*arrowhead*).

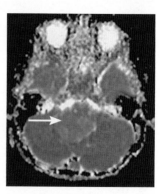

Axial DWI ADC map shows areas of decreased diffusion suggesting a higher-grade tumor (*arrow*).

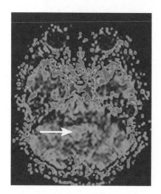

Cerebral blood volume map from dynamic susceptibility contrast perfusion imaging shows a hyperperfused portion of the tumor (*arrow*) consistent with high-grade anaplastic astrocytoma.

Answers

1. The differential of fourth ventricular masses include ependymoma, medulloblastoma (primitive neuroectodermal tumor), and atypical teratoid rhabdoid tumor.

2. Although not specific, ependymomas more commonly have calcification and hemorrhage than medulloblastomas and pilocytic astrocytomas. Cystic change can be commonly seen with all three tumors, especially with pilocytic astrocytomas. Squeezing out of the foramina is more typical of ependymomas.

3. There is an increased incidence of ependymomas in neurofibromatosis type 2.

4. Despite being a predominantly low-grade tumor, ependymomas have a generally poor prognosis with only 50%-60% 5-year survival rate.

5. Ependymomas most commonly occur in the posterior fossa in younger children and less commonly supratentorial in a periventricular location in older children. In adults, the spinal cord is the most common location.

Pearls

- Ependymomas are tumors arising from ependymal cells or rests commonly occurring in the fourth ventricle.
- Supratentorial ependymomas are usually periventricular, arising from ependymal rests.
- Ependymomas commonly have calcification, cysts, and hemorrhage.
- Infratentorial ependymomas are usually located within the fourth ventricle and have a tendency to squeeze out of the foraminas Luschka and Magendie.
- DWI and perfusion imaging can help distinguish higher-grade anaplastic varieties from low-grade classic ependymomas
- Spinal imaging prior to surgery is important to evaluate for drop metastasis.

Suggested Readings

Rumboldt Z, Camacho DL, Lake D, Welsh CT, Castillo M. Apparent diffusion coefficients for differentiation of cerebellar tumors in children. *AJNR Am J Neuroradiol.* 2008 Jan;27(6):1362-1369.

Spoto GP, Press GA, Hesselink JR, Solomon M. Intracranial ependymoma and subependymoma: MR manifestations. *AJNR Am J Neuroradiol.* 1990 May;11(1):83-91.

3-year-old female with unsteady gait

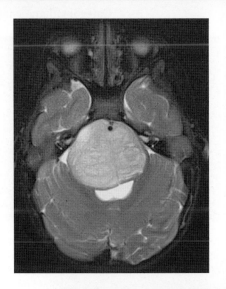

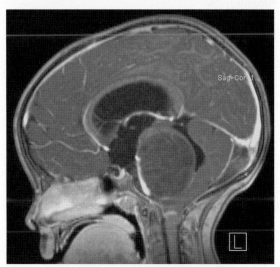

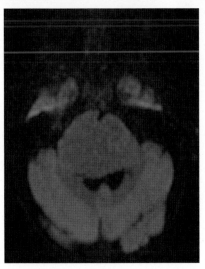

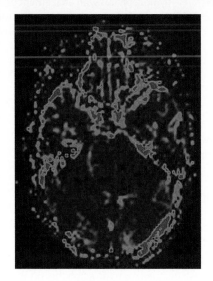

1. What is the differential diagnosis?

2. What are the typical MRI findings for this entity?

3. What is the typical histologic cell type of this tumor?

4. Which type of brainstem tumors have good prognosis?

5. What is the treatment for this disease?

Diffuse pontine glioma

Case ranking/difficulty: 🌶

Category: Intra-axial infratentorial

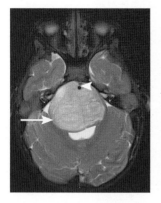

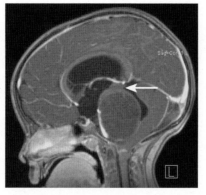

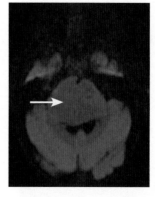

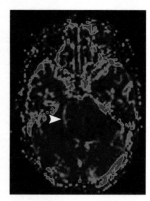

Axial T2 image shows diffuse expansile enlargement of the pons with increased T2 signal (*arrow*). There is encasement of the basilar artery (*arrowhead*).

Sagittal T1 postcontrast image shows no enhancing foci within the pontine mass. There is obstructive hydrocephalus with effacement of the cerebral aqueduct (*arrow*) causing enlargement of the third and lateral ventricles.

Axial b = 1000 DWI image shows no restricted diffusion of the pontine mass (*arrow*).

Axial CBV map from dynamic susceptibility contrast perfusion imaging shows no areas of increased perfusion. The linear structure of increased perfusion corresponds to a vessel (*arrowhead*).

Answers

1. The differential for diffuse T2 hyperintense swelling of the pons includes diffuse pontine glioma, acute disseminated encephalomyelitis, and osmotic demyelination.

2. Typical MRI findings of diffuse pontine glioma include diffuse T2 hyperintensity of the pons with mass-like expansion, and no enhancement. There is usually no uniform restricted diffusion or increased perfusion. When significantly large, the mass may encase the basilar artery and cause obstructive hydrocephalus on the fourth ventricle.

3. Typically diffuse pontine gliomas have been classified as fibrillary astrocytomas, with WHO grading varying from II to IV; however, all DPGs have poor prognosis.

4. All focal, exophytic, tectal, or cervicomedullary brainstem tumors have good prognosis approaching 100% long-term survival, although some have significant morbidity. This includes tumors associated with NF1. Diffuse pontine gliomas are the exception with poor prognosis and median survival of less than 1 year.

5. Corticosteroids are indicated to help with tumoral edema and symptoms in diffuse pontine glioma to improve quality of life. Radiation therapy can prolong survival by a few months. Chemotherapy has not been shown to be helpful. Surgery does not play a significant treatment role due to the location of the tumor.

Pearls

- Diffuse pontine gliomas (DPG) are biologically aggressive astrocytomas with poor prognosis in children; median survival is less than 1 year despite therapy.
- Other focal brainstem gliomas have an indolent course and generally good prognosis such as the exophytic pilocytic astrocytoma, tectal plate glioma, and brainstem tumors associated with NF1.
- Neuroimaging shows diffuse pontine swelling and uniform T2 hyperintensity.
- Enhancement or hemorrhage is atypical.
- Encasement of the basilar artery may be seen.

Suggested Readings

Löbel U, Sedlacik J, Reddick WE, et al. Quantitative diffusion-weighted and dynamic susceptibility-weighted contrast-enhanced perfusion MR imaging analysis of T2 hypointense lesion components in pediatric diffuse intrinsic pontine glioma. *AJNR Am J Neuroradiol.* 2011 Feb;32(2):315-322.

Sedlacik J, Winchell A, Kocak M, Loeffler RB, Broniscer A, Hillenbrand CM. MR imaging assessment of tumor perfusion and 3D segmented volume at baseline, during treatment, and at tumor progression in children with newly diagnosed diffuse intrinsic pontine glioma. *AJNR Am J Neuroradiol.* 2013 Jul;34(7):1450-1455.

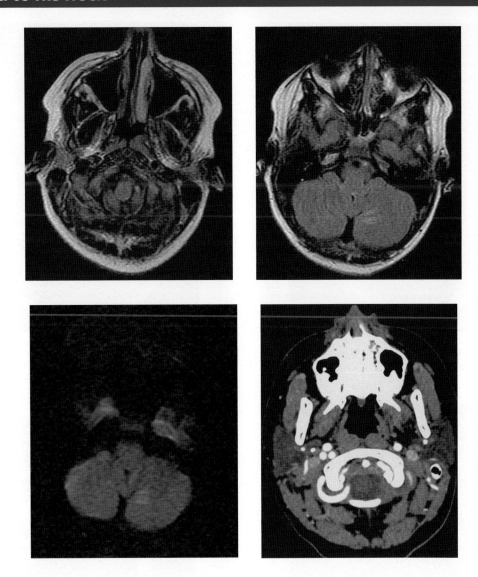

1. What is the most common cause of this finding?

2. If no clinical history of trauma, what is the possibility etiology?

3. What are possible clinical presentations?

4. What finding determines treatment options?

5. What is a medical treatment option in extracranial vertebral artery dissection?

Case ranking/difficulty: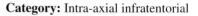

Category: Intra-axial infratentorial

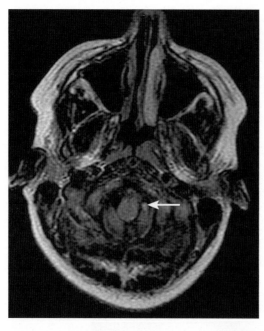

Axial FLAIR image demonstrates hyperintensity in the left V4 vertebral artery (*white arrow*).

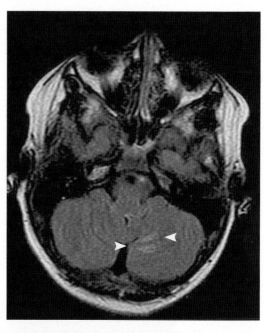

Axial FLAIR image demonstrates a focal area of FLAIR hyperintensity involving the left cerebellar hemisphere in the posterior inferior cerebellar artery distribution (*white arrowheads*).

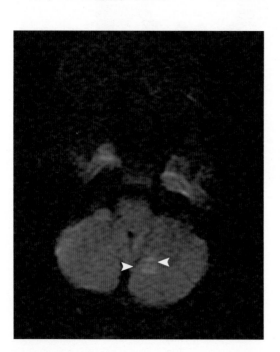

DWI image demonstrates restricted diffusion in the left cerebellar hemisphere in the PICA distribution (*white arrowheads*), consistent with acute infarct.

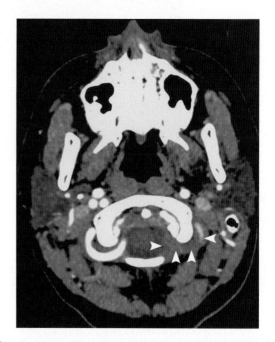

Axial postcontrast CT angiography shows occlusion of the distal V3, proximal V4 junction with tapering (*arrowheads*), indicating dissection in this teenager with a history of trauma.

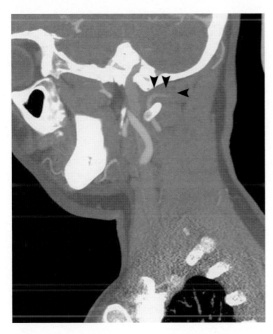

Sagittal MIP CTA image demonstrates smooth tapering of the left V3 vertebral artery, consistent with dissection (*arrowheads*).

Answers

1. Blunt trauma is the most common cause of vertebral artery dissection.

2. Spontaneous vertebral artery dissection may be associated with fibromuscular dysplasia (15%) or underlying connective tissue disease (Ehlers-Danlos syndrome, Marfan syndrome, autosomal dominant polycystic kidney disease, and osteogenesis imperfecta type 1).

3. Most frequent clinical manifestation of vertebral artery dissection is headache or neck pain accompanied or followed by posterior circulation ischemia (57%-84% of patients). Rare clinical manifestations include isolated head or neck pain, cervical spinal cord ischemia, cervical nerve root impingement, and Horner syndrome.

4. Patients with intracranial involvement of vertebral artery dissection should be treated by surgery or endovascular treatment, rather than antiplatelet therapy, especially with subarachnoid hemorrhage or large infarcts.

5. Extracranial vertebral artery dissection can be treated with antiplatelet agents to prevent artery-to-artery embolization and posterior circulation infarcts.

Pearls

- Blunt trauma is the most common cause of vertebral artery dissection.
- Spontaneous vertebral artery dissection may be associated with underlying connective tissue disease and fibromuscular dysplasia.
- It is important to determine whether the dissection extends into the intracranial V4 segment, due to different treatment options and prognosis.
- Intracranial dissections are prone to rupture with subarachnoid hemorrhage, with significant increase in mortality.
- CT/CTA is often the first imaging modality, demonstrating posterior fossa ischemia, subarachnoid hemorrhage, occluded vertebral artery, or mural thrombus.
- MRI/MRA is more sensitive in small posterior fossa ischemia, and also able to demonstrate intraluminal thrombus and intraluminal hemorrhage.
- Treatment for extracranial dissection is antiplatelet therapy to prevent artery-to-artery embolization and posterior circulation infarcts.
- Intracranial dissection, especially with subarachnoid hemorrhage or large infarcts, requires endovascular treatment or surgery.

Suggested Readings

Rodallec MH, Marteau V, Gerber S, Desmottes L, Zins M. Craniocervical arterial dissection: spectrum of imaging findings and differential diagnosis. *Radiographics*. 2008 Oct;28(6):1711-1728.

Vertinsky AT, Schwartz NE, Fischbein NJ, Rosenberg J, Albers GW, Zaharchuk G. Comparison of multidetector CT angiography and MR imaging of cervical artery dissection. *AJNR Am J Neuroradiol*. 2008 Oct;29(9):1753-1760.

53-year-old male with a severe headache and visual changes followed by a loss of consciousness

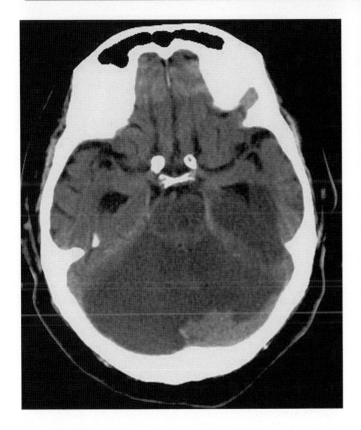
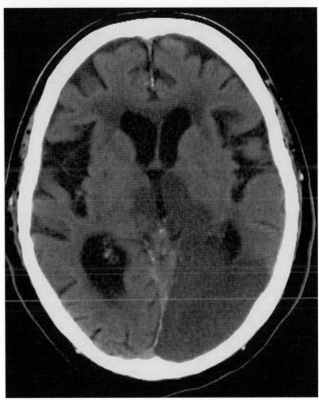

1. Where is the abnormality located?

2. What is the arterial distribution involved with this pattern?

3. What is the differential diagnosis?

4. What are risk factors for this disease?

5. What is the treatment for this entity?

Case ranking/difficulty: **Category:** Intra-axial infratentorial

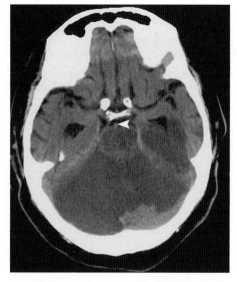

Axial CT shows hypodensity of the pons, left temporal lobe, and cerebellum. There is increased density of the basilar artery (*arrowhead*), which supplies these vascular territories.

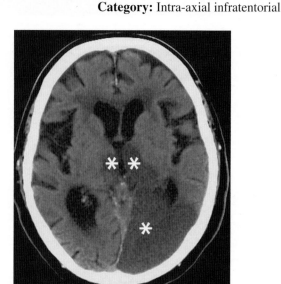

Axial CT image shows hypodensity of the bilateral medial thalami and left occipital temporal lobe from posterior circulation infarct (*asterisks*).

Answers

1. The abnormality involves the cerebellum, thalami, left occipital lobe, left temporal lobe, and portions of the brainstem.

2. The abnormality involves the basilar artery territory. Small portions of the left cerebellar hemisphere remain unaffected likely due to the left posterior inferior cerebellar artery, which originates from the vertebral artery.

3. The differential diagnosis includes basilar occlusion, artery of Percheron infarct, and dural venous sinus thrombosis. The artery of Percheron is a variant of the posterior circulation where a solitary trunk (Percheron) supplies the paramedian thalami and rostral midbrain.

4. Basilar artery occlusion risk factors include atherosclerosis, hyperlipidemia, propagation of clot secondary to dissection, and meningitis.

5. In the acute setting, mechanical thrombectomy has shown success with regard to improving mortality and overall outcome.

Pearls

- Basilar artery occlusion results in infarction of the cerebellum, brainstem, posterior temporal lobes, portions of the internal capsules, thalami, and occipital lobes.
- This is a neurointerventional emergency because of infarction of the brainstem.
- High density within the basilar artery is a nonspecific sign for thrombosis.
- Top of the basilar syndrome occurs when only the distal basilar artery is occluded, which results in infarction of the thalami, posterior limbs of internal capsules, and midbrain.
- CTA is helpful to visualize the thrombus.
- Mortality of basilar artery thrombosis is two to three times higher than internal carotid artery occlusion.

Suggested Readings

Cormier PJ, Long ER, Russell EJ. MR imaging of posterior fossa infarctions: vascular territories and clinical correlates. *Radiographics*. 1992 Nov;12(6):1079-1096.

Kostanian V, Cramer SC. Artery of Percheron thrombolysis. *AJNR Am J Neuroradiol*. 2007 May;28(5):870-871.

Puetz V, Sylaja PN, Hill MD, et al. CT angiography source images predict final infarct extent in patients with basilar artery occlusion. *AJNR Am J Neuroradiol*. 2009 Nov;30(10):1877-1883.

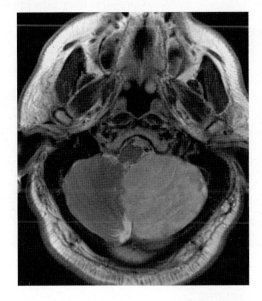
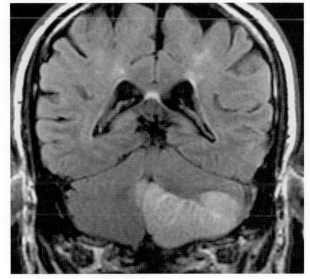

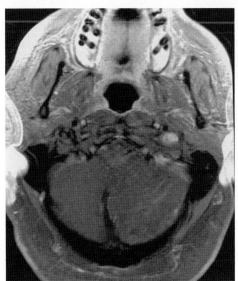

1. Where is the abnormality located?

2. What are the classic imaging findings for this entity?

3. What is the differential diagnosis?

4. What is the etiology for this finding?

5. What is the treatment for this entity?

Case ranking/difficulty: 🍂

Category: Intra-axial infratentorial

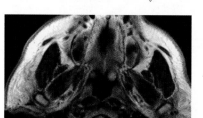

Axial T2 image shows swelling involving the inferior left cerebellar hemisphere and vermis (*arrow*) with mass effect on the medulla.

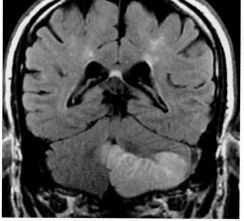

Coronal FLAIR image shows the high signal is seen involving the lower left cerebellar hemisphere (*arrow*) with associated regional mass effect.

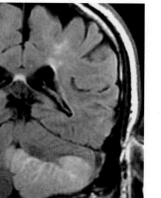

Axial T1 postcontrast shows linear sulcal enhancement of the left cerebellar hemisphere (*arrows*). This is likely from "luxury perfusion."

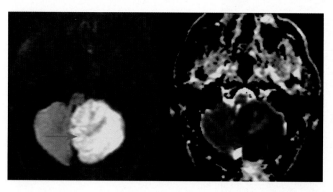

Axial DWI b-1000 and ADC map demonstrate restricted diffusion (*green arrow*) with corresponding low signal on ADC map (*blue arrow*) within the lower left cerebellar hemisphere.

Answers

1. The abnormality is located within the left cerebellar hemisphere.

2. The classic imaging findings for this entity on CT include obscuration of the cerebellar folia and low density within the affected cerebellar parenchyma. On MR, there is high signal on the T2 images with corresponding T1 low signal following the signal of edema. Specifically, diffusion-weighted imaging (DWI) is the most sensitive and specific MRI sequence for detecting acute infarcts, which will demonstrate increased signal with corresponding decreased signal on ADC ("restricted diffusion").

3. The differential diagnosis includes cerebellar infarction, metastasis, cerebellitis, astrocytoma, and dysplastic gangliocytoma.

4. PICA infarction is typically from atherosclerotic occlusion.

5. The treatment for this entity is typically supportive care, but consideration can be given to thrombolytic therapy with progressive basilar involvement. Surgical intervention may be necessary in cases of hydrocephalus or upward transtentorial herniation with resection of cerebellar tissue.

Pearls

- PICA supplies the inferior cerebellar hemispheres, inferior vermis, tonsils, and lateral medulla.
- The fourth ventricle may be effaced secondary to mass effect; upward transtentorial herniation may occur.
- PICA infarcts are the most common cerebellar infarcts associated with hemorrhagic transformation.
- The most common etiology in PICA infarcts is thrombosis related to atherosclerotic disease.
- Lateral medullary (Wallenberg) syndrome involves ipsilateral Horner syndrome, ipsilateral face loss of temperature and sensation with contralateral body loss of temperature and sensation.

Suggested Readings

Cano LM, Cardona P, Quesada H, Mora P, Rubio F. [Cerebellar infarction: prognosis and complications of vascular territories]. *Neurologia*. 2012 Nov;27(6):330-335.

Kim MJ, Chung J, Kim SL, et al. Stenting from the vertebral artery to the posterior inferior cerebellar artery. *AJNR Am J Neuroradiol*. 2012 Feb;33(2):348-352.

34-year-old male with headaches, status post fusiform aneurysm coiling, and vessel sacrifice

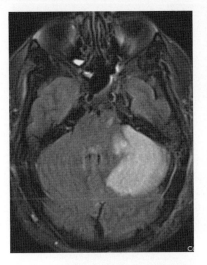
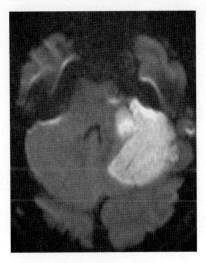

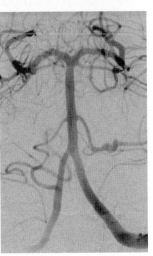
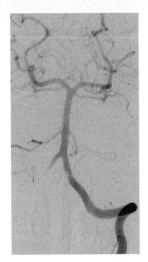

1. What is the differential diagnosis?

2. What are the typical MRI findings for this entity?

3. What structures are supplied by this artery?

4. What are the clinical symptoms for this finding?

5. What symptom helps differentiate this arterial territory infarct from the more common PICA infarct?

Case ranking/difficulty: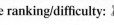

Category: Intra-axial infratentorial

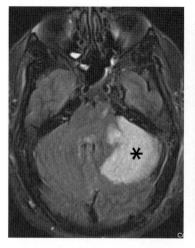

Axial FLAIR image shows increased T2 signal of the left anterior inferior cerebellum extending to the left middle cerebellar peduncle (*asterisk*) in the expected left AICA territory.

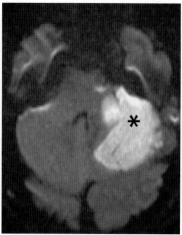

Axial DWI b = 1000 image shows diffusion restriction of the left anterior inferior cerebellum and middle cerebellar peduncle (*asterisk*).

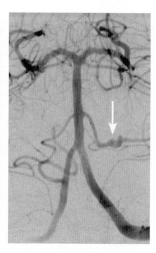

AP view of left vertebral artery injection DSA shows a fusiform aneurysm of the left AICA (*arrow*).

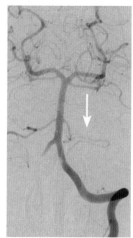

AP view of left vertebral artery injection DSA shows coiling of the left AICA aneurysm with sacrifice of the left AICA (*arrow*).

Answers

1. The differential for mass-like swelling of the anterior inferior cerebellar hemisphere includes cerebellitis, neoplasm, and acute infarct of the anterior inferior cerebellar artery (AICA) territory.

2. Typical MRI findings for acute infarct include T2 hyperintensity, T1 hypointensity, and DWI increased signal, and decreased ADC corresponding with cytotoxic edema.

3. The AICA supplies the anterior inferior cerebellum along the petrosal margin, the middle cerebellar peduncle, inferolateral pons and upper medulla, and fourth ventricular choroid plexus at the foramen of Luschka. Labyrinthine branch of the AICA supplies the vestibulocochlear structures and facial nerve.

4. Patients with AICA infarct present with dysarthria, Horner syndrome, and ipsilateral limb ataxia. Inner ear symptoms are also noted such as hearing loss, vertigo, and tinnitus.

5. Hearing loss is a clinical symptom that can differentiate an AICA from a PICA infarct due to labyrinthine branch supply to the inner ear from the AICA.

Pearls

- AICA supplies the anterior inferior cerebellar hemisphere along the petrosal surface.
- Middle cerebellar peduncle, inferior lateral pons and upper medulla, and fourth ventricular choroid plexus are also supplied by AICA.
- Labyrinthine branch supplies the inner ear, with hearing loss helping clinically differentiate from PICA infarct.
- Variations in AICA are common, including common PICA/AICA trunk.

Suggested Reading

Chang HM, Linn FH, Caplan LR. Bilateral anterior inferior cerebellar artery territory infarcts. *J Neuroimaging*. 1998 Jan;8(1):42-44.

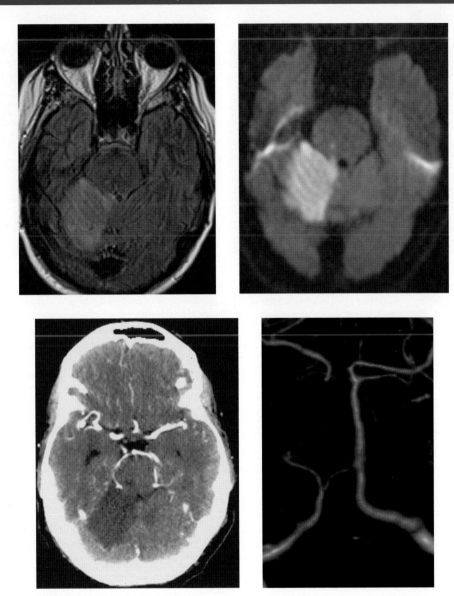

1. What is the differential diagnosis?

2. What are the typical MRI findings for this entity?

3. What structures are supplied by this artery?

4. What are the clinical symptoms for this finding?

5. What is Horner syndrome?

Case ranking/difficulty:

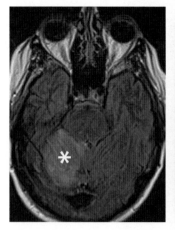

Axial FLAIR image shows T2 hyperintensity and swelling of the right superior cerebellum (*asterisk*).

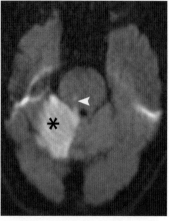

Axial DWI b = 1000 image shows diffusion restriction of the right superior cerebellum (*asterisk*) and dorsal pons (*arrowhead*).

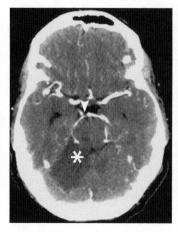

Axial CT angiography shows severe stenosis of the proximal right superior cerebellar artery (*arrowhead*) with associated hypodensity of the cerebellum and dorsal pons from acute infarct (*asterisk*).

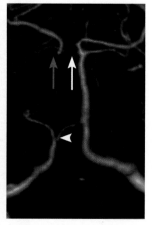

3D reformation of the posterior arterial circulation from CT angiography shows severe stenosis of the right superior cerebellar artery (*white arrow*). There is incidental fetal origin of the right posterior cerebral artery (*red arrow*) and normal variant hypoplasia of the distal right vertebral artery after the origin of the right PICA (*arrowhead*).

Answers

1. The differential for mass-like swelling of the superior cerebellum includes cerebellitis, traumatic edema, neoplasm, and superior cerebellar artery (SCA) infarct.

2. Typical MRI findings for acute infarct include T2 hyperintensity, T1 hypointensity, and DWI hyperintensity correlating with decreased ADC from cytotoxic edema.

3. The SCA supplies the superior cerebellum and dorsal lateral pons.

4. Clinical presentation of SCA infarction includes dysarthria, ipsilateral ataxia, and Horner syndrome.

5. Horner syndrome includes ptosis (drooping eyelid), miosis (constricted pupils), and anhidrosis (ipsilateral decreased sweating) from sympathetic dysfunction.

Pearls

- Superior cerebellar artery (SCA) supplies the superior cerebellum and dorsal lateral pons.
- Clinical symptoms include ataxia, dysarthria, and Horner syndrome.
- Isolated SCA infarct is rare and typically associated with basilar tip infarction.

Suggested Readings

Cano LM, Cardona P, Quesada H, Mora P, Rubio F.[Cerebellar infarction: prognosis and complications of vascular territories]. *Neurologia*. 2012 Nov;27(6):330-335.

Cho TH, Berthezene Y, Mechtouff L, Derex L, Nighoghossian N. Evolving basilar artery stenosis with watershed ischemia. *J Neuroimaging*. 2013 Sep.

51-year-old female with slurred speech, upper extremity weakness, dysphagia, and shortness of breath

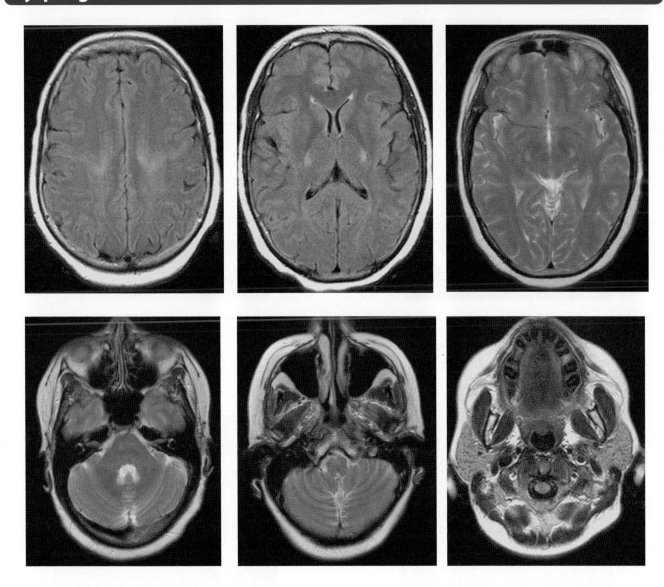

1. What is the structure demonstrating pathology in these images?

2. Which sequence is the most specific for T2 hyperintensity along this tract?

3. What is the method of inheritance in this disease?

4. What are the clinical presentations of this disease?

5. What is the prognosis for this disease?

Case ranking/difficulty:

Category: Intra-axial supratentorial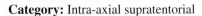

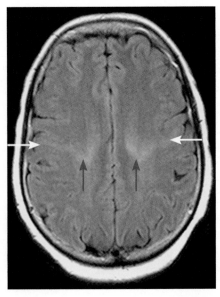

Axial FLAIR image at the level of the corona radiata shows hyperintensity of the corticospinal tract in the subcortical white matter of the primary motor cortex (*white arrows*) and extending to the corona radiata (*red arrows*).

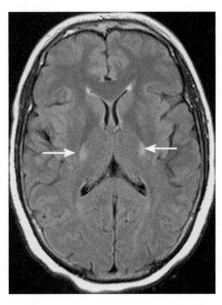

Axial FLAIR image at the ganglionic level shows hyperintensity of the posterior limb of the internal capsule (*white arrows*).

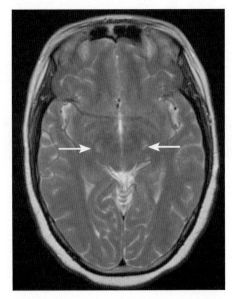

Axial T2 image of the superior midbrain shows symmetric hyperintensity of the corticospinal tract in the cerebral peduncles (*white arrows*).

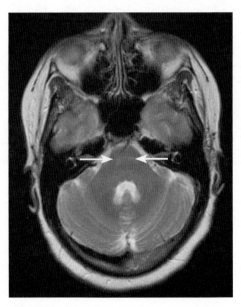

Axial T2 image of the pons shows corticospinal hyperintensity (*white arrows*).

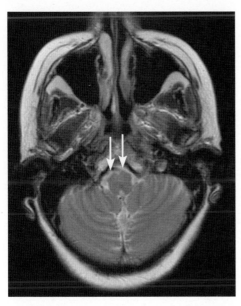

Axial T2 image at the medulla shows hyperintensity of the pyramids (*white arrows*).

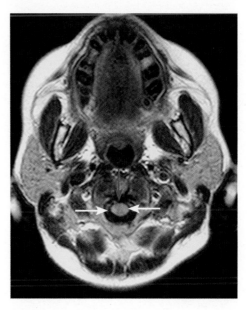

Axial FLAIR of the upper cervical cord shows hyperintensity of the lateral corticospinal tract (*white arrows*) and anterior corticospinal tract (*red arrow*).

Answers

1. The corticospinal tract begins superiorly at the motor and primary proprioception cortex, through the central corona radiata, posterior limb of the internal capsule, cerebral peduncles, pons, pyramid of the medulla, and into the lateral and anterior portions of the spinal cord. The corticobulbar tract runs with the corticospinal tract but is situated primarily in the genu of the internal capsule and more medial portions of the cerebral peduncle, separating from the corticospinal tract to innervate cranial nerve nuclei. The corticospinal tract is involved in ALS.

2. Although T1 signal changes have been reported in ALS, proton density is the most specific with regard to T2 hyperintense signal. Spin echo T2 is also more specific than FLAIR hyperintensity or DWI decreased diffusion as hyperintensity on FLAIR and DWI can be seen in normal individuals especially on 3T imaging.

3. Although the majority of ALS is sporadic, most of the genetic mutations have been described in familial forms on the ALS1 gene (Cu/Zn superoxide dismutase) located on 21q. A rare juvenile form is associated with the ALS2 gene on 2q.

4. ALS classically presents with both upper motor neuron (hyperreflexia, spasticity, and Babinski) and lower motor neuron (hyporeflexia, fasiculations, weakness, and atrophy). Variations include bulbar signs (dysphagia and dysarthria) as well as hypoxia and arrhythmia, which have a more rapid deterioration from brain stem involvement.

5. There is no current effective treatment for ALS, with all patient eventually progressing and deteriorating. Some patients have rapid progression to death within a few years while others can live for several decades.

Pearls

- T2 hyperintensity of the corticalspinal tract is typical of ALS.
- FLAIR imaging is sensitive but not specific as there is normal FLAIR hyperintensity of the corticalspinal tract especially on 3T.
- DWI is nonspecific with normal anisotropy of the corticalspinal tract.
- T2 and proton density are more specific for pathology.

Suggested Readings

Agosta F, Chiò A, Cosottini M, et al. The present and the future of neuroimaging in amyotrophic lateral sclerosis. *AJNR Am J Neuroradiol*. 2010 Nov;31(10):1769-1777.

da Rocha AJ, Maia AC, Valério BC. Corticospinal tract MR signal-intensity pseudonormalization on magnetization transfer contrast imaging: a potential pitfall in the interpretation of the advanced compromise of upper motor neurons in amyotrophic lateral sclerosis. *AJNR Am J Neuroradiol*. 2012 May;33(5):E79-E80.

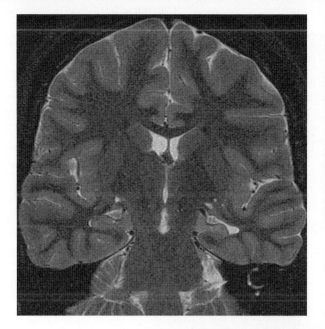
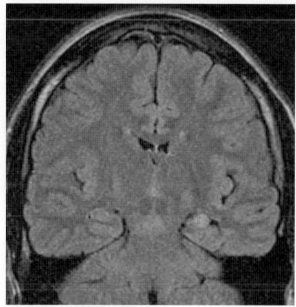
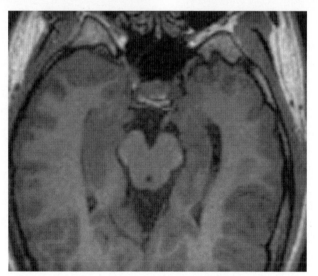

1. What is the differential diagnosis?

2. What are associated secondary findings of this entity?

3. What are typical MRI findings of this entity?

4. What is the likely etiology of this entity?

5. What is the treatment for this disease?

Case ranking/difficulty:    **Category:** Intra-axial supratentorial

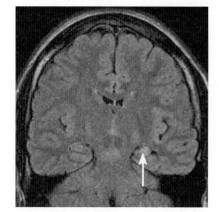

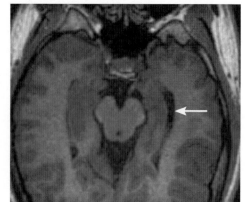

Coronal STIR image through the body of the hippocampi shows atrophy of the left hippocampus (*arrow*) with associated enlargement of the temporal horn (*arrowhead*).

Coronal FLAIR image shows increased signal of the smaller left hippocampus (*arrow*).

Axial T1 SPGR reformatted obliquely through the hippocampi shows left hippocampal atrophy and enlargement of the left temporal horn (*arrow*).

Answers

1. The differential diagnosis for increased T2 signal of the hippocampus includes status epilepticus, herpes encephalitis, cortical dysplasia, and mesial temporal sclerosis (MTS). Volume loss is primarily seen with MTS.

2. Associated secondary findings of MTS include ex-vacuo enlargement of the ipsilateral temporal horn and choroid fissure with atrophy of the ipsilateral mammillary body and fornix.

3. MTS typically shows decreased size of the hippocampus with increased T2 signal from sclerosis and loss of the internal architecture. 20% of MTS is bilateral.

4. There is lack of consensus whether MTS is caused by developmental factors or is acquired. The "two-hit" theory suggests that any primary insult to the hippocampus (infection, seizures, ischemia) with the predisposition of genetics or other developmental anomalies (associated tumors) is required to develop MTS.

5. MTS is the most common finding for temporal lobectomy for complex partial seizures. Surgery is indicated for medically refractory seizures or intolerable side effects of the medication.

Pearls

- Most common cause of complex partial seizures in young adults.
- Coronal FLAIR and T2 imaging increase sensitivity.
- Volumetrics increase sensitivity.
- 20% bilateral.
- Hippocampal atrophy, increased T2, and loss of internal architecture.
- Secondary signs: ipsilateral temporal horn and choroid fissure dilation, ipsilateral fornix, and mammillary body atrophy.

Suggested Readings

Coan AC, Kubota B, Bergo FP, Campos BM, Cendes F. 3T MRI quantification of hippocampal volume and signal in mesial temporal lobe epilepsy improves detection of hippocampal sclerosis. *AJNR Am J Neuroradiol*. 2014 Jan;35(1):77-83.

Howe KL, Dimitri D, Heyn C, Kiehl TR, Mikulis D, Valiante T. Histologically confirmed hippocampal structural features revealed by 3T MR imaging: potential to increase diagnostic specificity of mesial temporal sclerosis. *AJNR Am J Neuroradiol*. 2010 Oct;31(9):1682-1689.

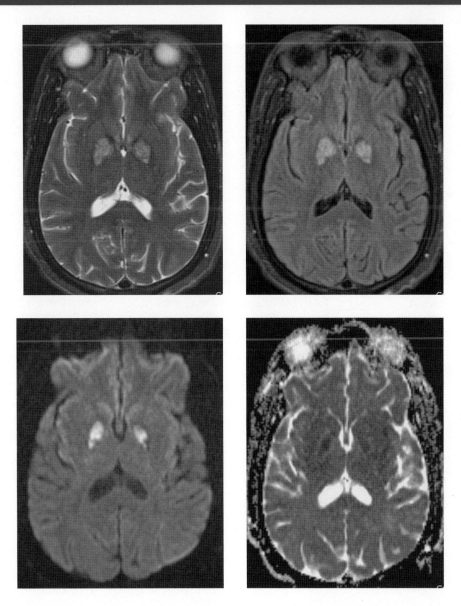

1. What is the most common cause of accidental toxic exposure?

2. What CNS structures are most commonly involved?

3. What is the pathophysiology of this disease?

4. What is the differential diagnosis of this finding?

5. What is the treatment for this disease?

Case ranking/difficulty:

Category: Intra-axial supratentorial

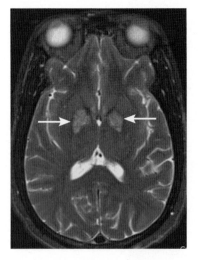

Axial T2 image shows increased symmetric T2 hyperintensity of the bilateral globi pallidi (*arrows*).

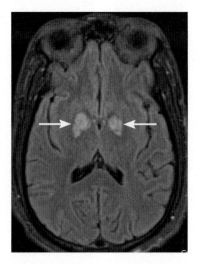

Axial FLAIR image at the level of the basal ganglia shows increased T2 signal of the globi pallidi (*arrows*).

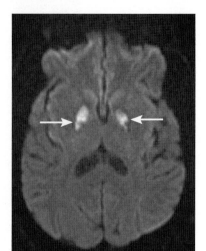

Axial DWI b = 1000 shows bright signal of the bilateral globi pallidi (*arrows*).

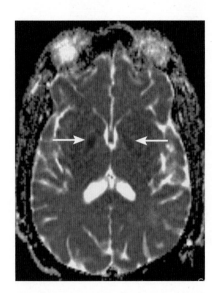

Axial ADC map shows dark signal of the bilateral globi pallidi (*arrows*) consistent with diffusion restriction and cytotoxic edema.

Answers

1. Carbon monoxide poisoning is the most common cause of accidental toxicity, especially in winter months in North America and Europe.

2. The globi pallidi are most commonly involved in a symmetric distribution with carbon monoxide poisoning followed by confluent deep cerebral white matter.

3. Carbon monoxide has over 200× binding affinity with hemoglobin than oxygen, not allowing appropriate oxygen delivery to cells.

4. The differential for bilateral, symmetric globi pallidi cytotoxic edema includes toxic metabolic processes such as carbon monoxide poisoning and mitochondrial disease such as Leigh disease. Other causes of anoxic injury include drowning. Creutzfeldt-Jakob can also show bilateral deep gray nuclei restricted diffusion.

5. Hyperbaric oxygen or 100% oxygen if hyperbaric chamber is not available within the first 6 hours may reduce neuropsychiatric sequelae.

Pearls

- Carbon monoxide poisoning typically occurs in winter months and is the most common nonaccidental toxicity in Europe and North America.
- The most common CNS site of abnormality is the globi pallidi followed by deep cerebral white matter in a bilateral symmetric distribution.
- Involvement of the deep gray nuclei, fornix, and hippocampi can also be seen.
- Acute lesions demonstrate T2 hyperintensity and restricted diffusion, with variable enhancement.
- Affected parenchyma progress to cystic encephalomalacia in the chronic stage.

Suggested Readings

Beppu T. The role of MR imaging in assessment of brain damage from carbon monoxide poisoning: a review of the literature. *AJNR Am J Neuroradiol.* 2014 Apr;35(4):625-631.

Sharma P, Eesa M, Scott JN. Toxic and acquired metabolic encephalopathies: MRI appearance. *AJR Am J Roentgenol.* 2009 Sep;193(3):879-886.

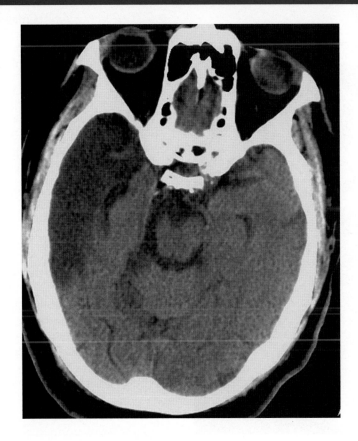

1. Where is the abnormality located?

2. In the acute/subacute setting, what findings are present?

3. Several months after the event, what findings are present?

4. What is the etiology for this finding?

5. What is the treatment for this entity?

Case ranking/difficulty: 🦠

Category: Intra-axial supratentorial

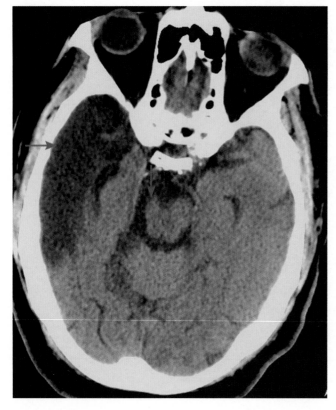

Axial CT image shows volume loss of the right cerebral peduncle (*red arrow*). There is encephalomalacia from previous large right MCA injury (*green arrow*).

Answers

1. The abnormality is located within the cerebral peduncle of the midbrain.

2. In Wallerian degeneration, the MR signal changes depend on the time from the event. Weeks 1 to 4, T1 and T2 are normal but DWI can show high signal. No contrast enhancement is seen.

3. Many months after injury, the diagnosis can be made by noting atrophy of the ipsilateral cerebral peduncle and pons.

4. Wallerian degeneration etiologies include infarction, hemorrhage, neoplasm, demyelination, trauma, and vascular malformations. Basically any process that cause neuronal damage, leading to anterograde axonal degeneration.

5. There is no specific treatment for Wallerian degeneration.

Pearls

- Anterograde axonal degeneration from proximal neuronal death.
- Best seen in the ipsilateral descending corticalspinal tract from proximal injury.
- DWI can have restricted diffusion acutely.
- T1 hyperintensity is noted in 4-14 weeks with myelin breakdown.
- T2 hyperintensity is noted in >14 weeks with gliosis.
- Atrophy best noted in the ipsilateral brainstem is seen in the chronic phase.
- Presence of restricted diffusion and T2 hyperintensity correlates with morbidity.

Suggested Readings

Ho ML, Moonis G, Ginat DT, Eisenberg RL. Lesions of the corpus callosum. *AJR Am J Roentgenol.* 2013 Jan;200(1):W1-W16.

Puig J, Pedraza S, Blasco G, et al. Wallerian degeneration in the corticospinal tract evaluated by diffusion tensor imaging correlates with motor deficit 30 days after middle cerebral artery ischemic stroke. *AJNR Am J Neuroradiol.* 2010 Aug;31(7):1324-1330.

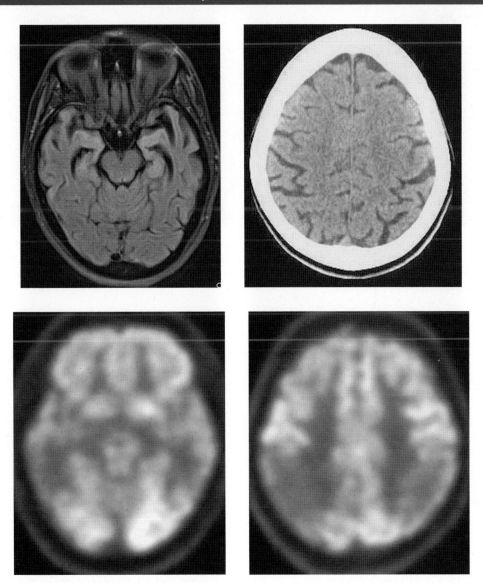

1. What is the differential diagnosis?

2. What comprises an abnormal amyloid ligand PET scan?

3. Which lobes are most affected in this disease?

4. What is seen on FDG PET imaging in this disease?

5. What percentage of patients are affected with this disease in the older than 85 years age group?

Case ranking/difficulty:

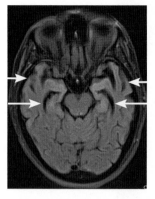

Axial FLAIR image demonstrates cortical atrophy most prominent in the temporal lobes and hippocampi (*arrows*).

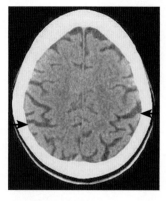

Axial CT image shows increased sulcal prominence from atrophy of the parietal lobes (*arrows*).

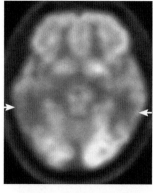

Axial PET FDG of the brain shows hypometabolism of the temporal lobes (*arrows*).

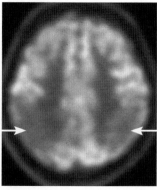

Axial PET FDG shows symmetric hypometabolism of the parietal lobes (*arrows*).

Answers

1. Differential diagnosis for nonreversible dementias includes Alzheimer, frontotemporal, dementia with Lewy bodies, vascular dementia, and corticobasal degeneration.

2. An abnormal florbetapir scan demonstrates increased uptake in the cortex with blurring of the gray-white differentiation. A normal amyloid scan demonstrates greater white matter uptake, with visualization of the gray-white interface.

3. Alzheimer predominantly affects the temporal and parietal lobes with greater atrophy.

4. Decreased uptake in the parietal and temporal lobes can be seen on FDG PET in Alzheimer disease.

5. Up to 45% of people older than 85 year of age have late-onset Alzheimer disease, which is the most common cause of dementia.

Pearls

- Late-onset Alzheimer disease is very common and the greatest risk factor is advanced age with up to 45% of people greater than 85 years of age demonstrating this disease.

- Early-onset Alzheimer (<60 years) is uncommon and may be associated with familial forms (5-10%).
- Definitive diagnosis requires brain biopsy with visualization of beta amyloid plaques in the cortex and intracellular neurofibrillary tangles.
- The role of imaging is to support the clinical diagnosis by excluding other causes, evaluate for degree of atrophy with volumetric imaging, and provide specificity with PET.
- Cortical atrophy is classically in the temporal and parietal lobes with hypometabolism of these regions on PET FDG or SPECT.
- PET florbetapir, which has high sensitivity of binding to beta amyloid, can show increased abnormal uptake in the cortex over normal uptake in the white matter
- Amyloid angiopathy with multiple hemorrhages can be seen in 80%-90% of Alzheimer patients.

Suggested Readings

Guo H, Song X, Vandorpe R, et al. Evaluation of common structural brain changes in aging and Alzheimer disease with the use of an MRI-based brain atrophy and lesion index: a comparison between T1WI and T2WI at 1.T and 3T. *AJNR Am J Neuroradiol.* 2014 Mar;35(3):504-512.

Kantarci K. Molecular imaging of Alzheimer disease pathology. *AJNR Am J Neuroradiol.* 2014 Jun;35(6 suppl): S12-S17.

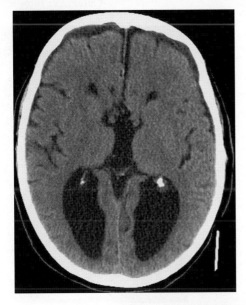
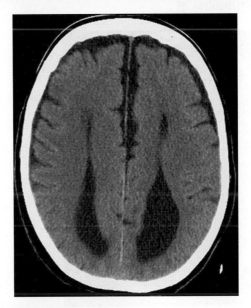
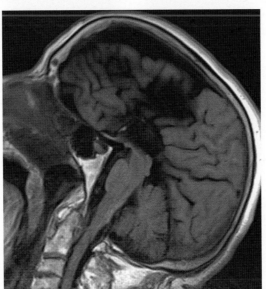

1. Where is the abnormality located?

2. What are the classic imaging findings for this entity?

3. What malformations are associated with this entity?

4. What is the etiology of this entity?

5. What is the treatment for this entity?

Case ranking/difficulty: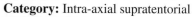

Category: Intra-axial supratentorial

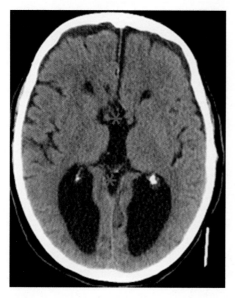

Axial CT image shows colpocephaly with nonvisualization of the genu and splenium of the corpus callosum (*asterisks*).

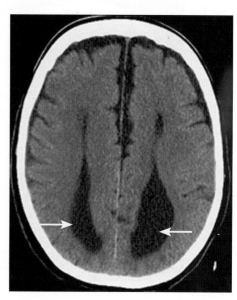

Axial CT image shows colpocephaly with a "tear drop" appearance to the lateral ventricular bodies (*arrows*).

3. Callosal dysgenesis may be associated with Aicardi syndrome, Chiari II malformation, pericallosal lipoma, migration anomalies, and Dandy-Walker malformation. Callosal dysgenesis is the most common finding in CNS malformations.

4. CC agenesis is a congenital process and thought to be a failure of axons to reach midline and cross to the contralateral hemisphere. Large, abnormal Probst bundles medial to the lateral ventricle are the result.

5. No treatment is needed.

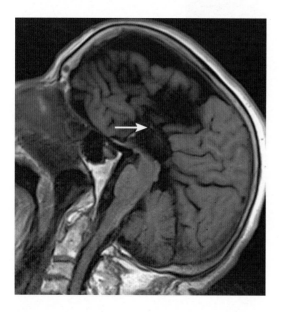

Sagittal T1 image shows absence of the corpus callosum (*white arrow*) and radiating appearance of the gyri.

Answers

1. The morphology of the lateral ventricles is abnormal from callosal agenesis.

2. Corpus callosum (CC) agenesis classic imaging findings are colpocephaly—lateral ventricular "tear drop" appearance (with a parallel orientation), and radiating pattern of the central gyri.

Pearls

- An embryonic insult during formation of the CC may result in dysgenesis to agenesis.
- Sagittal midline image demonstrates a central gyri with a radiating pattern.
- Axial images show abnormal parallel alignment of the lateral ventricles with a "tear drop" appearance (colpocephaly).
- CC dysgenesis has associations with midline lipomas, interhemispheric cysts, facial anomalies, azygous ACA, and cortical maldevelopment.

Suggested Reading

Ho ML, Moonis G, Ginat DT, Eisenberg RL. Lesions of the corpus callosum. *AJR Am J Roentgenol*. 2013 Jan;200(1):W1-W16.

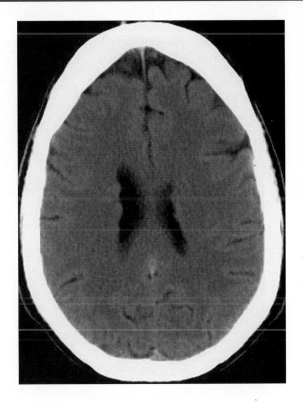
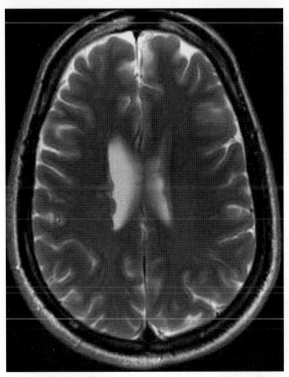

1. Where is the abnormality located?

2. What are the classic imaging findings for this entity?

3. What is the differential diagnosis?

4. What is the etiology of this entity?

5. What is the treatment for this entity?

Case ranking/difficulty:

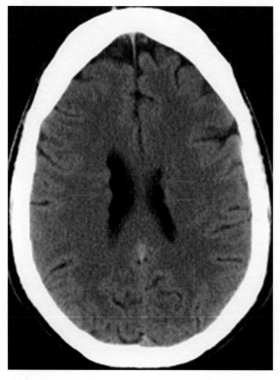

Axial CT image shows focal nodules along the subependymal lining of the lateral ventricles (*arrows*).

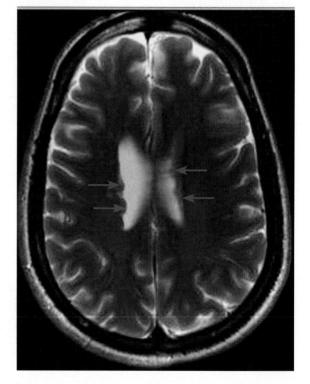

Axial T2 images show the nodules isointense to cortical gray matter (*arrows*).

Answers

1. The abnormality is located along the ependymal lining.

2. The classic imaging findings for this entity are lesions that have the same attenuation on CT or intensity on MR as gray matter.

3. The differential diagnosis includes tuberous sclerosis, heterotopic gray matter, and metastasis.

4. Heterotopic gray matter (HGM) is a congenital migration anomaly where gray matter is located within the white matter. Periventricular heterotopias are often genetic.

5. The treatment for this entity is medical aimed at seizure control. Surgery may be needed with nodule removal when intractable seizures are present.

Pearls

- Heterotopic gray matter (HGM) is a migration anomaly where gray matter is located within the white matter.
- This arrest in migration may occur from the start along the ventricular lining to the cortex.
- Subependymal heterotopia is associated with callosal agenesis, Chiari II, polymicrogyria, and basilar cephaloceles.
- HGM may be band like in morphology.
- If enhancement is present consider tumor or tubers.
- If calcifications are present consider subependymal or cortical tubers.

Suggested Readings

Barkovich AJ, Chuang SH, Norman D. MR of neuronal migration anomalies. *AJR Am J Roentgenol.* 1988 Jan;150(1):179-187.

Mitchell LA, Simon EM, Filly RA, Barkovich AJ. Antenatal diagnosis of subependymal heterotopia. *AJNR Am J Neuroradiol.* 2000 Feb;21(2):296-300.

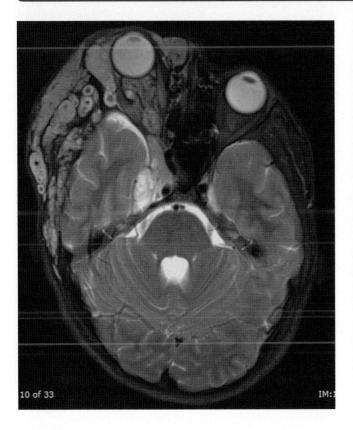
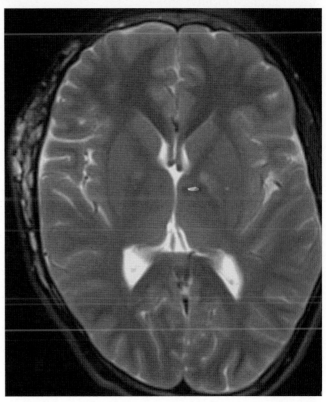

1. What is the genetic inheritance of this disease?

2. What are characteristic brain findings in this disease?

3. What are characteristic tumors and bony involvement for this disease?

4. What is the best imaging modality in the diagnosis and follow-up NF1?

5. Where are the foci of abnormal signal intensities in the brain located in this disease?

Case ranking/difficulty: 🌶

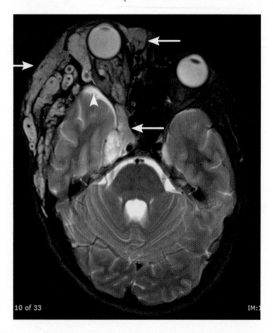

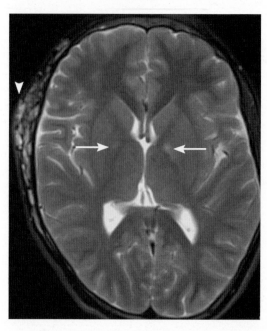

Axial T2 image demonstrates extensive, ropy T2 hyperintense lesions consistent with plexiform neurofibromas along the right side of the face extending to the intra- and extraconal space of the right orbit and along the right Meckel cave (*white arrows*). Noted is right sphenoid wing dysplasia (*white arrowhead*). Target appearance is a characteristic finding for plexiform neurofibromas in NF1 (*red arrowhead*).

Axial T2 image at the level of the basal ganglia shows bilateral foci of abnormal signal intensity of the globi pallidi (*arrows*). Again noted is the right facial plexiform neurofibroma extending to the temporal scalp (*arrowhead*).

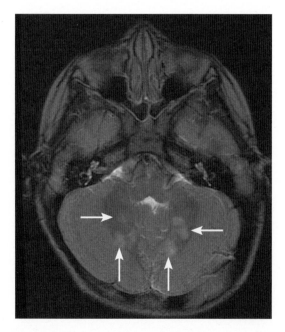

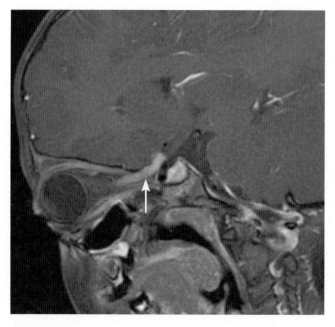

Axial T2 image of a 2-year-old female with NF1 shows multiple bilateral foci of abnormal signal intensity in the deep cerebellar white matter and dentate nuclei (*arrows*).

Oblique T1 postcontrast in a 4-year-old male with NF1 shows an enhancing optic nerve glioma extending through the orbital canal (*arrow*).

Answers

1. NF 1 is caused by mutation or deletion of the NF1 gene located on chromosome 17q11.2, causing interruption of neurofibromin protein production. This can be from autosomal dominant familial inheritance (50%) or new sporadic mutation (50%).

2. NF1 changes involving the brain include focal T2 hyperintense lesions termed foci of abnormal signal intensity or unidentified bright objects in the deep gray matter and periventricular white matter, brainstem gliomas, and optic nerve gliomas.

3. Classic radiographic findings include plexiform neurofibromas, sphenoid wing dysplasia, optic nerve gliomas, and white matter changes (myelin vacuolization).

4. Neurofibromatosis type 1 (NF1) or von Recklinghausen disease presents with multisystem genetic disorders including cutaneous, neurological, and orthopedic manifestations. STIR imaging is helpful to evaluate for neurofibromas throughout the body, foci of abnormal signal intensity within the brain, brain stem, and optic nerve gliomas.

5. Typical locations for NF1 foci of abnormal signal intensity include the globi pallidi, deep cerebellar white matter and dentate nuclei, hippocampi, brainstem, and periventricular white matter. There are amorphous foci of typically nonenhancing T2 hyperintensity without significant mass effect.

Pearls

- Neurofibromatosis type 1 (NF1) is the most common neurocutaneous disease.
- Mutation of NF1 gene in chromosome 17q11.2, causing disruption of neurofibrin, a tumor suppressor.
- Autosomal dominant inheritance (50%) or new mutation (50%).
- Present with cutaneous, neurological, and skeletal manifestations.
- Highly associated with learning disability and autism.
- Classic radiographic findings include plexiform neurofibromas, sphenoid wing dysplasia, optic nerve/optic pathway/brainstem glioma, and white matter changes (myelin vacuolization).
- Plexiform neurofibromas are ropy tumors with increased T2 signal and central T2 hypointensity forming a "target sign" with variable enhancement.
- Optic nerve gliomas demonstrate diffuse or focal thickening of the optic nerve with variable enhancement.
- Focal areas of signal intensity (FASI) or unidentified bright objects (UBO) are seen involving the deep cerebellar white matter, dentate nuclei, brainstem, hippocampi, globi pallidi, and periventricular white matter, thought to represent hamartomas.
- Surgical resection, radiation, or chemotherapy reserved for symptomatic patients and progressing masses.

Suggested Readings

Jacquemin C, Bosley TM, Svedberg H. Orbit deformities in craniofacial neurofibromatosis type 1. *AJNR Am J Neuroradiol*. 2003 Sep;24(8):1678-1682.

Lim R, Jaramillo D, Poussaint TY, Chang Y, Korf B. Superficial neurofibroma: a lesion with unique MRI characteristics in patients with neurofibromatosis type 1. *AJR Am J Roentgenol*. 2005 Mar;184(3):962-968.

Patel NB, Stacy GS. Musculoskeletal manifestations of neurofibromatosis type 1. *AJR Am J Roentgenol*. 2012 Jul;199(1):W99-W106.

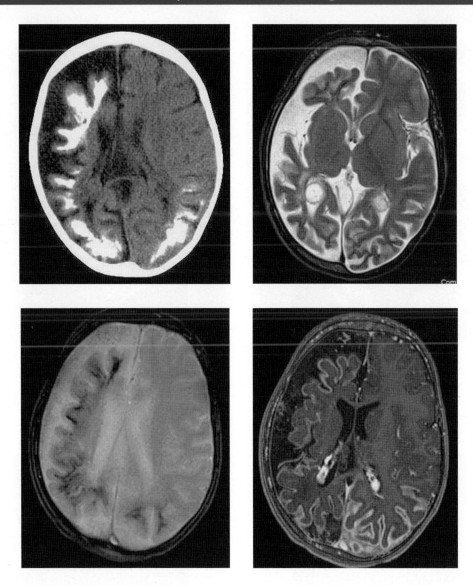

1. What is the differential diagnosis?

2. What are the characteristic radiographic features?

3. What is the typical clinical profile?

4. Where are typical locations for leptomeningeal enhancement?

5. What is the treatment option?

Case ranking/difficulty: 🌰

Category: Intra-axial supratentorial

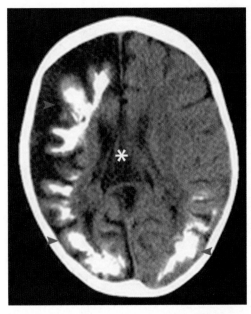

CT image of the brain demonstrates severe atrophy of the right cerebral hemisphere with extensive cortical/subcortical calcifications in the right cerebral hemisphere and left parieto-occipital lobe (*red arrowheads*). Incidentally noted is cavum septum pellucidum (*white asterisk*).

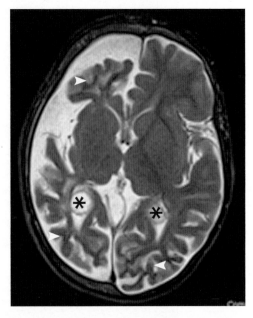

Axial T2 image demonstrate severe atrophy of the right cerebral hemisphere with T2 hypointensity involving cortical/subcortical white matter of the right fronto-parieto-occipital and left parieto-occipital lobes (*white arrowheads*). Bilateral choroidal cysts are noted (*black asterisks*).

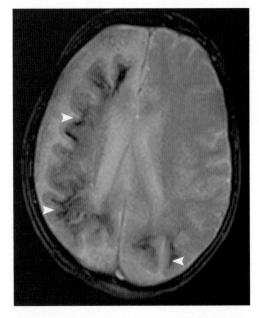

GRE image demonstrates hypointensity without blooming involving the right cerebral hemisphere and left occipital cortical/subcortical white matter (*white arrowheads*), consistent with calcifications seen in the prior CT.

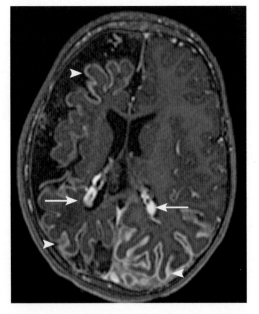

Postcontrast T1 image demonstrates extensive leptomeningeal enhancement involving right cerebral cortical sulci and left parieto-occipital sulci (*white arrowheads*) as well as avid enhancement of the choroid plexi bilaterally (*white arrows*). Note the relative lack of cortical veins of the atrophied right cerebral hemisphere compared to the contralateral normal brain parenchyma.

Answers

1. The differential diagnosis for a combination of cerebral calcification, cerebral hemiatrophy, and leptomeningeal enhancement includes Sturge-Weber, Klippel-Trenaunay-Weber, cerebral AVM, and meningioangiomatosis. All can have thickened leptomeningeal enhancement with calcification.

2. In Sturge Weber, serpentine pial enhancement corresponds to leptomeningeal angiomatosis, in combination with lack of cortical veins and progressive venous stasis, leads to cortical atrophy and subsequent calcification. The ipsilateral choroid plexus is typically enlarged.

3. The typical clinical profile for Sturge-Weber syndrome is a port-wine stain of the face, ipsilateral glaucoma, and seizures in an infant.

4. In Sturge-Weber, leptomeningeal enhancement from pial angiomatosis can involve any pial surface but is most commonly posterior (parieto-occipital) and unilateral. Bilateral involvement is seen in 20% of cases.

5. There is no curative treatment for Sturge-Weber syndrome. Treatment of seizures can include hemispherectomy. Low-dose aspirin may help decrease frequency of stroke-like episodes.

Pearls

- Rare sporadic congenital vascular malformation, with increased levels of endothelial proliferation, and failure of development of fetal cortical veins.
- Increasing venous stasis leads to decreased cortical perfusion.
- Clinical diagnosis based on presence of hemifacial port-wine stain, usually along the V1 and V2 distributions, and ocular choroidal angiomas.
- Usually present with seizures and hemiparesis,
- Radiographic features include hemispheric gyral/subcortical white matter calcifications (tram-track gyral calcification) associated with brain atrophy, serpentine leptomeningeal enhancement, and ipsilateral engorged choroid plexi.
- Absence of pial angiomas at age 1 year can reliably exclude the future development of abnormal leptomeningeal vessels.
- Approximately 90% of infants with facial port-wine stains do not have intracranial lesions and would be expected to develop normally.

Suggested Reading

Nozaki T, Nosaka S, Miyazaki O, et al. Syndromes associated with vascular tumors and malformations: a pictorial review. *Radiographics*. 2013;33(1):175-195.

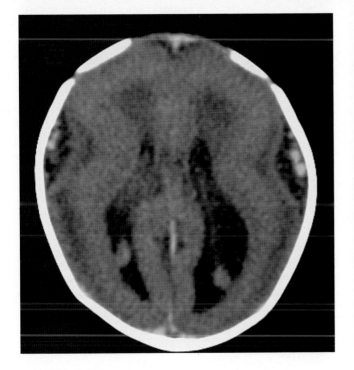 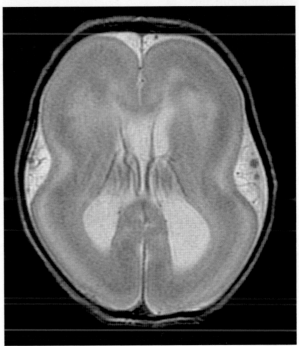

1. What is the differential diagnosis for this finding?

2. What is the pathogenesis of this finding?

3. What is the classic radiographic description?

4. What are clinical characteristics of patients demonstrating only band heterotopia?

5. In prenatal US or fetal MRI what must be known about the patient prior to diagnosing lissencephaly?

Case ranking/difficulty:

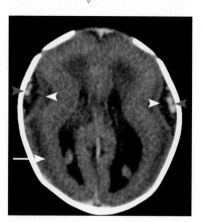

Axial CT image demonstrates hourglass configuration of cerebral hemispheres with smooth cortical surface and shallow sylvian fissures (*white arrowheads*) with lateralized middle cerebral vessels (*green arrowheads*). Also noted is symmetric subcortical gray matter thick band heterotopia (*white arrow*).

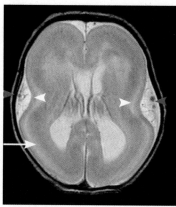

Axial T2 image demonstrates hourglass configuration of cerebral hemispheres with smooth cortical surface and shallow sylvian fissures (*white arrowheads*) with lateralized middle cerebral vessels (*green arrowheads*). Also noted is continuous subcortical hypointense band consistent with heterotopic gray matter (*white arrow*).

Answers

1. Differential diagnosis includes cobblestone lissencephaly (usually associated with congenital muscular dystrophies), other migrational abnormalities (band heterotropia), simplified gyral pattern, and intrauterine infections. This severe form is consistent with Miller-Dieker syndrome, a type I lissencephaly.

2. Classic lissencephaly (type 1) results from undermigration of neuron secondary to syndromic (Miller-Dieker, or Norman-Roberts syndrome), x-linked, or isolated forms secondary to in utero toxin exposure or congenital infection.

3. Classic radiographic features include hourglass or figure eight configuration with smooth cortical surface, shallow sylvian fissures with lateral displacement of the middle cerebral vessels. Subcortical gray matter and thick band heterotopia may be seen.

4. Patients with only band heterotopia are overwhelmingly female and with mild symptoms. This is associated with the x-linked DCX gene with mild phenotype in females with isolated band heterotopia. Male children of these females have more severe lissencephaly with frontal predominance.

5. Findings suggesting lack of sulcation must be correlated with gestational age to diagnose lissencephaly versus normal immature brain.

Pearls

- Severe malformation of the cerebral cortex from impaired neuronal migration during third to fourth months of gestation.
- Divided into two types: Classic (type 1) and cobblestone (type 2) lissencephaly.
- **Classic lissencephaly** results from undermigration; may be syndromic, x-linked, or isolated.
  - Typical radiographic features include hourglass (figure eight) configuration with smooth surface and shallow sulci involving bilateral cerebral hemispheres as well as lateral displacement of the middle cerebral vessels; may be associated with band heterotopia.
  - Miller-Dieker syndrome can be differentiated from isolated lissencephaly by presence of facial dymorphism and severe lissencephaly.
- **Cobblestone lissencephaly** results from overmigration leading to disorganized underlayered and irregular cortex, usually associated with congenital muscular dystrophies.
  - Typical radiographic features include cobblestone appearance with severe ventriculomegaly associated with hypomyelination, vermian hypogenesis, kinked brainstem, cerebellar polymicrogyria or cysts, cephalocele, corpus callosum hypogenesis, and hydrocephalus.

Suggested Reading

Ghai S, Fong KW, Toi A, Chitayat D, Pantazi S, Blaser S. Prenatal US and MR imaging findings of lissencephaly: review of fetal cerebral sulcal development. *Radiographics*. 2006;26(2):389-405.

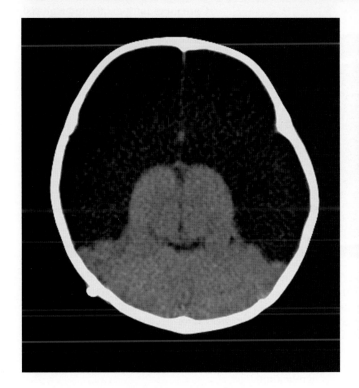 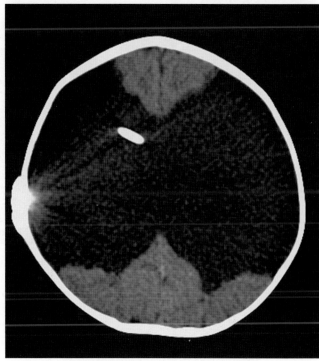

1. What is the differential diagnosis?

2. What is the possible cause of this disease?

3. What are the typical radiographic features?

4. What are treatment options?

5. What cerebral cortex is typically intact, if any?

Case ranking/difficulty:

Category: Intra-axial supratentorial

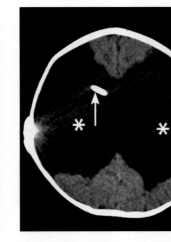

Axial CT demonstrates fluid filled in cranial vault (*white asterisks*) with intact falx cerebri (*white arrowhead*), thalami (*green asterisk*), and cerebellar hemisphere (*blue asterisk*).

Axial CT demonstrates fluid-filled cranial vault (*white asterisks*). There is residual brain parenchyma in the frontal and occipital lobes (*green asterisks*). VP shunt is noted (*white arrow*)

Axial T2-weighted image fetal MRI demonstrates fluid-filled cranial vault (*white asterisks*) with intact falx cerebri (*black arrowhead*), thalami (*green asterisk*), and occipital lobe (*blue asterisk*).

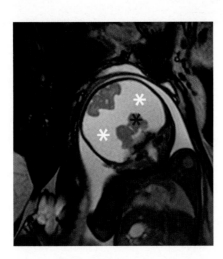

Fetal MRI demonstrates fluid-filled cranial vault (*white asterisks*). There is residual brain parenchyma in the frontal lobes (*green asterisks*) with intact thalami (*blue asterisk*).

Answers

1. Differential diagnosis for hydranencephaly includes severe hydrocephalus, severe bilateral open lip schizencephaly, and alobar holoprosencephaly.

2. Occlusion of bilateral supraclinoid internal carotid arteries is the favored etiology. Other possible etiologies include intrautero infection, maternal carbon monoxide or butane exposure, and thromboembolism from a deceased monochorionic twin.

3. Classic radiographic features include fluid-filled cranial vault, absent cerebral mantle, partially or completely intact falx cerebri, intact thalami, brainstem, and cerebellum.

4. Hydranencephaly patients have a poor prognosis, usually dying in infancy. Supportive treatment with ventriculostomy placement is suggested for macrocephaly.

5. Residual supratentorial cortex seen in hydranencephaly can include structures that can be supplied by the posterior cerebral artery, including the occipital lobes, and paramedian parietal and posterior frontal lobes.

Pearls

- Congenital brain defect secondary to massive brain infarction.
- Postnatal presentations include macrocephaly, developmental failure, calvarial translumination, seizure, or neurological function limited to brainstem.
- Radiographic features are the same in both pre- and postnatal imaging.
- Classic radiographic features include fluid-filled cranial vault, absent cerebral mantle, partially or completely intact falx cerebri, intact thalami, brainstem, and cerebellum.

Suggested Readings

Gentry M, Connell M. Hydranencephaly. *Ultrasound Q.* 2013 Sep;29(3):267-268.

Poe LB, Coleman LL, Mahmud F. Congenital central nervous system anomalies. *Radiographics.* 1989 Sep;9(5):801-826.

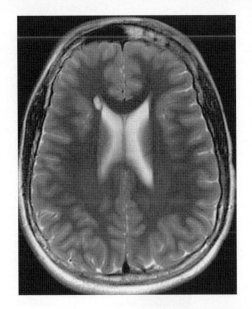
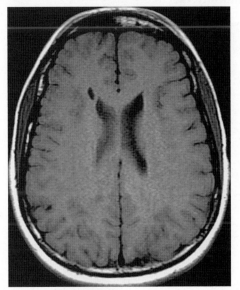
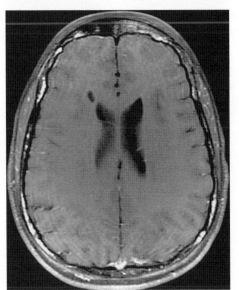

1. Where is the abnormality located?

2. What are the classic imaging findings for this entity?

3. What is the differential diagnosis?

4. What is the etiology of this entity?

5. What is the treatment for this entity?

Case ranking/difficulty: 🥉

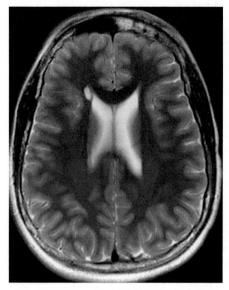

Axial T2 image shows a well-circumscribed lesion of high T2 signal within the white matter adjacent to the right frontal horn (*arrow*).

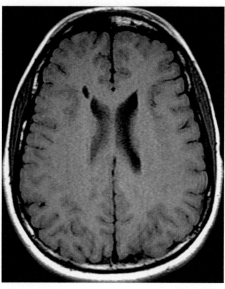

Axial T1 image shows a well-circumscribed lesion of low signal within the white matter adjacent to the right frontal horn (*arrow*).

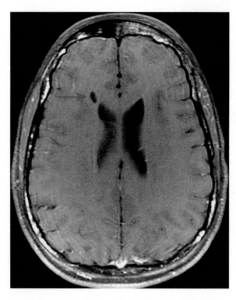

Axial T1 postcontrast image demonstrates no abnormal enhancement (*arrow*).

Answers

1. The abnormality is located within the white matter adjacent to the right frontal horn.

2. Neuroglial cysts follow CSF on CT and all MRI sequences. Therefore, they are low T1, high T2 signal with low density on CT. Also, no associated enhancement is seen.

3. The differential diagnosis includes perivascular space, porencephalic cyst, and neuroglial cyst.

4. Neuroglial cysts are also known as glioependymal cysts and are congenital, benign neuroepithelial-lined lesions. They are thought to be the sequestered lining of the embryonic neural tube.

5. No treatment is needed for this entity.

Pearls

- Neuroglial cyst (NGC) and glioependymal cyst are benign epithelial-lined lesions.
- NGC can be seen anywhere along the neural axis but are more common within the brain parenchyma (most commonly frontal lobe).
- These lesions are usually well circumscribed, round, and unilocular.
- If multiloculated, consider perivascular space.
- If cyst communicates with a ventricle, consider porencephaly.
- If contrast enhancement is seen, consider tumor.

Suggested Reading

Osborn AG, Preece MT. Intracranial cysts: radiologic-pathologic correlation and imaging approach. *Radiology*. 2006 Jun;239(3):650-664.

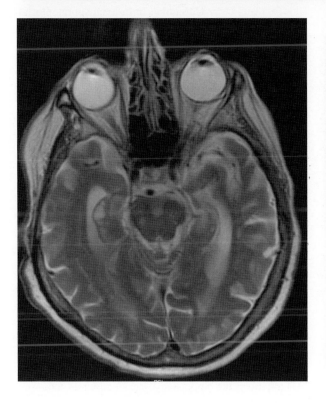 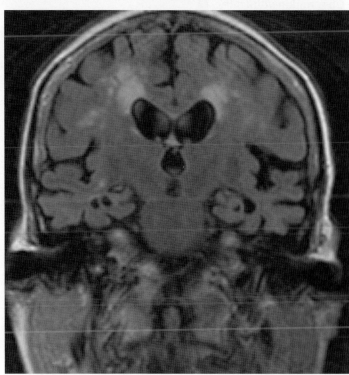

1. Where is the abnormality located?

2. What are the classic imaging findings for this entity?

3. What is the differential diagnosis?

4. What is the etiology of this entity?

5. What is the treatment for this entity?

Case ranking/difficulty: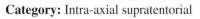

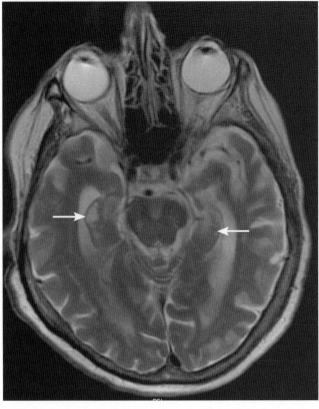

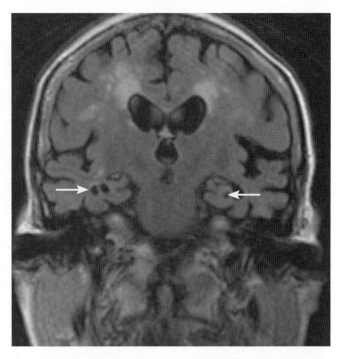

Coronal FLAIR shows the hippocampal lesions suppress, following CSF signal (*arrows*).

Axial T2 image shows well-defined, subcentimeter high T2 signal lesions within the hippocampal gyri appearing as a "string of cysts."

Answers

1. A string of cystic lesions is noted along the bilateral hippocampi.

2. Hippocampal sulcus remnants (HSR) on MRI have corresponding high T2 signal and low T1 and FLAIR signal, following CSF. HSR do not show contrast enhancement or restriction on DWI.

3. The differential diagnosis includes hippocampal sulcus remnant, mesial temporal sclerosis, and choroidal fissure cyst.

4. HSR is thought to be a partial lack of fusion of the hippocampal sulcus as the cornu ammonis and dentate gyrus fold to form the characteristic hippocampal gyrus. These may become more prominent with volume loss and are more easily seen on high-resolution imaging.

5. No treatment is needed for this entity.

Pearls

- Hippocampal sulcus remnants (HSR), also called hippocampal sulcal cavities, are a common finding and are likely the result of incomplete folding of the hippocampus along the vestigial sulcus.
- Seen as string of CSF cysts along the lateral margin of the hippocampus.
- If focal increased FLAIR signal consider infarct and encephalitis.
- Consider mesial temporal sclerosis with increased T2/FLAIR signal and hippocampal volume loss.

Suggested Reading

van Veluw SJ, Wisse LE, Kuijf HJ, et al. Hippocampal T2 hyperintensities on 7 Tesla MRI. *Neuroimage Clin*. 2013 Jan;3(3):196-201.

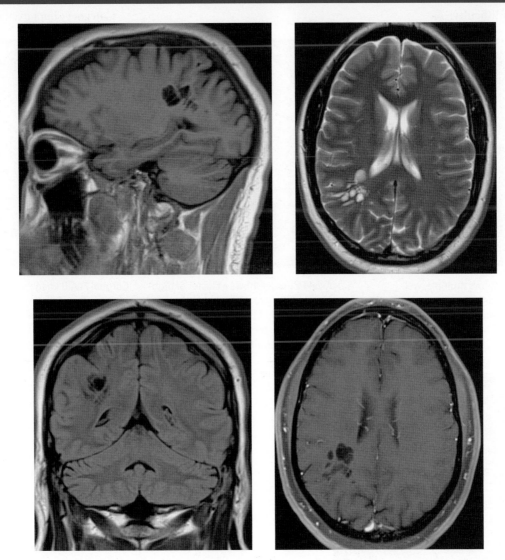

1. Where is the abnormality located?

2. What are the classic imaging findings for this entity?

3. What is the differential diagnosis?

4. What is the etiology of this entity?

5. What is the treatment for this entity?

Case ranking/difficulty: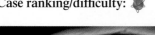

Category: Intra-axial supratentorial

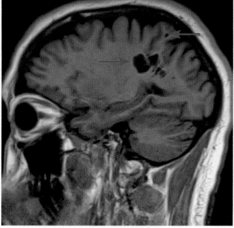

Sagittal T1 image shows multiple, well-circumscribed low-signal structures within the white matter of the right parietal lobe (*arrows*).

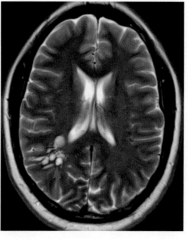

Axial T2 image shows a cluster of high-signal cystic structures within the white matter of the right parietal lobe (*arrow*). Note the radial orientation to the lateral ventricle.

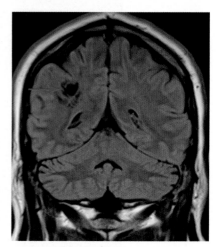

Coronal FLAIR image demonstrates suppression of the cystic lesions following CSF (*arrow*).

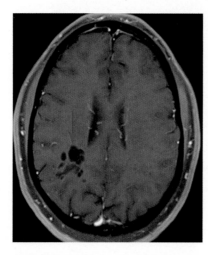

Axial T1 postcontrast image shows no enhancement within the right parietal lobe white matter cystic lesions (*arrow*).

Answers

1. The abnormality is located within the subcortical white matter of the right parietal lobe.

2. On imaging, perivascular spaces (PVS) always follow CSF signal on all pulse sequences. Therefore, these are low T1 and high T2 signals with suppression on FLAIR. These spaces do not restrict diffusion or enhance.

3. The differential diagnosis includes lacunar infarction, perivascular spaces, cystic neoplasm, cryptococcoma, and neurocysticercosis.

4. PVS is thought to be developmental, from accumulation of interstitial fluid between the penetrating vessel and pia.

5. No treatment is needed for this entity.

Pearls

- Perivascular spaces (PVS) are also known as Virchow-Robin spaces.
- Follows CSF on all pulse sequences and do not enhance.
- 25% have some minimal increased surrounding FLAIR signal.
- White matter and deep gray nuclei location.
- The most common site involves the lower basal ganglia.
- Radial orientation to the ventricle in the deep white matter.
- As age increases, the size of PVS enlarges.
- These spaces are usually 2 to 5 mm in size.

Suggested Readings

Osborn AG, Preece MT. Intracranial cysts: radiologic-pathologic correlation and imaging approach. *Radiology*. 2006 Jun;239(3):650-664.

Kwee RM, Kwee TC. Virchow-Robin spaces at MR imaging. *Radiographics*. 2007;27(4):1071-1086.

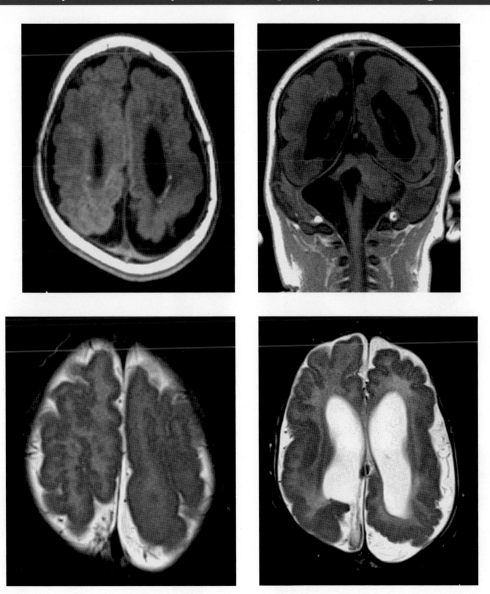

1. What is the incidence for this disease?

2. What is the typical clinical presentation?

3. What are characteristic radiographic findings?

4. What is the differential diagnosis?

5. What are common late sequelae of this disease?

Case ranking/difficulty: 🌑

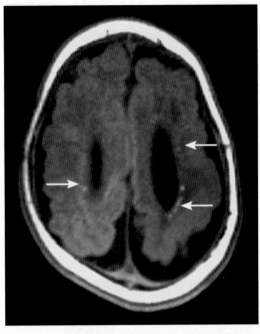

Axial T1 image demonstrates multiple punctate foci of T1 hyperintensity in bilateral periventricular white matter (*white arrows*), consistent with periventricular calcifications.

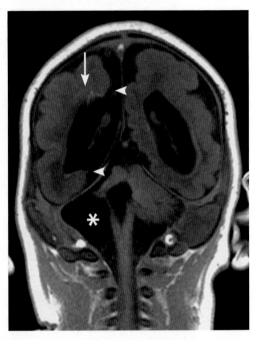

Coronal T1 image demonstrates foci of T1 hyperintensity in right periventricular white matter (*white arrows*), consistent with periventricular calcifications. There is open-lip schizencephaly in the right parietal lobe (*white arrowhead*). Also noted is right cerebellar hypoplasia (*asterisk*).

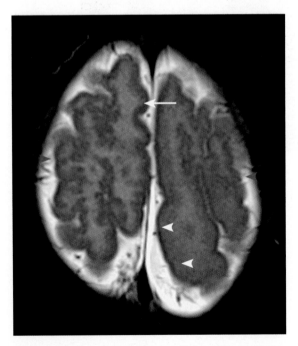

Axial T2 image demonstrates diffuse migrational anomalies with pachygyria (*white arrow*), lissencephaly (*white arrowhead*), and polymicrogyria (*red arrowheads*).

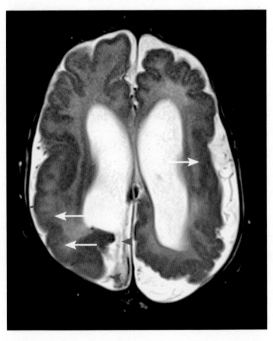

Axial T2 image demonstrates pachygyria in the left frontoparietal cortices (*arrows*). Again noted is the right parietal schizencephalic cleft (*red arrowheads*).

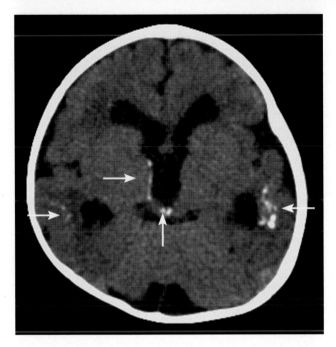

Noncontrast CT image from another infant with congenital CMV demonstrates periventricular calcifications (*arrows*).

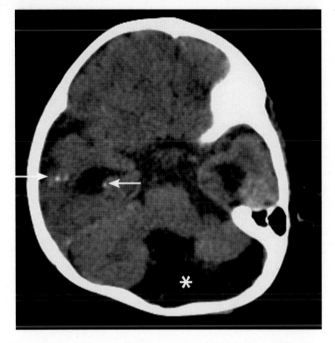

Noncontrast CT image demonstrates periventricular calcifications (*white arrows*) and hypoplasia of the left cerebellum (*asterisk*).

Answers

1. Congenital CMV infection is the most common serious viral infection affecting approximately 1% of all newborns in the United States.

2. Only 10% of infected infants are symptomatic at birth. Most common systemic signs of disease involvement include prematurity, hepatosplenomegaly, jaundice, petechiae, chorioretinitis, and intrauterine growth retardation. CNS involvement includes microcephaly, seizure, hypo- or hypertonia, and late findings of sensorineural hearing loss.

3. Classic CNS radiographic findings include periventricular calcifications, cortical malformations ranging from agyria, pachygyria, diffuse polymicrogyria, focal cortical dysplasia, and schizencephaly. Delayed myelination and cerebellar hypoplasia are commonly seen.

4. Differential diagnosis of congenital CMV infection includes other TORCH infections, pseudo-TORCH syndrome, and congenital lymphocytic choriomeningitis.

5. Sensorineural hearing loss is the most common late sequela; however, other CNS sequelae include seizures, lack of coordination, mental disability, and microcephaly.

Pearls

- Most common cause of intrauterine infection with congenital brain damage in the United States.
- Usually asymptomatic (90%); only 10% of patients have signs and symptoms at birth.
- Classic clinical presentations: microcephaly, seizure, chorioretinitis, petechiae, deafness, and hepatosplenomegaly.
- Classic brain findings: periventricular calcifications, cortical malformation ranging from agyria, pachygyria, diffuse polymicrogyria, focal cortical dysplasia, and schizencephaly, in addition to delayed myelination and cerebellar hypoplasia.
- Degree of intracranial abnormalities depends on gestational age at time of infection.
- Sensorineural hearing loss is the most common late sequela.

Suggested Readings

Malinger G, Lev D, Zahalka N, et al. Fetal cytomegalovirus infection of the brain: the spectrum of sonographic findings. *AJNR Am J Neuroradiol*. 2003 Jan;24(1):28-32.

Teissier N, Fallet-Bianco C, Delezoide AL, et al. Cytomegalovirus-induced brain malformations in fetuses. *J Neuropathol Exp Neurol*. 2014 Feb;73(2):143-158.

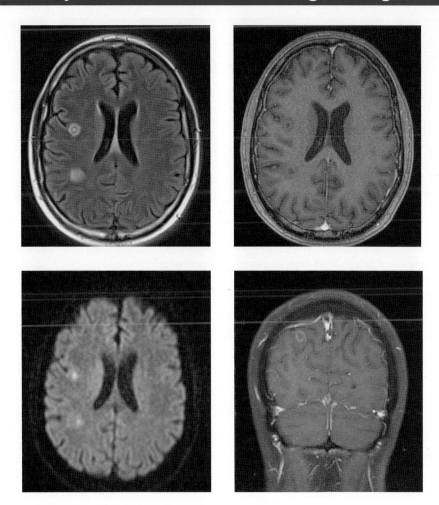

1. What is the differential diagnosis for this finding?

2. What is an imaging sign helpful to distinguish between ring-enhancing etiologies such as abscess and metastatic disease?

3. What is the cause of T2 hypointensity in the periphery of these lesions?

4. What vascular distribution is more common for these lesions?

5. What organism(s) has more likelihood of angioinvasion?

Case ranking/difficulty: **Category:** Intra-axial supratentorial

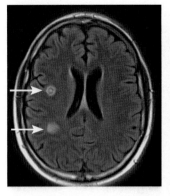

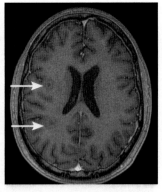

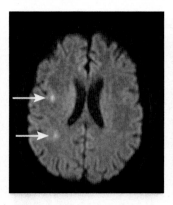

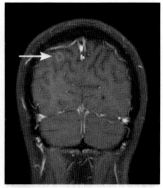

Axial FLAIR image shows two rounded ring-like lesions in the right frontal parietal lobe, at the gray-white junction. Note the T2 hypointense rim and minimal surrounding edema of the lesion (*white arrows*).

Axial T1 postcontrast image shows rim enhancement (*white arrows*) which is relatively faint, likely due to immunosuppressed state.

Axial DWI b = 1000 shows central diffusion restriction (*white arrows*) suggesting abscesses.

Coronal T1 postcontrast demonstrates another posterior parietal faint ring-enhancing lesion at the gray-white junction (*white arrow*).

Answers

1. The differential for multiple ring-enhancing lesions includes both fungal and bacterial abscesses, toxoplasmosis, and metastatic disease.

2. Abscesses can show central restricted diffusion from pyogenic material. Likewise, metastases can show peripheral restricted diffusion from hypercellularity and central facilitated diffusion in areas of necrosis.

3. T2 hypointense rims coinciding with peripheral enhancement correlate histologically with the abscess capsule. It is thought that paramagnetic free radicals formed by macrophages give the susceptibility effect of decreased T2 signal. It has been suggested that iron is a significant component of this paramagnetic effect in fungal abscesses.

4. The anterior circulation is involved more often from hematogenous seeding of abscesses, with the gray-white junction most commonly involved.

5. Angioinvasion has typically been described with invasive aspergillosis and mucormycosis in the immunocompromised. This has also been described to a lesser extent with candidiasis.

Pearls

- Think about fungal disease in immunocompromised patients!
- MRI findings of hematogenous fungal disease are not distinguishable from bacterial causes.
- Postcontrast images can show meningeal enhancement or nodular and ring appearance in the parenchyma.
- Ring-enhancing lesions may show less than expected enhancement and edema in immunocompromised patients.
- Central diffusion restriction and a rim of T2 hypointensity may be seen with fungal abscesses, helping distinguish from metastatic disease.
- Aspergillosis and mucormycoses can be angioinvasive, causing mycotic aneurysms and hemorrhagic infarcts.

Suggested Readings

Boes B, Bashir R, Boes C, Hahn F, McConnell JR, McComb R. Central nervous system aspergillosis. Analysis of 26 patients. *J Neuroimaging*. 1994 Jul;4(3):123-129.

Mathur M, Johnson CE, Sze G. Fungal infections of the central nervous system. *Neuroimaging Clin N Am*. 2012 Nov;22(4):609-632.

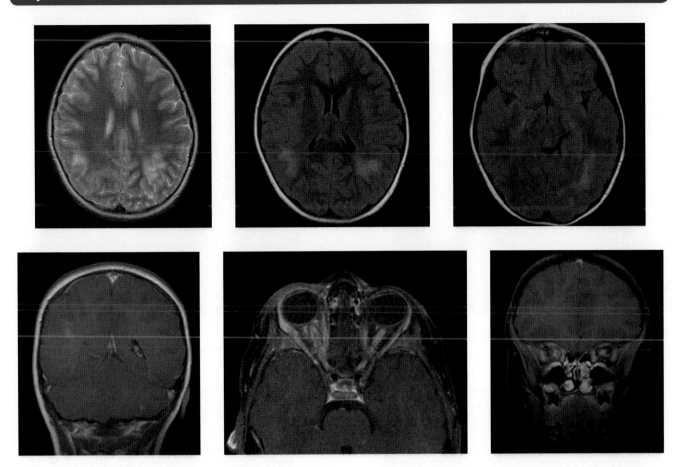

1. What is the differential diagnosis for this finding?

2. What other findings can be seen with this disease?

3. What is the treatment for this disease?

4. What is the prognosis of this disease?

5. How well does imaging correlate with disease progress?

Case ranking/difficulty:

Category: Intra-axial supratentorial

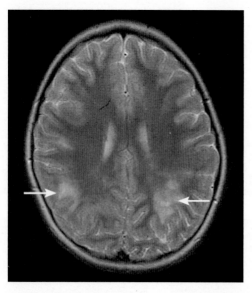

Axial T2 image shows bilateral patchy asymmetric white matter hyperintensities (*white arrows*).

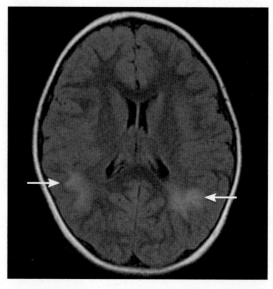

Axial FLAIR image shows patchy white matter hyperintensities (*white arrows*) that do not extend to the callosal septal interface.

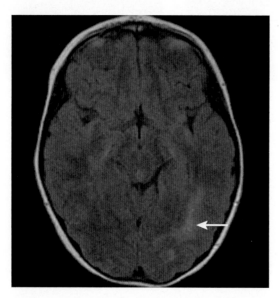

Axial FLAIR image demonstrates left temporal subcortical white matter T2 hyperintensity (*white arrow*).

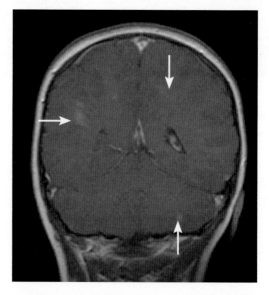

Coronal postcontrast image shows vague amorphous enhancement of the white matter lesions (*white arrows*) without significant T1 hypointensity of the involved areas. Note an isolated lesion of the left cerebellum.

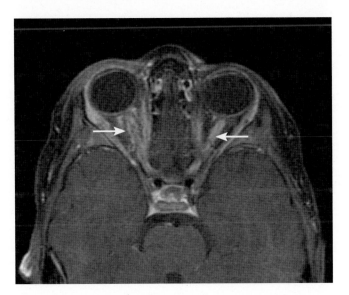

Axial T1 postcontrast image through the orbits shows bilateral thickening and enhancement of the optic nerves (*white arrows*). This is consistent with optic neuritis.

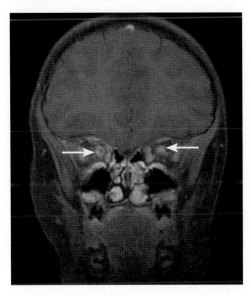

Coronal T1 postcontrast through the orbital apex shows the bilateral enlargement and enhancement of the optic nerves (*white arrows*).

Answers

1. Differential diagnosis for bilateral patchy white matter lesions with vague enhancement includes demyelinating processes such as ADEM and MS. With the bilateral posterior distribution in this case, PRES could be considered.

2. ADEM can also have basal ganglia involvement in half of cases and spinal cord involvement in 30% of cases. Cranial nerve involvement with edema and enhancement is also described.

3. Immunosuppression from corticosteroids is the typical first-line treatment for ADEM. Patients who do not respond to steroid therapy may benefit from plasmapheresis or IVIG.

4. 50%-60% of patients with ADEM will recover with adequate treatment without permanent deficit. Up to 30% can have persistent sequelae, primarily seizures. 10%-20% of cases of ADEM lead to fatality.

5. With ADEM, imaging findings typically lag the clinical symptoms. The initial imaging at presentation may be normal.

Pearls

- ADEM is a monophasic, immune-mediated inflammatory demyelination 1-2 weeks after viral or bacterial infection, as well as immunization.
- Bilateral patchy white matter involvement is typical, with variable enhancement.
- Central white matter is not usually involved like MS.
- Half of cases have basal ganglia involvement.
- Cranial nerve involvement with enhancement can be seen.
- Spinal cord involvement can be seen in 30%.
- The majority make a full recovery with treatment. Less than 1/3 have neurologic sequelae or progress to fatality.

Suggested Readings

Honkaniemi J, Dastidar P, Kähärä V, Haapasalo H. Delayed MR imaging changes in acute disseminated encephalomyelitis. *AJNR Am J Neuroradiol.* 2002 Feb;22(6):1117-1124.

Marin SE, Callen DJ. The magnetic resonance imaging appearance of monophasic acute disseminated encephalomyelitis: an update post application of the 2007 consensus criteria. *Neuroimaging Clin N Am.* 2013 May;23(2):245-266.

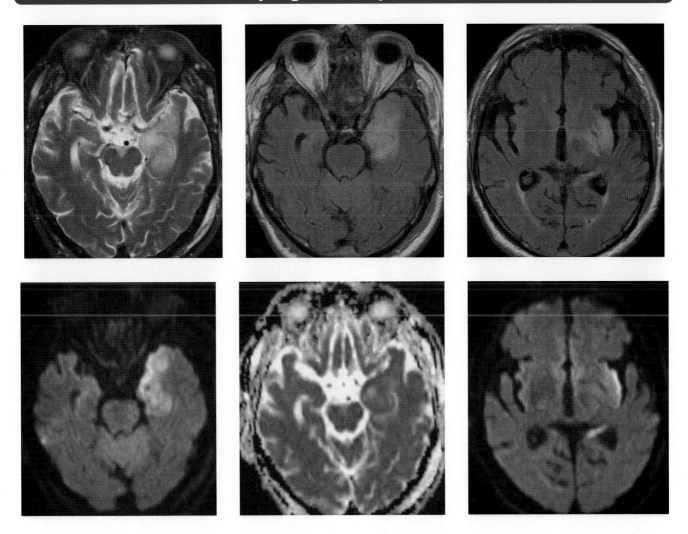

1. What is the differential for these MRI findings?

2. What is the usual anatomy affected in this disease?

3. What is the prognosis of this disease?

4. What are typical MRI findings on different pulse sequences for this disease?

5. Which population groups have a higher risk of this disease?

Case ranking/difficulty: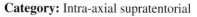

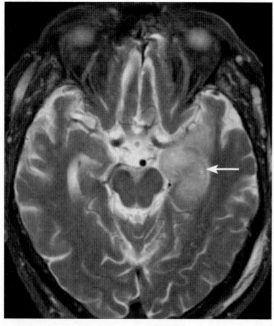

Axial T2 image through the midbrain shows sulcal effacement from swelling and T2 hyperintensity of the medial temporal lobe (*white arrow*).

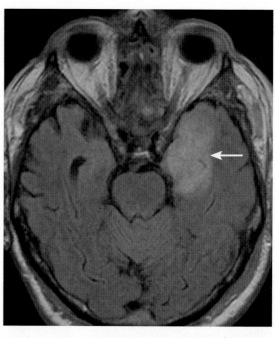

Axial FLAIR image shows hyperintensity with sulcal effacement of the medial temporal lobe (*white arrow*).

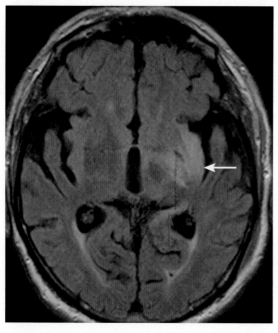

Axial FLAIR image shows further involvement with T2 hyperintensity of the insular cortex and subthalamic nuclei (*white arrow*). Note involvement of the tail of the hippocampus (*red arrow*).

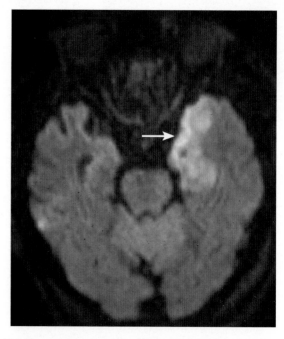

Axial DWI b = 1000 image shows increased cortical and subcortical signal of the left medial temporal lobe (*white arrow*).

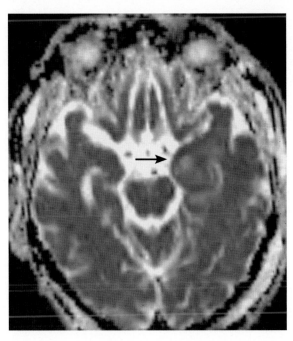

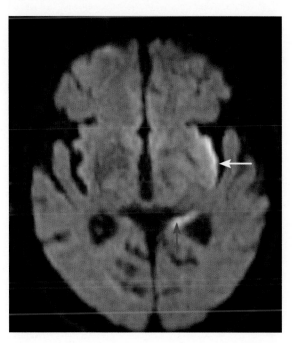

Axial ADC map at the level of the midbrain shows decreased diffusion involving primarily the cortex of the medial temporal lobe (*black arrow*).

Axial DWI b = 1000 image also shows diffusion restriction of the left insular cortex (*white arrow*) and hippocampal tail (*red arrow*).

Answers

1. The differential for medial temporal lobe swelling includes herpes encephalitis, acute stroke, and limbic encephalitis (which does not consistently cause restricted diffusion). Neurosyphilis has also been reported to involve the medial temporal lobes as a herpes encephalitis mimicker.

2. Herpes encephalitis usually involves the medial temporal lobes, insular cortex, and inferior frontal lobes. The disease can be bilateral but asymmetric.

3. Untreated herpes encephalitis can have up to 70% mortality. Even with acyclovir treatment, a majority (2/3) of patients will have some neurologic sequelae. Treatment with acyclovir should be initiated rapidly in patients with suspected herpes encephalitis.

4. In herpes encephalitis, swelling of the medial temporal lobe causes increased signal on T2 and FLAIR, which can be more sensitive than T2. Enhancement is variable early in the disease; however, gyral enhancement a week after presentation is more typical. DWI images typically show bright cortical signal with corresponding decreased signal on ADC, indicating restricted diffusion.

5. Herpes encephalitis has a bimodal distribution occurring more often in people less than 20 and older than 50 years of age. 1/3 of cases occur in the less than 20 demographic, who also tend to have better prognosis than patients older than 50. There is no gender or ethnic predilection.

Pearls

- Herpes encephalitis typically involves the medial temporal lobes, insular cortex, and inferior frontal lobes.
- Cortical diffusion restriction is typical with variable enhancement early in the disease course.
- Sparing of the deep white matter and basal ganglia is commonly seen.
- Any pathology involving the medial temporal lobe with the typical clinical history of fever and headaches must include herpes in the differential.
- If herpes encephalitis is suspected, urgent communication with the clinical team is necessary to quickly start antiviral therapy (acyclovir), as untreated herpes encephalitis is often fatal.

Suggested Readings

Küker W, Nägele T, Schmidt F, Heckl S, Herrlinger U. Diffusion-weighted MRI in herpes simplex encephalitis: a report of three cases. *Neuroradiology*. 2004 Feb;46(2):122-125.

Noguchi T, Yoshiura T, Hiwatashi A, et al. CT and MRI findings of human herpesvirus 6-associated encephalopathy: comparison with findings of herpes simplex virus encephalitis. *AJR Am J Roentgenol*. 2010 Mar;194(3):754-760.

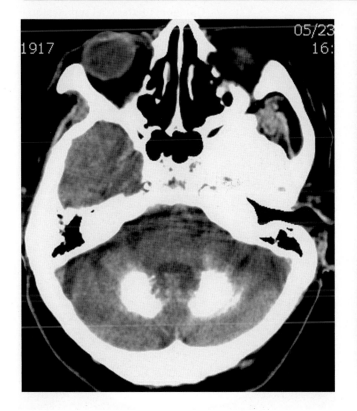 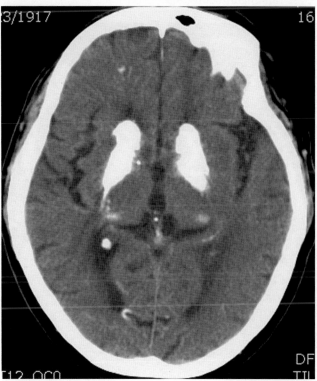

1. Where is the abnormality located?

2. What are the classic imaging findings for this entity?

3. What is the differential diagnosis?

4. What brain structures can this entity involve?

5. What is the most common source of the high attenuation?

Case ranking/difficulty:

Category: Intra-axial supratentorial

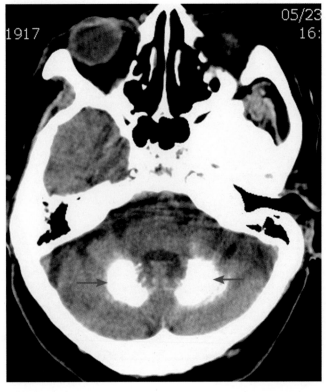

Axial CT shows symmetric high density in the dentate nuclei (*arrows*).

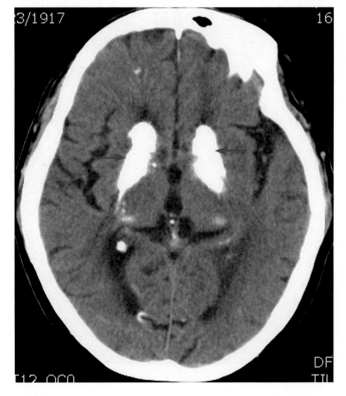

Axial CT shows symmetric high density in the basal ganglia bilaterally (*arrows*).

Answers

1. Symmetric high density is seen in the basal ganglia and the dentate nuclei.

2. Symmetric, bilateral high density within the basal ganglia, especially in a young adult.

3. The differential diagnosis includes hypoparathyroidism, pseudohypoparathyroidism, Fahr disease, mineralizing microangiopathy from prior injury, and normal calcification in the middle aged to elderly.

4. Fahr disease may involve the basal ganglia (caudate nucleus and lentiform nucleus), dentate nuclei, thalami, subcortical white matter, and centrum semiovale.

5. The most common source of the high attenuation is calcium deposition.

Pearls

- Fahr disease is also called bilateral striopallidodentate calcinosis.
- The key to this diagnosis on CT is the symmetric high density (calcification) of the basal ganglia in the absence of hypercalcemia.
- Bilateral, symmetric basal ganglia calcifications in a young adult (<40) or children are usually not normal.
- Calcifications are readily seen on CT.
- Dentate nuclei commonly are calcified.

Suggested Readings

Avrahami E, Cohn DF, Feibel M, Tadmor R. MRI demonstration and CT correlation of the brain in patients with idiopathic intracerebral calcification. *J Neurol*. 1994 May;241(6):381-384.

Govindarajan A. Imaging in Fahr's disease: how CT and MRI differ? *BMJ Case Rep*. 2013 Nov 27;2013.

Hegde AN, Mohan S, Lath N, Lim CC. Differential diagnosis for bilateral abnormalities of the basal ganglia and thalamus. *Radiographics*. 2011;31(1):5-30.

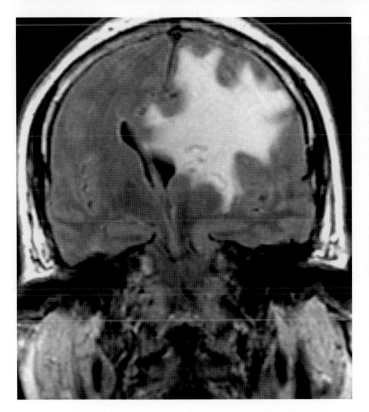 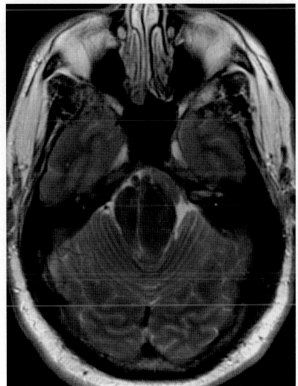

1. What are the key imaging findings?

2. What are causes for intracranial herniation?

3. What clinical symptoms are associated with left uncal herniation?

4. What is Kernohan notch phenomenon?

5. Where do Duret hemorrhages occur?

Case ranking/difficulty: 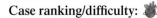   **Category:** Intra-axial supratentorial

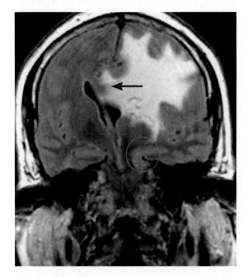

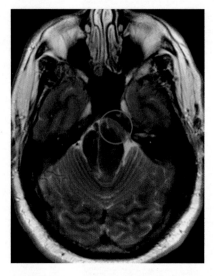

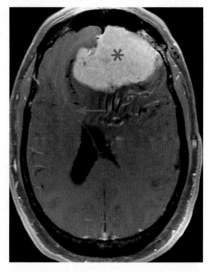

Coronal FLAIR image shows left frontal lobe vasogenic edema with resultant subfalcine herniation from left to the right (*arrow*) with left uncal herniation (*circle*).

Axial T2 image shows left uncal herniation with uncus located in the left anterior prepontine cistern (*circle*).

Axial T1 postcontrast image shows left frontal lobe enhancing extraaxial mass (*asterisk*) causing subfalcine herniation to the right (*arrow*).

Answers

1. The key imaging findings is significant vasogenic edema, resulting in rightward subfalcine herniation and left uncal herniation.

2. Chiari malformation, diffuse cerebral edema, CNS mass lesions, hydrocephalus, and intracranial hemorrhage are causes of intracranial herniation.

3. Mass effect on the ipsilateral third cranial nerve with resultant dilation of the pupil and failed constriction with light stimulus due to malfunction of the parasympathetic fibers. The third cranial nerve compression will also result in the ipsilateral eye to deviate "down and out," from retained function of the lateral rectus and superior oblique muscles from cranial nerves VI and IV, respectively.

4. Kernohan notch phenomenon is a result of transtentorial herniation causing contralateral compression of the midbrain over the tentorium (Kernohan notch), which in turn causes hemiparesis ipsilateral to the transtentorial herniation but contralateral to Kernohan notch.

5. Duret hemorrhages are microbleeds in the medulla or pons in patients with rapid herniation. They are typically in the midline and possibly due to laceration of pontine perforators or draining veins.

Pearls

- Uncal herniation is an emergent finding.
- Look for effacement of the suprasellar and prepontine cistern.
- Subfalcine herniation typically precedes transtentorial herniation.
- With a "blown pupil" look for ipsilateral uncal herniation.
- With uncal herniation, the tentorium cerebelli may create mass effect on the cerebral peduncle, which may lead to ipsilateral hemiparesis.

Suggested Reading

Mejía Kattah J, Vilá Barriuso E, García Bernedo C, Gallart Gallego L. [Kernohan-Woltman notch phenomenon secondary to a cranial epidural hematoma]. *Rev Esp Anestesiol Reanim.* 2014 Jun-Jul;61(6):332-335.

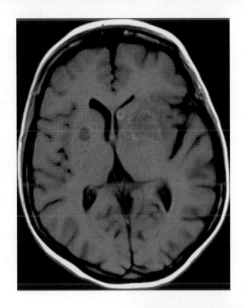
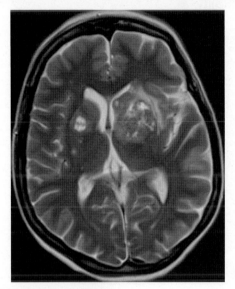
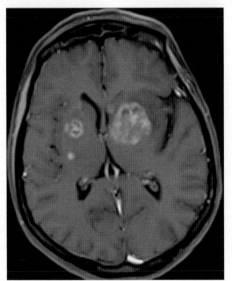

1. Where is the abnormality located?

2. What are the classic imaging findings for this entity?

3. What is the differential diagnosis?

4. What are the most common etiologies of this finding?

5. What is the treatment for this entity?

Case ranking/difficulty: 🥀

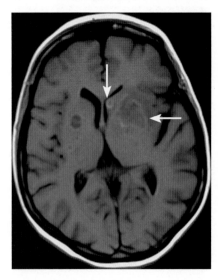

Axial T1 image shows bilateral heterogeneous lesions within both basal ganglia. These lesions show T1 shortening, which may correspond to blood products (*arrows*).

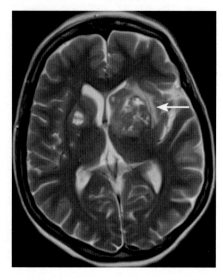

Axial T2 image shows heterogeneous appearance of the lesions with mild edema adjacent to the largest lesion in the left basal ganglia (*arrow*).

4. The most common etiologies include lung, melanoma, and breast carcinoma.

5. The treatment for CNS metastases is dependent on the primary carcinoma, but usually disseminated disease is treated with whole brain radiation and/or chemotherapy.

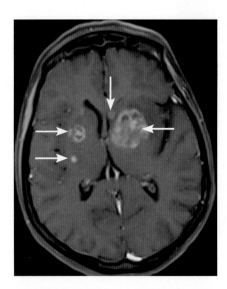

Axial T1 postcontrast image shows multiple, bilateral heterogeneously enhancing lesions within both basal ganglia (*arrows*). Also note that there is regional mass effect resulting from the left basal ganglia lesion with effacement of the anterior horn of the left lateral ventricle and mild midline shift.

Answers

1. The abnormality is located within the basal ganglia.

2. Metastasis can affect any part of the brain. The imaging appearance is variable and depends on the primary tumor. Classically, the lesions enhance and are multiple.

3. The differential diagnosis includes metastasis, abscess, and demyelinating disease.

Pearls

- Suspect metastasis with multiple lesions.
- Most commonly involves the supratentorial brain.
- The most common etiologies include lung, melanoma, and breast carcinoma.
- 50% of CNS metastases are solitary.
- 50% of all brain tumors.
- History of primary carcinoma.
- Consider infectious etiology in immunocompromised patients.

Suggested Readings

Tang YM, Ngai S, Stuckey S. The solitary enhancing cerebral lesion: can FLAIR aid the differentiation between glioma and metastasis? *AJNR Am J Neuroradiol*. 2006 Mar;27(3):609-611.

Toh CH, Wei KC, Ng SH, Wan YL, Lin CP, Castillo M. Differentiation of brain abscesses from necrotic glioblastomas and cystic metastatic brain tumors with diffusion tensor imaging. *AJNR Am J Neuroradiol*. 2011 Oct;32(9):1646-1651.

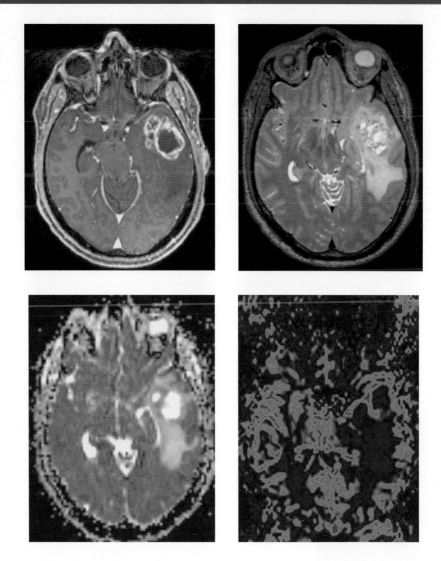

1. What is the differential diagnosis?

2. What does the adjacent T2 hyperintensity of the white matter represent?

3. What does the central nonenhancing component represent?

4. What is the prognosis for this disease?

5. What can be seen with perfusion and diffusion imaging?

Case ranking/difficulty: 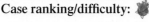   **Category:** Intra-axial supratentorial

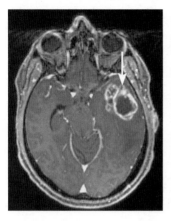

Axial T1 postcontrast image shows an irregular ring-enhancing lesion in the left temporal lobe (*arrow*).

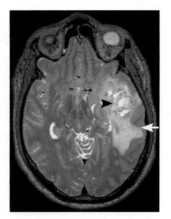

Axial T2 image shows the heterogeneous nature of the lesion with a rim of T2 hypointensity (*black arrowhead*) and adjacent white matter T2 hyperintensity (*white arrow*), typically representing a combination of vasogenic edema and tumor infiltration in this case of GBM. Note the mass effect on the midbrain.

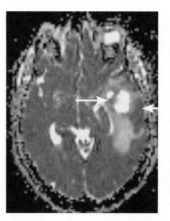

Axial DWI ADC map shows areas of peripheral decreased ADC from hypercellular portions of the tumor (*arrows*).

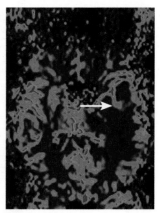

Axial relative cerebral blood volume map from dynamic susceptibility contrast perfusion imaging shows a rim of hyperperfusion largely correlating with the enhancing components (*arrow*).

4. Prognosis remains dismal for glioblastoma multiforme, with most cases resulting in death within 12 months.

5. A hallmark of GBM is central necrosis with hypercellular, viable tumor at the periphery, which shows increased perfusion and decreased diffusion, similar to other high-grade neoplasms.

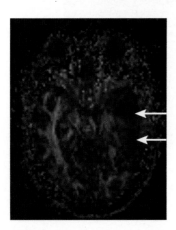

Axial fractional anisotropy map shows a loss of anisotropy of Meyer loop likely from tumor infiltration (*arrows*).

Answers

1. The differential for ring-enhancing mass-like lesions includes glioblastoma, abscess, CNS lymphoma, solitary metastasis, and tumefactive demyelination.

2. The adjacent white matter T2 hyperintensity of glioblastomas typically represents a combination of vasogenic edema and tumor infiltration.

3. The central nonenhancing components of glioblastomas are typically necrotic portions which have outgrown its blood supply.

Pearls

- Glioblastoma multiforme (GBM) is the most common primary brain neoplasm in adults.
- Heterogeneous enhancement, sometimes in a ring with central necrosis, can be seen.
- The enhancing component may demonstrate decreased T2 signal and decreased ADC, as well as increased perfusion from hypercellular portions of the tumor.
- There is typically adjacent white matter T2 hyperintensity, which represents vasogenic edema and tumor infiltration.
- Centrally necrotic areas will not have central restricted diffusion, which can be seen with abscesses.

Suggested Readings

Hirai T, Murakami R, Nakamura H, et al. Prognostic value of perfusion MR imaging of high-grade astrocytomas: long-term follow-up study. *AJNR Am J Neuroradiol.* 2008 Sep;29(8):1505-1510.

Young GS, Setayesh K. Spin-echo echo-planar perfusion MR imaging in the differential diagnosis of solitary enhancing brain lesions: distinguishing solitary metastases from primary glioma. *AJNR Am J Neuroradiol.* 2009 Mar;30(3):575-577.

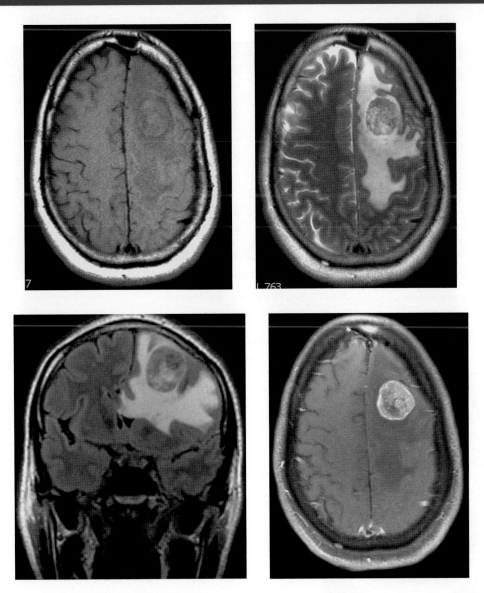

1. Where is the abnormality located?

2. What are the classic imaging findings?

3. What is the differential diagnosis?

4. Which part of the brain does this entity commonly involve?

5. What are the most common primary etiologies in adults with this entity?

Case ranking/difficulty:

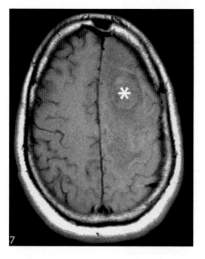

Axial T1 image shows a heterogeneous lesion within the left frontal lobe, cortical/subcortical location in the superior frontal gyrus (*asterisk*).

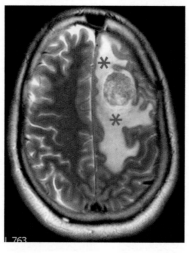

Axial T2 image shows the heterogeneous lesion with significant adjacent T2 hyperintensity in the white matter, likely from vasogenic edema (*asterisks*).

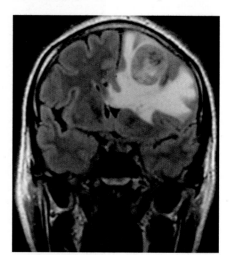

Coronal FLAIR image shows the left frontal mass and associated edema causing left to right midline shift (*asterisk*).

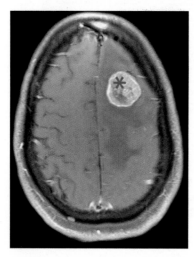

Axial T1 postcontrast image shows heterogeneous contrast enhancement within the left frontal lobe lesion (*asterisk*).

Answers

1. The abnormality is located within the left frontal lobe.

2. The imaging appearance of parenchymal metastasis is variable. Therefore, there is no classic appearance, as it depends on the primary tumor. The majority of lesions enhance with different patterns from solid enhancement to a "ring" pattern with variable adjacent edema. There is a predilection for the gray-white junction with relatively circumscribed masses.

3. The differential diagnosis includes glioblastoma, metastasis, and abscess.

4. Metastasis can affect any part of the brain. Most commonly it involves the supratentorial brain.

5. CNS metastases are most commonly from lung, melanoma, and breast carcinoma.

Pearls

- At least 50% of brain tumors are from metastasis.
- The most common etiologies include lung, melanoma, and breast carcinoma.
- 50% of intracranial metastasis presents as a solitary lesion.
- The imaging appearance is variable and lesions enhance with different patterns from solid enhancement to a "ring" pattern.
- With history of primary carcinoma or significant risk factors for cancer, metastasis should be favored.
- If there is no diagnosis of a primary carcinoma, then consider body CT in search of the primary tumor.
- Consider infectious etiology in immunocompromised patients.

Suggested Readings

Tang YM, Ngai S, Stuckey S. The solitary enhancing cerebral lesion: can FLAIR aid the differentiation between glioma and metastasis? *AJNR Am J Neuroradiol.* 2006 Mar;27(3):609-611.

Toh CH, Wei KC, Ng SH, Wan YL, Lin CP, Castillo M. Differentiation of brain abscesses from necrotic glioblastomas and cystic metastatic brain tumors with diffusion tensor imaging. *AJNR Am J Neuroradiol.* 2011 Oct;32(9):1646-1651.

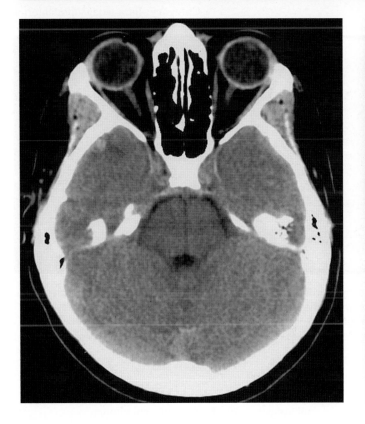
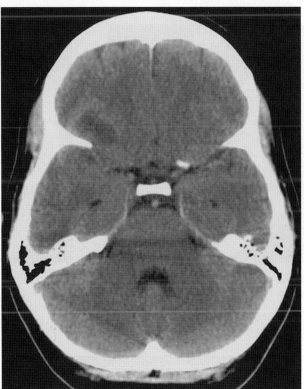

1. Where is the abnormality located?

2. Which MRI sequence is specifically useful for this type of injury?

3. What is the differential diagnosis?

4. What other CNS findings can be associated with this type of injury?

5. What is the source of the high attenuation?

Case ranking/difficulty:

Category: Intra-axial supratentorial

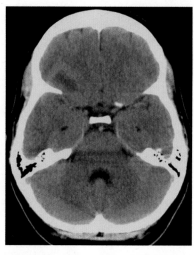

Axial CT shows focus of hyperattenuation within the anterior right temporal lobe with surrounding vasogenic edema (*arrow*).

Axial CT image shows focus of hypoattenuation within the inferior right frontal lobe (*arrow*).

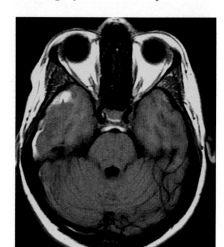

Axial T1 image shows focus of high signal within the anterior right temporal lobe corresponding with blood products (*green arrow*). Also seen is a small right subdural hematoma (*red arrow*).

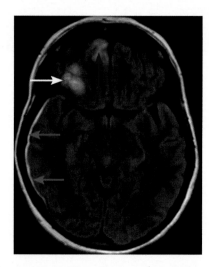

Axial FLAIR image shows foci of high signal within the inferior right frontal lobe (*white arrow*) and involving the right gyrus rectus, not visible on the CT (*blue arrow*). Right subdural hematoma again noted (*red arrows*).

Answers

1. The abnormality is located in the right temporal and inferior frontal lobes.

2. Although the entity is likely visible on all pulse sequences, T2* imaging, such as gradient echo (GRE), is useful for visualizing small foci of traumatic blood due to the induced artifact of "blooming" (makes the foci of blood appear larger, hence easier to detect).

3. The differential diagnosis includes high-density metastasis, cortical contusion, and glioma.

4. Brain contusions may be associated with subarachnoid hemorrhage, epidural hematoma, subdural hematoma, diffuse axonal injury, and skull fractures.

5. The high attenuation is secondary to hemorrhage.

Pearls

- Brain contusions occur with deceleration injury of the brain against the skull.
- Contusions are classified with calvarial fracture, coup, and contrecoup injury.
- Common sites are the anterior temporal and frontal lobes.
- With contusions less than 5 mm, edema may not be seen on CT.
- Look for small foci of subarachnoid blood and small subdural hematomas.
- Use GRE and SWI MRI sequences to detect trauma-associated hemorrhage.

Suggested Reading

Aiken AH, Gean AD. Imaging of head trauma. *Semin Roentgenol.* 2010 Apr;45(2):63-79.

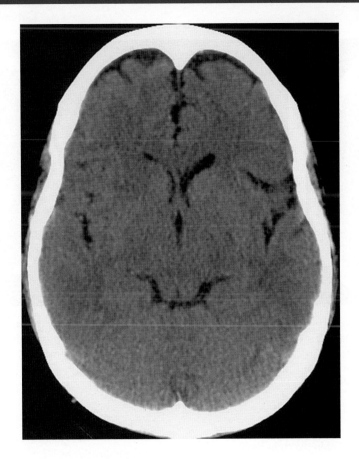

1. Where is the abnormality located?

2. Which MRI sequence is the most accurate for the diagnosis of this entity?

3. What is the differential diagnosis?

4. What are presenting symptoms for this lesion?

5. What is the treatment for this entity?

Case ranking/difficulty: 🦠

Category: Intra-axial supratentorial

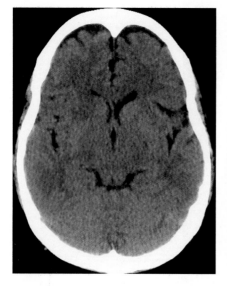

Axial CT image shows an area of low attenuation within the right basal ganglia affecting the head of caudate nucleus, anterior limb of the internal capsule, and anterior lateral lentiform nucleus (*arrow*).

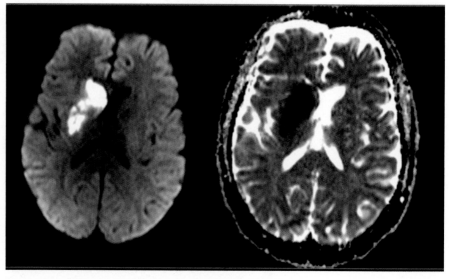

Axial DWI and ADC map shows high signal seen within the right basal ganglia on the diffusion-weighted image (*green arrow*) with corresponding low signal on the ADC image (*red arrow*). This is consistent with cytotoxic edema.

Answers

1. The abnormality is located within the right basal ganglia.

2. MRI with diffusion-weighted imaging has the highest sensitivity and specificity for acute infarct.

3. The differential diagnosis includes CVA, abscess, and metastasis.

4. Patients with basal ganglia infarcts usually present with contralateral muscular weakness.

5. TPA (tissue plasminogen activator) thrombolysis can be delivered systemically through IV or directly intra-arterial with microcatheters. Mechanical catheter thrombolysis is also another treatment option.

Pearls

- The majority of infarcts are caused by occlusion of a blood vessel resulting in ischemia (80%).
- The middle cerebral artery (MCA) is the most commonly affected vessel.
- Basal ganglia (BG) derive their blood supply from the lenticulostriate arteries.
- Restricted diffusion must be confirmed with low signal on ADC.

- Bilateral basal ganglia (BG) infarcts consider toxic/metabolic causes.
- Cortical infarcts may have gyriform enhancement.
- Ring-like enhancement consider tumor or abscess.
- Look for gray matter involvement in the MCA distribution to confirm BG infarct related to MCA vessel occlusion.

Suggested Readings

de Lucas EM, Sánchez E, Gutiérrez A, et al. CT protocol for acute stroke: tips and tricks for general radiologists. *Radiographics*. 2008 Oct;28(6):1673-1687.

Saenz RC. The disappearing basal ganglia sign. *Radiology*. 2005 Jan;234(1):242-243.

Tomura N, Uemura K, Inugami A, Fujita H, Higano S, Shishido F. Early CT finding in cerebral infarction: obscuration of the lentiform nucleus. *Radiology*. 1988 Aug;168(2):463-467.

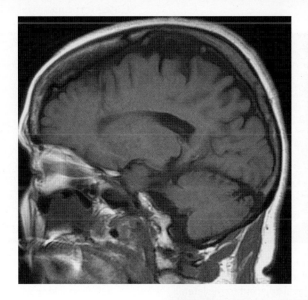
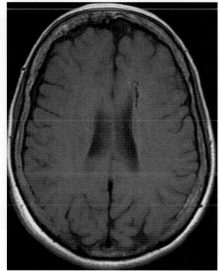
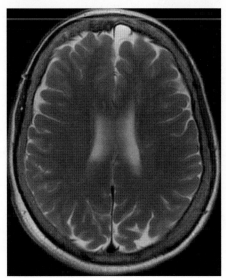

1. Where is the abnormality located?

2. What are the classic imaging findings for this entity?

3. What MR sequences are helpful to visualize this entity?

4. What are presenting symptoms for this lesion?

5. What is the treatment for this entity?

Case ranking/difficulty: 🍂

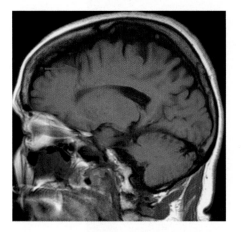

Sagittal T1 image shows a frontal lobe vascular structure (*arrow*) with branching extending to the level of the left lateral ventricle (upside down umbrella shape).

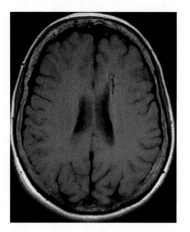

Axial T1 image demonstrates the vascular malformation that is low signal adjacent to the lateral ventricle (*arrow*).

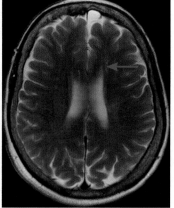

Axial T2 image shows the faint vascular malformation within the left frontal lobe white matter with branching pattern (*arrow*).

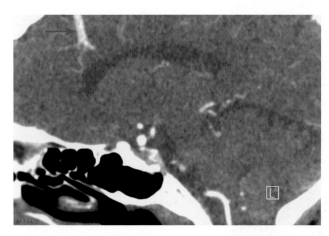

Sagittal CT with contrast better demonstrates the vascular malformation (*arrow*) within the frontal lobe white matter. Morphologically, it has an upside down "umbrella" or "medusa head" appearance.

Pearls

- Developmental venous anomaly (DVA) is a congenital vascular malformation.
- It is the most common type of vascular malformation seen at autopsy.
- The most common location is adjacent to the frontal horns.
- Morphologically, it has an upside down "umbrella" or "Medusa head" appearance.
- Multiple DVAs can be seen with blue rubber-bleb nevus syndrome.
- Postcontrast imaging and SWI make detection easier.
- If vasogenic edema is seen consider metastasis versus DVA associated with cavernous malformation and/or recent hemorrhage.

Answers

1. The abnormality is located within the frontal lobe.

2. A large vein within the parenchyma resembling an upside down "umbrella."

3. On MRI, T1 PD, FLAIR, and T2 the signal intensity is variable. The lesions are more readily seen with the use of contrast or susceptibility-weighted imaging (SWI) on MRI.

4. Developmental venous anomalies are usually asymptomatic but can, on occasion, be associated with headaches.

5. No treatment is usually necessary for this entity.

Suggested Readings

Fushimi Y, Miki Y, Togashi K, Kikuta K, Hashimoto N, Fukuyama H. A developmental venous anomaly presenting atypical findings on susceptibility-weighted imaging. *AJNR Am J Neuroradiol*. 2008 Aug;29(7):E56.

Robert T, Villard J, Oumarou G, Daniel RT, Pollo C, Uské A. Intracerebellar hemorrhage caused by developmental venous anomaly, from diagnosis to treatment. *J Neurol Surg A Cent Eur Neurosurg*. 2013 Dec;74(suppl 1): e275-e278.

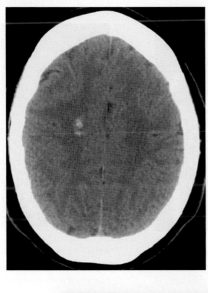
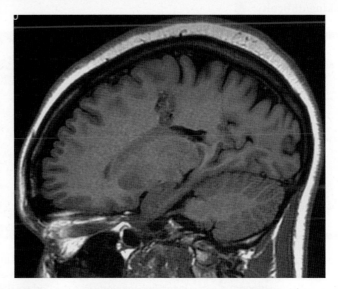
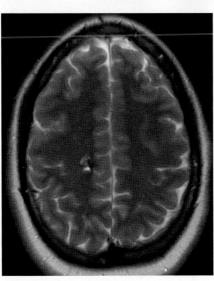
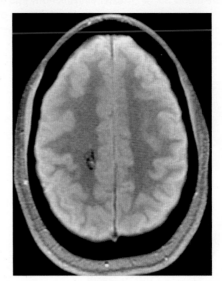

1. Where is the abnormality located?

2. What are the classic imaging findings for this entity?

3. What other findings are associated with this entity?

4. What is the imaging method of choice?

5. What is the treatment for this entity?

Case ranking/difficulty:

Category: Intra-axial supratentorial

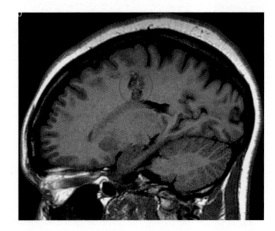

Axial CT image shows high attenuation representing calcification vs subacute blood products in the subcortical white matter of the posterior right frontal lobe (*circle*). There is no significant vasogenic edema.

Sagittal T1 image shows mixed signal intensity within the posterior right frontal lobe lesion extending inferiorly into the body of the right lateral ventricle (*circle*). There is central isointense signal to white matter and peripheral low signal intensity.

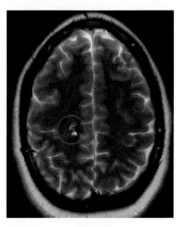

Axial T2 image shows central high signal is present within the posterior right frontal lobe lesion with peripheral low signal intensity (*circle*). Central high signal is likely late subacute blood products within a cystic locule. There is no significant vasogenic edema.

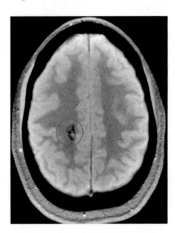

Axial gradient echo shows blooming artifact primarily lining the lesion (*circle*) consistent with hemosiderin rim. Cavernous malformations can grow in size with repeated hemorrhages.

Answers

1. There is a focal lesion within the subcortical white matter of the right frontal lobe.

2. Classic findings for cavernous malformation include calcified "popcorn" lesion seen on noncontrast CT containing different stages of blood degradation on MRI. Larger lesions demonstrate central cystic locules with possible fluid-fluid levels and a hemosiderin rim. No vasogenic edema is seen unless hemorrhage is present.

3. Other vascular malformations may be present, most notably developmental venous anomaly. Cavernous malformations may be singular (sporadic) or multiple (familial).

4. MRI with susceptibility weighted or gradient echo sequences to evaluate for multiple lesions.

5. Larger, symptomatic lesions with higher risk of rehemorrhage can be removed surgically.

Pearls

- Cavernous malformations may occur in combination with other vascular malformations, particularly developmental venous anomalies.
- "Popcorn" calcifications typical on noncontrast CT.
- Hemorrhagic lesions can have varying ages of blood products on MRI.
- Have no vasogenic edema unless recent hemorrhage is present.
- Larger lesions may have central cystic locules with fluid-fluid levels.
- May have minimal to no enhancement.
- Typically not seen on DSA ("angiographically occult").
- Patients often asymptomatic, however can present with seizures when hemorrhage is present.

Suggested Readings

Ginat DT, Meyers SP. Intracranial lesions with high signal intensity on T1-weighted MR images: differential diagnosis. *Radiographics*. 2012;32(2):499-516.

Vilanova JC, Barceló J, Smirniotopoulos JG, et al. Hemangioma from head to toe: MR imaging with pathologic correlation. *Radiographics*. 2010 Jul;24(2):367-385.

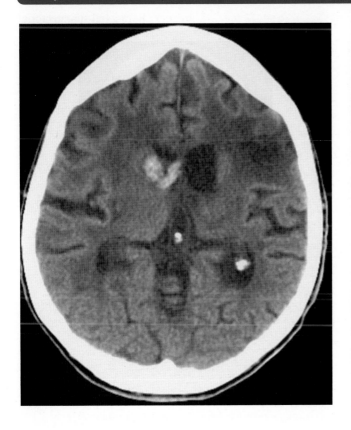
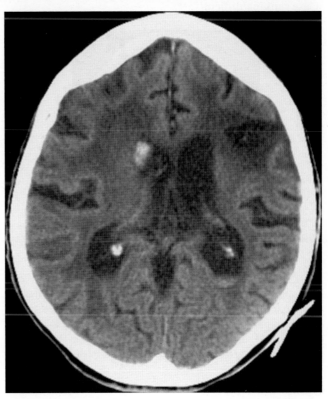

1. Where is the abnormality?

2. What is the differential diagnosis?

3. What are the most common locations for this entity?

4. Which vessels supply the basal ganglia?

5. What structures are usually supplied by the recurrent artery of Heubner?

Case ranking/difficulty: **Category:** Intra-axial supratentorial

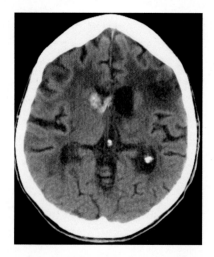

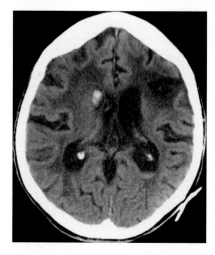

Axial CT image shows high density within the right caudate head (*green arrow*). Similar high density is identified within the anterior horn of the right lateral ventricle (*red arrow*). There is encephalomalacia of the left frontal lobe. There are significant confluent areas of low attenuation involving the periventricular white matter likely from hypertensive arteriolosclerosis.

Axial CT image shows a fluid-fluid level that is high density within the dependent posterior horn of the left lateral ventricle (*red arrow*). The right caudate hemorrhage is again seen (*circle*).

Answers

1. The abnormality is located within the right basal ganglia and lateral ventricles.

2. The differential diagnosis includes vascular malformation, tumor-related hemorrhage, and hypertensive hemorrhage.

3. Most common locations for hypertensive hemorrhages are the basal ganglia followed by the thalamus, pons, and cerebellum.

4. Branches of the A1-segment of the anterior cerebral artery (medial lenticulostriate arteries) supply the anterior inferior parts of the basal nuclei and the anterior limb of the internal capsule. Branches of the M1-segment of the middle cerebral artery (lateral lenticulostriate arteries) supply the superior part of the head and the body of the caudate nucleus, most of the globus pallidus, putamen, and the posterior limb of the internal capsule.

5. It supplies the head of caudate, anterior portion of the lentiform nucleus, and anterior limb of the internal capsule. It originates from the proximal ACA and is the largest branch vessel of the proximal ACA typically seen on angiography.

Pearls

- Hypertension is the most common cause for spontaneous intracranial hemorrhage in the elderly population.
- Hypertensive hemorrhage most commonly involves the basal ganglia, thalamus, pons, and cerebellum.
- Second most common cause of stroke (10%-20% of stroke patients).
- Check the dependent portions of the lateral ventricles for blood.
- Check the position of the septum pellucidum to evaluate for midline shift.
- Midline shift (subfalcine herniation) is seen prior to transtentorial herniation.

Suggested Readings

Lin WM, Yang TY, Weng HH, et al. Brain microbleeds: distribution and influence on hematoma and perihematomal edema in patients with primary intracerebral hemorrhage. *Neuroradiol J*. 2013 Apr;26(2):184-190.

Zheng T, Wang S, Barras C, Davis S, Yan B. Vascular imaging adds value in investigation of basal ganglia hemorrhage. *J Clin Neurosci*. 2012;19(2):277-280.

Zheng W, Zhang C, Hou D, Cao C. Comparison on different strategies for treatments of hypertensive hemorrhage in the basal ganglia region with a volume of 25 to 35 ml. *Acta Cir Bras*. 2012 Oct;27(10):727-731.

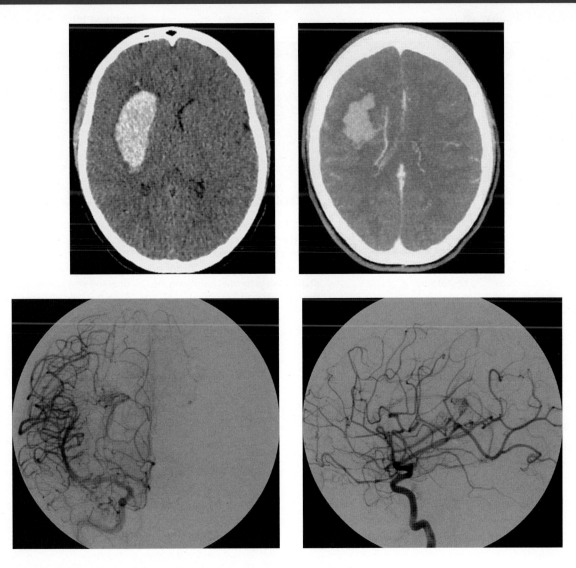

1. What is the differential diagnosis?

2. How do patients with this abnormality typically present?

3. What are the three basic vascular components of this lesion?

4. What is the key finding on digital subtraction angiography for arteriovenous shunting?

5. What is an associated syndrome at risk for development of AVMs?

Case ranking/difficulty:

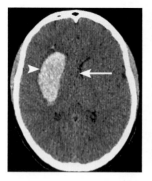

Axial CT image shows a large hemorrhage (*arrowhead*) centered in the right basal ganglia with mild midline shift (*arrow*).

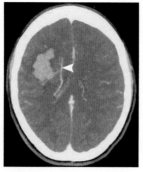

Axial MIP image from CT angiography shows a prominent draining vein (*arrowhead*) medial to the hematoma.

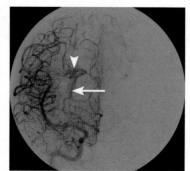

Frontal radiograph of a right internal carotid artery injection shows a tangle of vessels consistent with nidus (*arrowhead*) with an early draining vein (*arrow*) emptying into the basal vein of Rosenthal.

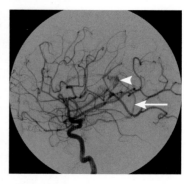

Lateral radiograph of a right internal carotid artery injection shows a tangle of vessels consistent with nidus (*arrowhead*) with an early draining vein (*arrow*) emptying into the basal vein of Rosenthal.

Answers

1. Differential diagnosis for an intraparenchymal hemorrhage with associated abnormal vessels includes arteriovenous malformation (AVM), dural AV fistula, and possibly a high-grade neoplasm with significant neoangiogenesis causing shunting.

2. The typical profile is a young adult with headache and hemorrhage. 50% of AVMs present with headache and spontaneous hemorrhage.

3. The three basic components of AVMs are enlarged arterial feeders, compact nidus, and dilated draining veins. Intranidal aneurysms (>50%) and feeding artery aneurysms (10-15%) are associated but not necessary.

4. The early draining vein on DSA is the key finding for arteriovenous shunting without intervening capillary bed seen in AVMs and AV fistulas.

5. Although syndromic CNS AVMs are rare (2%), knowledge of associated syndromes including hereditary hemorrhagic telangiectasias, Klippel Trenaunay Weber, Wyburn-Mason, and capillary malformation-arteriovenous malformation syndrome is necessary in a patient with multiple vascular lesions.

Pearls

- Arteriovenous malformations (AVM) are abnormal pial vascular malformations with direct shunting from arterial to venous without intervening capillaries.
- 2% of cases are associated with syndromes such as hereditary hemorrhagic telangiectasia (Osler-Weber-Rendu).
- 50% present with hemorrhage, the remainder with seizure or focal deficit from vascular steal ischemia.
- Three basic components on imaging: enlarged arterial feeders, compact nidus of abnormal vessels, and dilated draining veins.
- >50% have intranidal aneurysm.
- Digital subtraction angiography best details the vascular architecture with visualization of the early draining vein from real-time imaging.
- Treatment includes embolization, surgery, and stereotactic radiosurgery.
- Spetzler-Martin scale assesses risk of surgery.

Suggested Readings

Dmytriw AA, Ter Brugge KG, Krings T, Agid R. Endovascular treatment of head and neck arteriovenous malformations. *Neuroradiology*. 2014 Mar;56(3):227-236.

Fiehler J, Illies T, Piening M, et al. Territorial and microvascular perfusion impairment in brain arteriovenous malformations. *AJNR Am J Neuroradiol*. 2009 Feb;30(2):356-361.

Mamourian A, Wallace R. When is an atypical DVA an AVM? *AJNR Am J Neuroradiol*. 2009 Feb;30(2):E24; author reply E25.

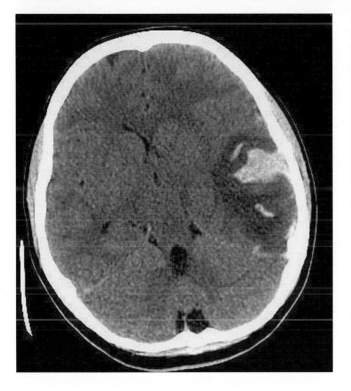
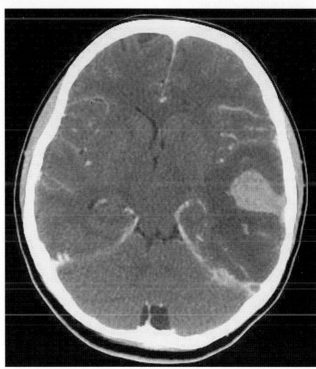

1. What is the differential diagnosis?

2. What is the most common clinical presentation?

3. What is the common age group with this diagnosis?

4. What are typical radiographic findings?

5. What is the most sensitive modality for diagnosis?

Case ranking/difficulty:

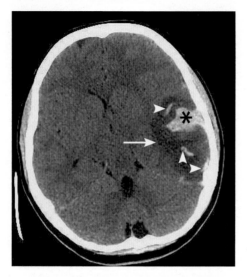

Axial CT image demonstrates dense tubular structures (dense cord sign) in the left parietal lobe, suggestive of thrombus in the cortical veins (*white arrowheads*). A hyperdense focus in the left parietal lobe (*black asterisk*) with surrounding vasogenic edema (*white arrow*) is consistent with intraparenchymal hemorrhage.

Answers

1. Hemorrhagic tumor, from primary neoplasm or metastasis, hemorrhagic arterial infarct, hypertensive hemorrhage, and amyloid angiopathy can be considered. Venous infarcts should be considered in young females, especially in a pattern not consistent with an arterial territory.

2. Most common presentation for cerebral venous infarct is headache. Clinical symptoms can be grouped into three clinical syndromes: isolated signs of intracranial hypertension, seizures or focal neurologic deficits, and multifocal signs including encephalopathy, stupor, or coma.

3. CVT is more common in young adult females.

4. Direct CT signs for cerebral venous thrombosis include "cord sign" (hyperdensity of thrombosed veins) and empty delta sign (lack of luminal enhancement in the sagittal sinus). On MRI, susceptibility artifact on T2* imaging can be seen of the thrombus and for hemorrhagic infarcts, which are predominantly T2 hyperintense and may be in a pattern outside typical arterial distributions.

5. MRI with contrast and MR venography is the most sensitive to evaluate for venous thrombosis and infarct. Contrast-enhanced vessels in conjunction with time of flight MRV help decrease false positives from noncontrast time of flight MRV, alone, which is highly sensitive to intraluminal flow dynamics.

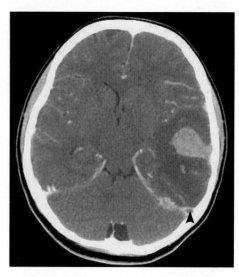

Axial CT venogram demonstrates intraluminal thrombus in the left transverse/sigmoid sinus junction (*black arrowhead*).

Pearls

- Cerebral venous infarction is relatively uncommon compared with arterial infarct.
- 20%-25% of cases are unable to identify an etiology.
- More common in females and young adults.
- Headache is the most common clinical presentation.
- CT is normal in up to 30% of cases.
- Direct CT signs of CVT: dense triangular clot sign, cord sign, and postcontrast empty delta sign.
- Indirect CT signs: intense contrast enhancement of the falx and tentorium, dilated transcerebral veins, small ventricles, and parenchymal abnormality.
- MRI with contrast and MR venography (MRV) are the most sensitive imaging modality to demonstrate thrombus and occluded dural sinus/vein (caution: TOF MRV is sensitive to flow heterogeneity with loss of signal, which may lead to false positive).
- Venous infarcts are T2 hyperintense, prone to hemorrhage with variable signal due to evolution of blood.
- The infarct may be outside of a typical arterial distribution, with variable restricted diffusion.

Suggested Readings

Buyck PJ, De Keyzer F, Vanneste D, Wilms G, Thijs V, Demaerel P. CT density measurement and H:H ratio are useful in diagnosing acute cerebral venous sinus thrombosis. *AJNR Am J Neuroradiol.* 2013 Aug;34(8):1568-1572.

Leach JL, Strub WM, Gaskill-Shipley MF. Cerebral venous thrombus signal intensity and susceptibility effects on gradient recalled-echo MR imaging. *AJNR Am J Neuroradiol.* 2007 May;28(5):940-945.

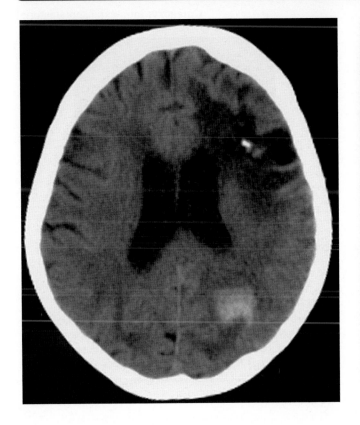 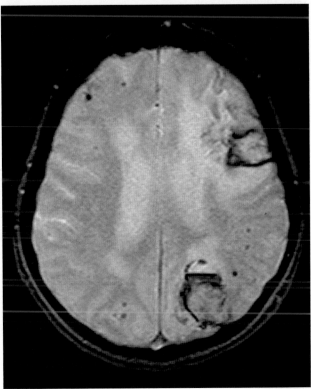

1. What is the differential diagnosis?

2. What are common clinical presentations of this disease?

3. What are typical radiographic features?

4. What is the best imaging modality?

5. What are other manifestations or associations of cerebral amyloid disease?

Case ranking/difficulty:

Category: Intra-axial supratentorial

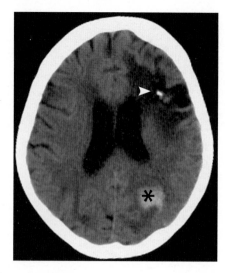

Axial CT brain image demonstrates a left parietal hematoma (*black asterisk*) with minimal surrounding vasogenic edema. Also noted is a dystrophic calcification in the left frontal lobe (*white arrowhead*) associated with encephalomalacia, related to prior hemorrhage.

Answers

1. In addition to amyloid angiopathy, differential diagnosis includes hypertensive hemorrhage, hemorrhagic infarct, bleeding metastasis or primary brain tumor, coagulopathy, or underlying vascular malformation.

2. Stroke-like symptoms can be seen in the acute setting, while dementia is more common in chronic settings.

3. Typical radiographic features include lobar hemorrhage in the cortex/subcortical white matter, which may extend to the ventricle or subarachnoid spaces, multiple hematomas of differing ages, and microhemorrhages.

4. MRI is modality of choice due to sensitivity to multiple ages of hematoma and microhemorrhages. GRE/SWI sequences are the most sensitive modality to detect microbleeds.

5. Cerebral amyloid angiopathy is the most common manifestation of cerebral amyloid disease, and is seen in up to 88% of Alzheimer patients. Other manifestations include uncommon focal amyloidoma and a rare diffuse white matter leukoencephalopathic form.

Pearls

- A cerebrovascular disorder secondary to deposition of amyloid beta peptide deposits within small- to medium-sized blood vessels of the brain and leptomeninges.

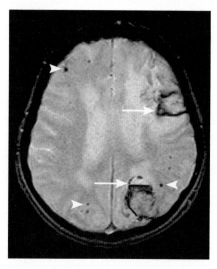

Axial GRE image demonstrates multiple punctate foci of susceptibility artifacts scattered in the bilateral cerebral hemispheres (*white arrowheads*). Also noted are a rim of susceptibility artifacts in the left frontal as well as layering fluid-fluid level in the left parietal lobe (*white arrows*). Multiple cortical hemorrhages in an elderly patient are compatible with amyloid angiopathy.

- Cerebral amyloid angiopathy (CAA) is the most common presentation of cerebral amyloid disease, which also includes uncommon focal amyloidoma and a rare diffuse white matter infiltrating form.
- Up to 88% Alzheimer patients have CAA.
- Stroke-like symptoms in the acute setting and dementia in the chronic setting.
- Radiographic features include lobar hemorrhage, usually in the cortical and subcortical white matter.
- In younger patients with inflammatory CAA may mimic PRES.
- Consider CAA in cases of normotensive demented elderly patients older than 60 years old with multiple episodes of intracranial hemorrhage.
- SWI is the most sensitive technique to detect chronic microbleeds.

Suggested Readings

Chao CP, Kotsenas AL, Broderick DF. Cerebral amyloid angiopathy: CT and MR imaging findings. *Radiographics.* 2009 Dec;26(5):1517-1531.

Haacke EM, DelProposto ZS, Chaturvedi S, et al. Imaging cerebral amyloid angiopathy with susceptibility-weighted imaging. *AJNR Am J Neuroradiol.* 2007 Feb;28(2):316-317.

Wagle WA, Smith TW, Weiner M. Intracerebral hemorrhage caused by cerebral amyloid angiopathy: radiographic-pathologic correlation. *AJNR Am J Neuroradiol.* 1990 May;5(2):171-176.

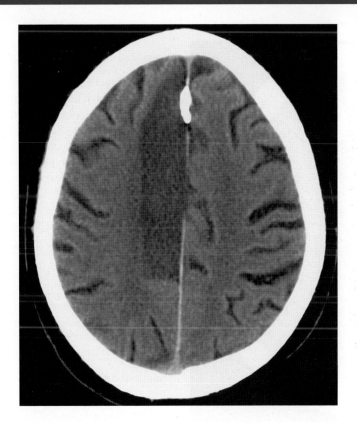

1. Where is the abnormality located?

2. What are the classic imaging findings for this entity?

3. What is the differential diagnosis?

4. What is the most common arterial distribution involved in this entity?

5. What is the treatment for this entity?

Case ranking/difficulty:

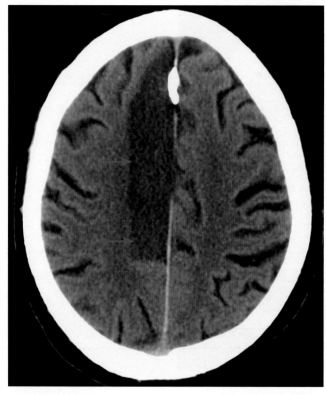

Axial CT shows low attenuation involving the gray matter and subcortical white matter with loss of the gray-white discrimination of the medial aspect of the superior frontal gyrus (*arrows*).

Pearls

- Anterior cerebral artery (ACA) is the least common "circle of Willis" vessel responsible for infarcts.
- Maximum cytotoxic edema occurs at 48 to 72 hours.
- DWI is highly sensitive and specific for acute infarct in the first 7-10 days.
- "Mohawk" sign is cytotoxic edema involving the medial frontal lobe corresponding to the ACA territory.
- May have gyriform enhancement secondary to "luxury perfusion."
- Susceptibility-weighted imaging may show "blooming" with acute clot and parenchymal hemorrhage.
- High FLAIR signal within the artery may be seen with slow flow and thrombus.
- CTA or MRA to evaluate for arterial thrombus/occlusion.

Suggested Readings

King S, Khatri P, Carrozella J, et al. Anterior cerebral artery emboli in combined intravenous and intra-arterial rtPA treatment of acute ischemic stroke in the IMS I and II trials. *AJNR Am J Neuroradiol.* 2008 Mar;28(10):1890-1894.

Moussouttas M, Boland T, Chang L, Patel A, McCourt J, Maltenfort M. Prevalence, timing, risk factors, and mechanisms of anterior cerebral artery infarctions following subarachnoid hemorrhage. *J Neurol.* 2013 Jan;260(1):21-29.

Park YW, Kim CH, Kim MO, Jeong HJ, Jung HY. Alien hand syndrome in stroke—case report & neurophysiologic study. *Ann Rehabil Med.* 2012 Aug;36(4):556-560.

Answers

1. The abnormality is located within the medial right frontal lobe, along the anterior cerebral artery distribution.

2. Anterior cerebral artery (ACA) infarcts have the same findings as other arterial strokes. CT signs of infarction include obscuration of the gray-white junctions and high density within the vessels. On MR, there is high signal on the T2 images (including PD and T2 FLAIR) with corresponding T1 low signal in cytotoxic edema. Diffusion-weighted imaging (DWI) demonstrates increased signal, corresponding with decreased ADC from restriction.

3. The differential diagnosis includes anterior cerebral artery infarction, metastasis, and cerebritis.

4. Anterior cerebral artery (ACA) infarcts are the least common "circle of Willis" vessel in infarcts. The most common etiology of ischemic stroke is MCA infarct.

5. The typical treatment for this entity is supportive care with consideration for thrombolytic therapy.

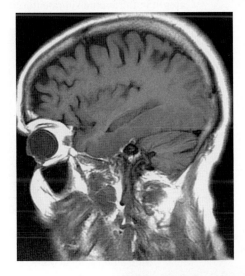
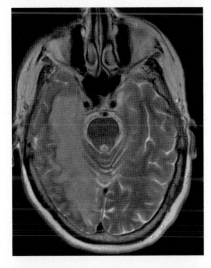
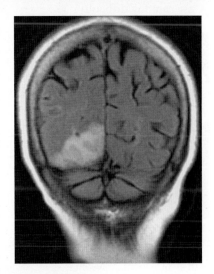

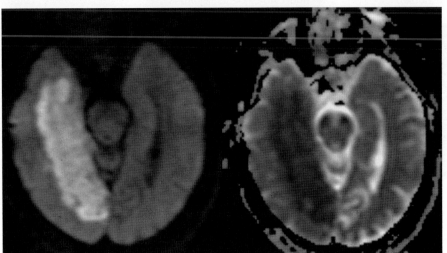

1. Where is the abnormality located?

2. What are the classic imaging findings for this entity?

3. What is the differential diagnosis?

4. What is the likely etiology of this entity?

5. What is the treatment for this entity?

Case ranking/difficulty:

Category: Intra-axial supratentorial

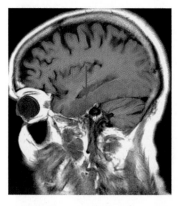

Sagittal T1 image shows the gyri of the inferior right temporal lobe with enlargement, gray-white blurring, and low signal (*arrow*).

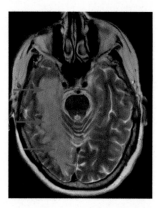

Axial T2 image shows the gyri of the right mesial temporal lobe and occipital lobe with high T2 signal consistent from cytotoxic edema (*arrows*).

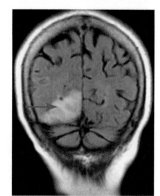

Coronal FLAIR shows the gyri of the right occipital lobe with high T2 signal from cytotoxic edema (*arrow*).

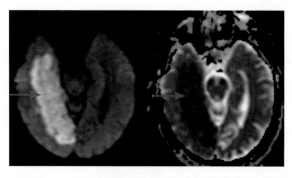

Axial DWI b-1000 and ADC show the gyri of the right temporal lobe and right occipital lobe with DWI high signal (*green arrow*) and corresponding low signal on the ADC map (*red arrow*) confirming cytotoxic edema and acute PCA infarct.

Answers

1. The abnormality is located within the right temporal lobe and occipital lobe.

2. CT signs of infarction include obscuration of the gray-white junctions, sulcal effacement, and high density within the vessels. With regard to acute stroke imaging, noncontrast MRI is more accurate than CT. On MR, there is high signal on the T2 images (including PD and T2 FLAIR) with corresponding T1 low signal. Specifically, diffusion-weighted imaging (DWI) is the most accurate imaging sequence for detecting acute infarcts.

3. The differential diagnosis includes infarction, metastasis, and cerebritis. Metastasis is typically multifocal and associated with vasogenic edema. Cerebritis of the temporal lobe is common with herpes simplex encephalitis.

4. The most common etiology of PCA infarcts is thrombosis related to atherosclerotic disease.

5. The treatment for this entity is typically supportive with consideration for thrombolytic therapy.

Pearls

- Posterior cerebral artery (PCA) infarcts account for 5%-10% of ischemic strokes.
- PCA high FLAIR signal can be seen with slow flow and thrombus.
- PCA supplies the medial occipital, temporal lobes, thalamus, hypothalamus, and posterior limb of the internal capsule.
- Herpes cerebritis should be considered with involvement of the temporal lobe, insular cortex, and inferior frontal lobe with deep white matter sparing.
- The most common etiology of PCA infarcts is thrombosis related to atherosclerotic disease.
- Transtentorial herniation may also cause bilateral PCA infarction secondary to compression between the temporal lobe and the tentorium.
- Infarction of the medial occipital lobe causes homonymous hemianopsia (a visual field defect involving either the left or right halves of the visual field).
- Consider CTA or MRA to evaluate for arterial thrombus/occlusion.

Suggested Readings

Cereda C, Carrera E. Posterior cerebral artery territory infarctions. *Front Neurol Neurosci.* 2012 Jul;30(30):128-131.

Förster A, Gass A, Kern R, Wolf ME, Hennerici MG, Szabo K. MR imaging-guided intravenous thrombolysis in posterior cerebral artery stroke. *AJNR Am J Neuroradiol.* 2011 Feb;32(2):419-421.

Seo KD, Lee KO, Choi YC, Kim WJ, Lee KY. Fluid-attenuated inversion recovery hyperintense vessels in posterior cerebral artery infarction. *Cerebrovasc Dis Extra.* 2013 Dec;3(1):46-54.

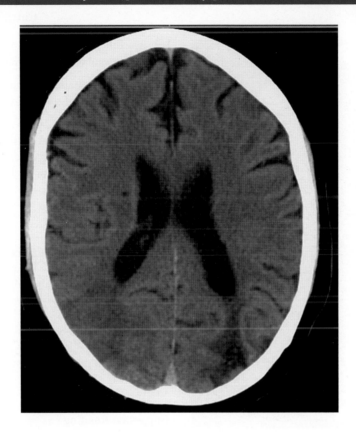

1. Where is the abnormality located?

2. What are the classic imaging findings for this entity?

3. What is the differential diagnosis?

4. What is the etiology of this entity?

5. What is the treatment for this entity?

Case ranking/difficulty: 🌑

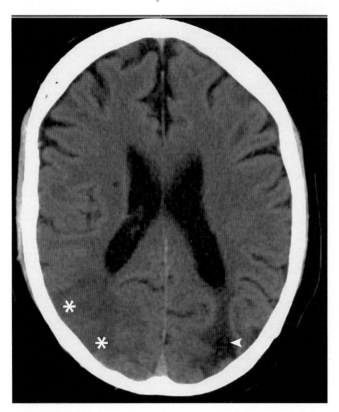

Axial CT image shows a wedge-shaped area of low attenuation located between the right occipital and parietal lobes, between the MCA and PCA arterial distribution (*asterisks*). Note there is an area of encephalomalacia within the left occipital lobe within the contralateral watershed territory (*arrowhead*).

Answers

1. The abnormality is located within the arterial watershed region between major vascular territories of the MCA and PCA involving the right parietal and occipital lobes.

2. Watershed infarcts are diagnosed on imaging based on their location either in wedge-shaped cortical infarcts between major vascular territories or in the deep white matter. The CT signs of infarction include hypodensity, obscuration of the gray-white junctions, and sulcal effacement. On MR, there is high signal on the T2 images (including PD and T2 FLAIR) with corresponding T1 low signal. Diffusion-weighted imaging (DWI) shows high signal corresponding with low signal on apparent diffusion coefficient (ADC) map.

3. The differential diagnosis includes border zone (watershed) infarct, embolic infarct, PRES, and cerebritis.

4. Watershed infarcts are typically secondary to vascular disease, arterial stenosis, hypotension, and hemodynamic compromise.

5. The treatment for this entity is typically supportive with correction of hypotension and consideration of antithrombolytics for occlusive disease.

> ### Pearls
>
> - Watershed infarcts are also called border zone infarcts.
> - Between major arterial territories (ACA, MCA, PCA) in the cortex and subcortical white matter.
> - Between perforating arteries (parasagittal deep white matter), "string of beads" appearance.
> - When watershed injuries are bilateral the etiology is usually secondary to hypotension.
> - Unilateral may be from vessel stenosis.

Suggested Reading

Mangla R, Kolar B, Almast J, Ekholm SE. Border zone infarcts: pathophysiologic and imaging characteristics. *Radiographics*. 2011 Oct;31(5):1201-1214.

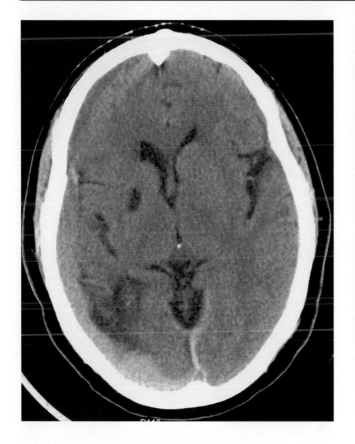
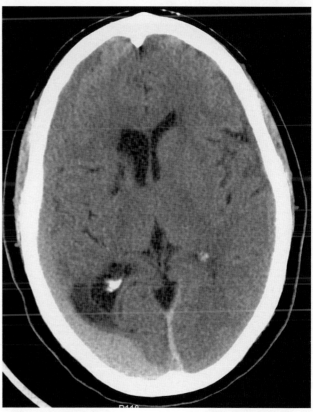

1. Where is the abnormality located?

2. What is the age of the injury?

3. What is the differential diagnosis?

4. What is the significance of mixed attenuation within this entity?

5. What injured anatomic structure is the cause of the high attenuation?

Case ranking/difficulty:

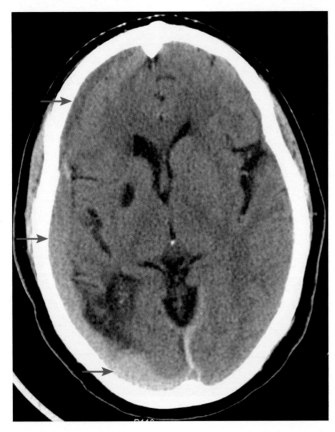

Axial CT image at the level of the basal ganglia demonstrates a right extraaxial fluid collection (*arrows*). The fluid is of mixed attenuation with higher density seen posteriorly.

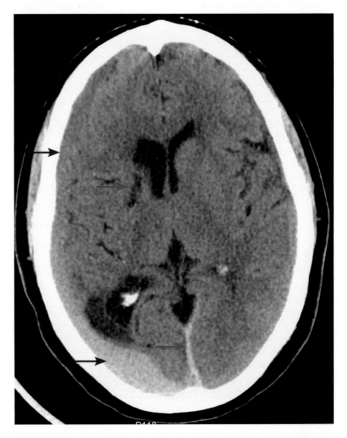

Axial CT image at the level of the basal ganglia demonstrates the extraaxial fluid collection extending along the posterior falx (*green arrow*). Mixed density right hemispheric crescentic SDH is again seen (*blue arrows*). A focal right chronic lacunar basal ganglia infarct is also noted (*red arrow*).

Answers

1. Given the appearance of the extraaxial collection (crescent shape) and because it crosses suture lines it is in the subdural space.

2. The layering hyperdensity may suggest an acute on subacute hemorrhage. The increased attenuation when compared to the brain parenchyma indicates there is an acute component.

3. The differential diagnosis for extraaxial hemorrhages includes subdural hematoma, epidural hematoma, and subarachnoid hemorrhage.

4. The significance of mixed attenuation involving SDH usually represents the presence of hyperacute blood in an acute hematoma or acute on chronic blood products.

5. The most common source for blood products seen in SDH is the bridging veins.

Pearls

- Subdural hematomas (SDH) occur most commonly secondary to trauma.
- Crescent in shape.
- SDH may be subdivided into three categories based on age: acute 1-7 days, subacute 1-3 weeks, and chronic older than 3 weeks.
- Mixed attenuation indicates rebleeding of a chronic injury or acute clotted and nonclotted blood products.
- Majority are caused by bridging vein injury.
- Contrecoup location most common.

Suggested Reading

Aiken AH, Gean AD. Imaging of head trauma. *Semin Roentgenol*. 2010 Apr;45(2):63-79.

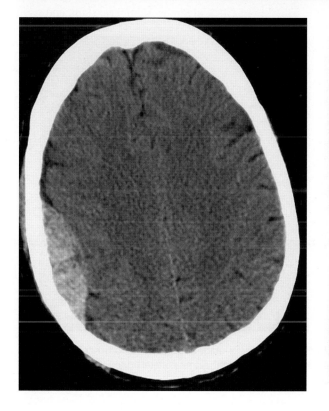

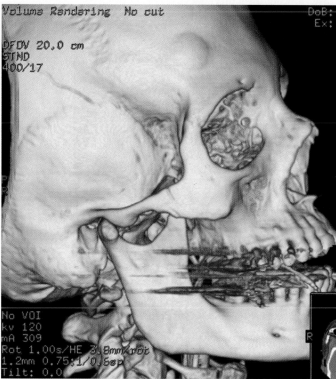

1. Where is the abnormality located?

2. What pathology is usually associated with this entity?

3. What is the differential diagnosis?

4. What is the significance of mixed attenuation within this entity?

5. What is the most common source of the high attenuation?

Case ranking/difficulty:

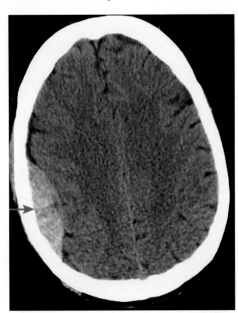

Axial CT image shows a lenticular (convex) extraaxial fluid collection adjacent to the right hemisphere (*arrow*).

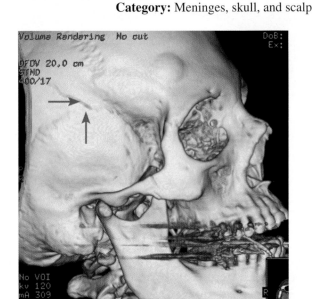

This 3D reconstructed image of the skull demonstrates a fracture (*green arrow*) traversing the right parietal bone, joining the squamosal suture (*red arrow*).

3. The differential diagnosis for extraaxial hemorrhage includes epidural hematoma, subdural hematoma, and subarachnoid hemorrhage.

4. Mixed attenuation within an epidural hematoma is usually indicative of mixed clotted and unclotted blood products. This may indicate an expanding hematoma.

5. The most common source of the high attenuation (blood) is arterial injury.

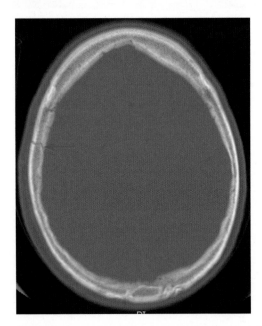

Axial CT bone window image demonstrates a fine fracture line traversing the right parietal bone (*arrow*) overlying the epidural hematoma.

Pearls

- Epidural hematomas (EDH) occur most commonly secondary to trauma.
- Lenticular shape.
- Bound by sutures.
- Can cross midline.
- High association with skull fracture.
- Primarily middle meningeal arterial injury, although can be from torn dural venous sinus in the minority of cases.

Answers

1. The abnormality is in the epidural space. This is evident given the characteristic lenticular shape.

2. EDH is usually associated with a skull fracture.

Suggested Reading

Aiken AH, Gean AD. Imaging of head trauma. *Semin Roentgenol.* 2010 Apr;45(2):63-79.

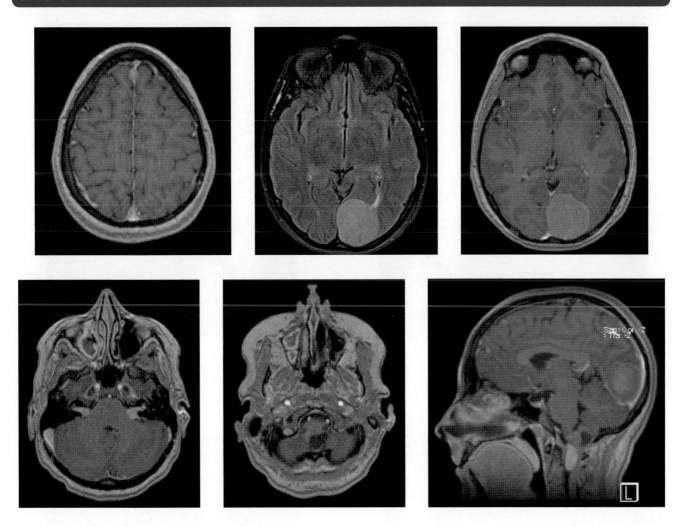

1. What is the differential diagnosis?

2. What are the characteristic radiographic findings for this disease?

3. Which chromosome has an abnormality in this disease?

4. What are criteria for the diagnosis of this disease?

5. What is the primary treatment option for this disease?

Case ranking/difficulty: 🍂

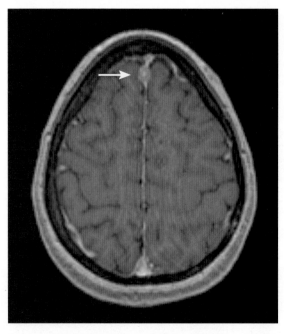

Axial T1 postcontrast image shows a small homogeneously enhancing lesion in the frontal falx consistent with meningioma (*arrow*).

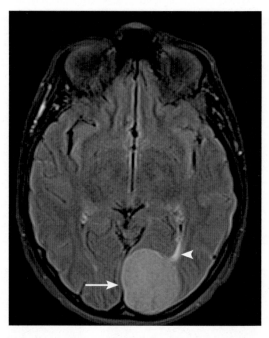

Axial FLAIR image shows a large extraaxial mass in the left occipital region (*arrow*) with homogeneous hyperintensity and well-circumscribed borders with little adjacent edema (*arrowhead*).

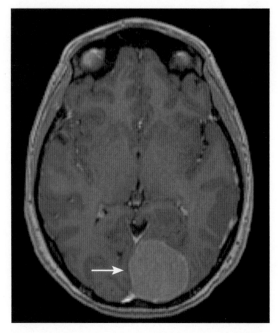

Axial T1 postcontrast image shows the extraaxial mass with homogeneous enhancement consistent with a meningioma (*arrow*).

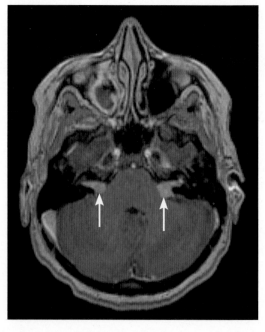

Axial T1 postcontrast image shows bilateral enhancing masses in the internal auditory canals (*arrows*), consistent with vestibular schwannomas, which is diagnostic of neurofibromatosis type 2.

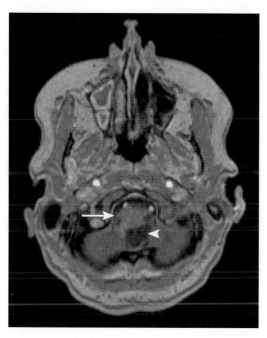

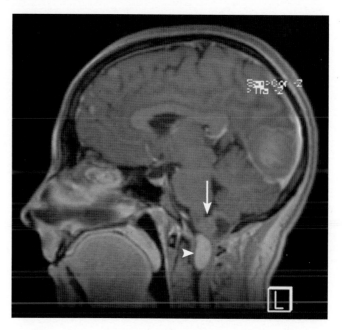

Axial T1 postcontrast image shows a mixed enhancing mass in the medulla (*arrow*) with a dorsal cyst (*arrowhead*) consistent with an ependymoma.

Sagittal postcontrast T1 image shows moderately enhancing mass in the medulla with a dorsal cyst (*arrow*) just superior to a homogeneous intensely enhancing mass at the cranial cervical junction consistent with a cervical meningioma (*arrowhead*).

Answers

1. The differential diagnosis for multiple enhancing primarily extraaxial masses includes neurofibromatosis 2, schwannomatosis, and multiple meningiomatosis.

2. The radiographic features represent the mnemonic "MISME" multiple inherited schwannomas, meningiomas, and ependymomas.

   Patients with suspected features of NF2 need a careful evaluation of other cranial nerves and entire neuraxis.

3. NF2 gene is located on chromosome 22q12 and encodes for the Merlin protein, with tumor suppression function.

4. Criteria for diagnosis for NF2 include bilateral vestibular schwannomas, or first degree relative with NF2 and one vestibular schwannoma, or first degree relative with NF2 and two of the following tumors: neurofibroma, meningioma, schwannoma, glioma, or posterior subcapsular lenticular opacity.

5. Surgical resection is the primary option for symptomatic tumors. Adjuvant chemotherapy has shown some decrease in tumor size in trials for unresectable tumor. Radiation therapy is controversial due to potential increased incidence of treatment-induced tumor.

Pearls

- Neurocutaneous syndrome; 50% autosomal dominant inheritance and 50% new mutation.
- Chromosome 22q12 abnormalities.
- Defect in Merlin gene, causing truncated Merlin protein production, a tumor suppression protein.
- "MISME"—multiple inherited schwannomas meningiomas and ependymomas.
- Less common than NF1, less cutaneous manifestation.
- Diagnostic criteria includes:
  - Bilateral vestibular schwannomas
  - First degree relative with NF2 and one vestibular schwannoma
  - First degree relative with NF2 and two of the following findings: neurofibroma, meningioma, glioma, schwannoma, or posterior subcapsular lenticular opacity.

Suggested Readings

Aboukais R, Zairi F, Baroncini M, et al. Intracranial meningiomas and neurofibromatosis type 2. *Acta Neurochir (Wien).* 2013 Jun;155(6):997-1001; discussion 1001.

Koontz NA, Wiens AL, Agarwal A, Hingtgen CM, Emerson RE, Mosier KM. Schwannomatosis: the overlooked neurofibromatosis? *AJR Am J Roentgenol.* 2013 Jun;200(6):W646-W653.

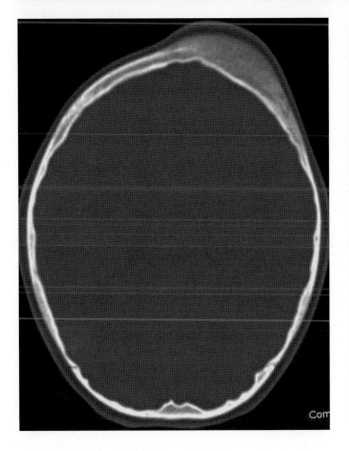
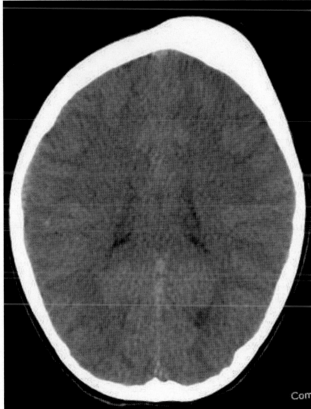

1. What is the differential diagnosis?

2. What are the classic imaging findings for this entity?

3. What are common locations for this disease?

4. What is the most common syndrome associated with this entity?

5. What are possible clinical findings in patients with this entity?

Case ranking/difficulty:

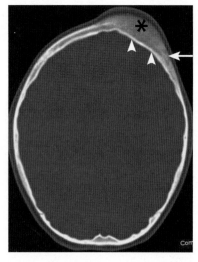

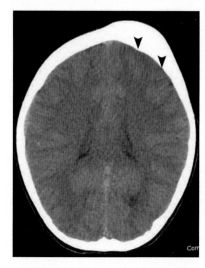

Axial CT image bone algorithm shows an expansile lesion primarily in the frontal bone with ground glass matrix (*asterisk*) and narrow zone of transition. There is crossing of the left coronal suture (*arrow*) with relative sparing of the inner table (*arrowheads*).

Axial CT brain window shows the sparing of the inner table and no significant mass effect to the underlying brain parenchyma (*arrowheads*).

Answers

1. The differential for an expansile bony lesion includes fibrous dysplasia (FD), blastic metastasis, nonossifying fibroma, Paget disease, and sclerosing osteomyelitis.

2. Classic findings for FD include an expansile bony lesion with narrow zone of transition and ground glass matrix. When the skull is affected, there is relative inner table sparing. Mixed lytic and sclerotic findings can be seen in "pagetoid" FD, and homogeneous sclerosis is seen in up to 1/3 of cases.

3. The three most common sites of monostotic FD involve the ribs, proximal femur, and craniofacial bones with the orbit, skull base, mandible, and maxilla commonly involved in craniofacial disease. Polyostotic forms may be monomelic, involving one side of an extremity.

4. 3% of cases of FD are associated with McCune-Albright syndrome, which has the classic triad of polyostotic FD, cafe-au-lait spots, and precocious puberty. Monostotic FD can occur in McCune-Albright syndrome. Mazabraud syndrome is a rare disease with polyostotic FD and muscular myxomas.

5. Presenting symptoms include swelling and deformity with pathological fractures contributing to pain. Cranial neuropathy can be seen along with proptosis from skull base and orbital involvement. Multiple endocrine disorders associated with polyostotic fibrous dysplasia can be seen with or without the setting of McCune-Albright syndrome. Increased risk of sarcomatous transformation has been described with radiation.

Pearls

- CT with bone algorithm helpful to assess bony matrix, and local extent of disease.
- MRI may have variable appearance and enhancement, which may confuse the diagnosis, but can be helpful for extent of disease and marrow involvement.
- Variable PET and bone scan uptake, although bone scan can be helpful in nonspecific evaluation of extent of polyostotic disease.
- Ground glass matrix classic.
- Mixed lytic and sclerosis in "pagetoid" FD.
- Homogenous sclerosis can also be seen.

Suggested Readings

Lui YW, Dasari SB, Young RJ. Sphenoid masses in children: radiologic differential diagnosis with pathologic correlation. *AJNR Am J Neuroradiol.* 2011 Apr;32(4):617-626.

Sirvanci M, Karaman K, Onat L, Duran C, Ulusoy OL. Monostotic fibrous dysplasia of the clivus: MRI and CT findings. *Neuroradiology.* 2002 Oct;44(10):847-850.

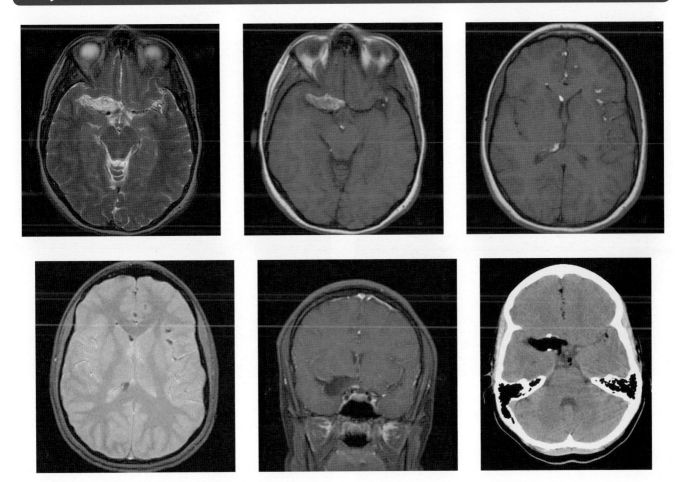

1. What is the biochemical makeup of the T1 bright substance?

2. What are typical MRI findings for this lesion?

3. How does this lesion develop?

4. What is a life-threatening consequence of this lesion?

5. What can cause chemical meningitis?

Case ranking/difficulty: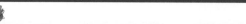

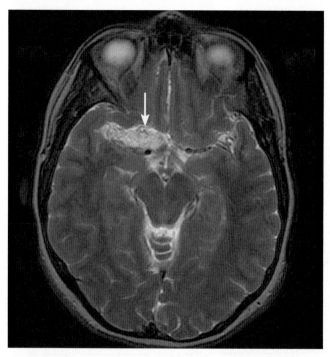

Axial T2 image at the suprasellar cistern shows a hyperintense, heterogeneous, extraaxial mass displacing the right MCA (*arrow*).

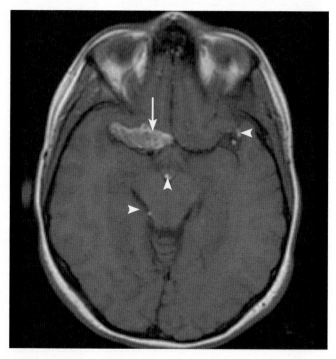

Axial T1 image at the suprasellar cistern shows T1 hyperintensity following fat of the extraaxial lesion (*white arrow*). There are also extraaxial foci of T1 hyperintensity suggesting rupture (*arrowheads*).

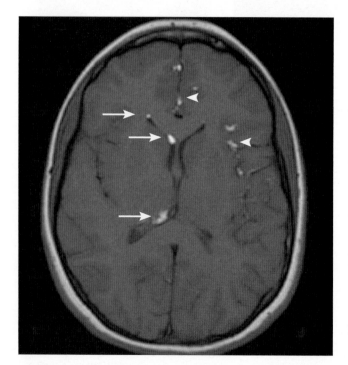

Axial T1 shows multiple extraaxial hyperintense fat droplets from rupture (*arrowheads*) in this patient with signs and symptoms of chemical meningitis. Note the fat fluid level of the droplet in the right lateral ventricle, which is nondependent (*arrows*).

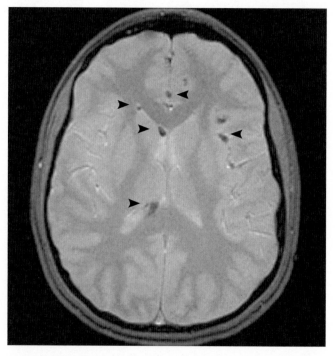

Axial gradient echo shows suppression of these subarachnoid fat droplets (*arrowheads*) from dermoid rupture.

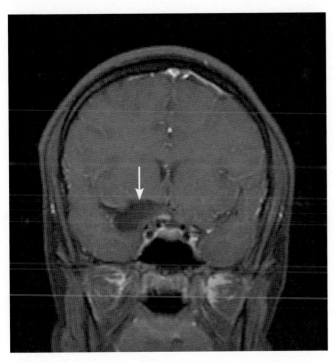

Coronal T1 postcontrast with fat suppression confirms the fatty nature of the mass (*arrow*); there is no central enhancement.

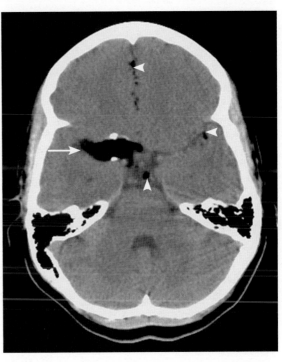

Axial CT image of the head at the suprasellar cistern confirms the low-density fatty nature of this extraaxial dermoid (*arrow*) and associated rupture into the subarachnoid space (*arrowheads*).

Answers

1. In this case of ruptured dermoid cyst, the T1 hyperintensity is from fat.

2. Dermoid cysts are extraaxial lesions that tend to be midline. There is typically heterogeneity within the cyst with fatty elements and sometimes fat-fluid levels both in the cyst and in the ventricles if there is rupture. Capsular enhancement is variable, but no internal enhancement is expected. There is decreased signal on sequences that naturally have fat suppression such as STIR or GRE.

3. Dermoid and epidermoid cysts are thought to arise from sequestered portions of surface ectoderm included within neural tube closure during third to fifth weeks of embryo development.

4. Chemical meningitis from dermoid cyst rupture is the most well-known potentially life-threatening sequela of this lesion. Chemical meningitis may vary from mild and self-limited to severe and life threatening. Seizures have also been described with dermoids with or without rupture. Larger masses may cause obstructive hydrocephalus. Malignant degeneration is a rare but described risk of dermoid and epidermoid cysts.

5. Causes of chemical meningitis can be blood products, post-neurologic surgery, and rupture of intracranial cystic neoplasms, such as epidermoid and dermoid cysts, craniopharyngiomas, and Rathke cleft cyst. Other reported causes include epidural injection of steroids or bupivacaine, and intrathecal injection of contrast material.

Pearls

- Chemical meningitis can be caused by various etiologies of intracranial biochemical irritation of the meninges and include blood products, post-neurological surgery, rupture of intracranial cystic tumors, and epidural medication.
- MR imaging of chemical meningitis may not be sensitive to detect meningeal enhancement in all cases, with clinical history and CSF analysis required.
- Dermoid cysts are congenital predominantly midline lesions that can rupture into the subarachnoid space.
- Fat suppression techniques can be helpful to confirm the fatty nature of the cyst to distinguish dermoids from epidermoids.
- Fat-fluid level within the ventricles and in the cyst is also helpful to confirm the presence of fat.
- Dermoids tend to be more heterogeneous than lipomas.

Suggested Readings

Burke JW, Podrasky AE, Bradley WG. Meninges: benign postoperative enhancement on MR images. *Radiology.* 1990 Jan;174(1):99-102.

Smirniotopoulos JG, Chiechi MV. Teratomas, dermoids, and epidermoids of the head and neck. *Radiographics.* 1995 Nov;15(6):1437-1455.

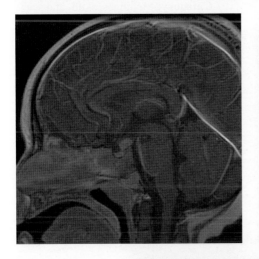
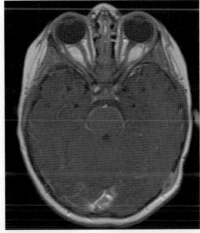
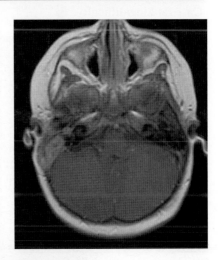

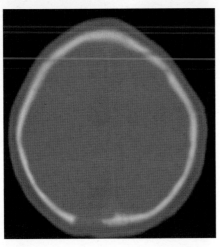
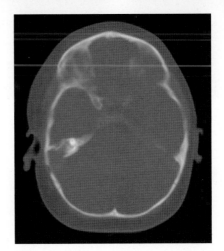

1. What is the differential diagnosis for the suprasellar lesion?

2. What is the differential of the calvarial lesions?

3. What is the prognosis of this disease?

4. What is the treatment for this disease?

5. What organ system is the most commonly involved?

Case ranking/difficulty:

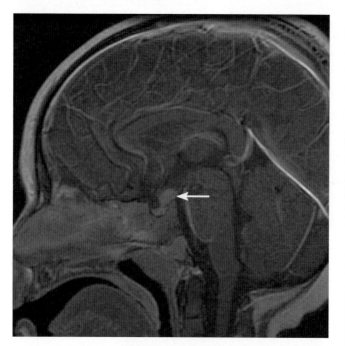

Sagittal T1 postcontrast of the midline shows a suprasellar enhancing mass involving the infundibulum (*arrow*).

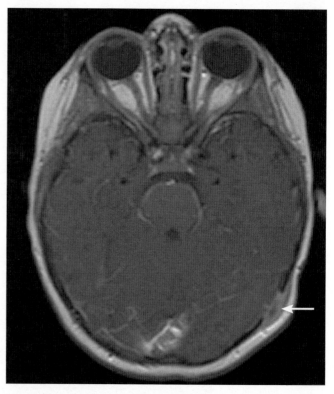

Axial T1 image postcontrast shows an enhancing soft tissue mass focally destroying the left parietal calvarium (*arrow*).

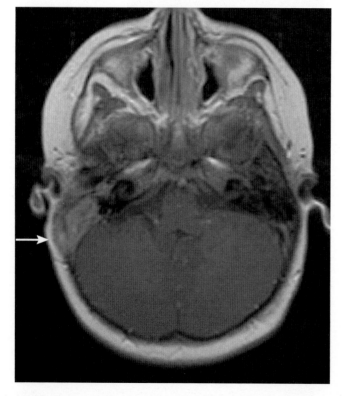

Axial T1 image postcontrast shows mass-like enhancement of the right temporal bone (*arrow*) in this patient with Langerhans cell histiocytosis.

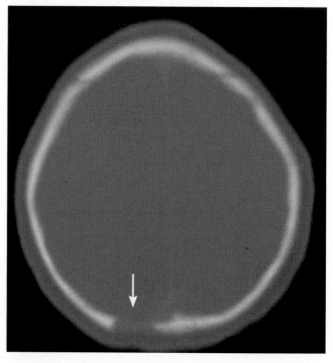

Axial CT image with bone windows shows a lytic lesion of the high right parietal calvarium with a "beveled edge" (*arrow*).

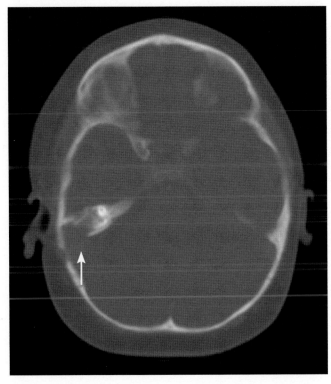

Axial CT image of the head with bone windows shows a lytic mass of the right temporal bone (*arrow*), a common location for Langerhans cell histiocytosis.

Multifocal multisystem—previously Letterer-Siwe disease with multiorgan involvement and 50% mortality even with aggressive chemotherapy.

4. Systemic steroids and/or chemotherapy are used in multifocal disease. Surgical excision and focal radiation can be used on isolated lesions.

5. Skeletal lesions are the most common manifestation of Langerhans cell histiocytosis.

Pearls

- Langerhans cell histiocytosis is an inflammatory or neoplastic process more commonly seen in children.
- LCH is in the differential of single or multiple bony lytic lesions in a child, especially with diabetes insipidus.
- CNS involvement of LCH (multifocal unisystem or Hand-Schüller-Christian) is typically seen in the pituitary stalk and hypothalamus with enhancement and mild T2 hyperintensity.
- Rare enhancing masses involving the choroid plexus, leptomeninges, and basal ganglia have been described.
- Rare cerebellar white matter demyelination has also been reported.

Answers

1. Differential of solid-enhancing masses of the pituitary stalk include Langerhans cell histiocytosis, germinoma, and lymphocytic hypophysitis.

2. With multiple lytic calvarial lesions in children, Langerhans cell histiocytosis followed by metastatic disease of childhood malignancies should be considered. TB can present with multiple bone lesions especially in endemic areas. Medulloblastoma does not usually metastasize to the bone, even late in the disease.

3. LCH was previously divided into three named subtypes, which are now classified by systemic involvement:

   Unifocal—previously eosinophilic granuloma, typically involves one or multiple lesions in the bone without extraskeletal involvement, with excellent prognosis.

   Multifocal unisystem—previously Hand-Schüller-Christian disease with 50% involvement of the pituitary stalk, as well as scalp and calvarial involvement. Diabetes insipidus, exophthalmos, and lytic bone lesions is considered the Hand-Schüller-Christian triad. Prognosis is variable with 30% of complete remission, 60% with chronic course, and 10% mortality.

Suggested Readings

Chung EM, Murphey MD, Specht CS, Cube R, Smirniotopoulos JG. From the archives of the AFIP. Pediatric orbit tumors and tumorlike lesions: osseous lesions of the orbit. *Radiographics.* 2008 Aug;28(4):1193-1214.

D'Ambrosio N, Soohoo S, Warshall C, Johnson A, Karimi S. Craniofacial and intracranial manifestations of langerhans cell histiocytosis: report of findings in 100 patients. *AJR Am J Roentgenol.* 2008 Aug;191(2):589-597.

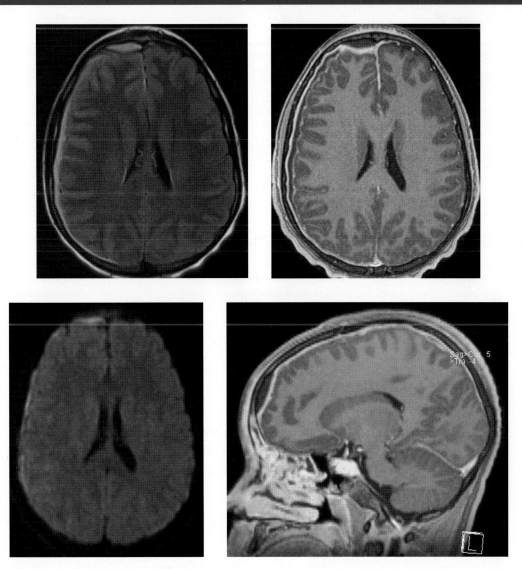

1. What is the differential diagnosis?

2. What imaging sequence has the greatest sensitivity for this disease?

3. What is the most common etiology of this disease in adults?

4. What is the most common etiology of this disease in infants?

5. What procedure is potentially lethal in this disease?

Case ranking/difficulty:

Category: Meninges, skull, and scalp

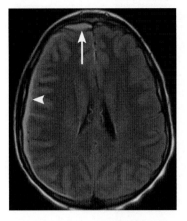

Axial FLAIR image shows hyperintense collections in the right frontal epidural space (*arrow*), which extends up to the anterior falx and a hemispheric subdural collection (*arrowhead*) with similar characteristics.

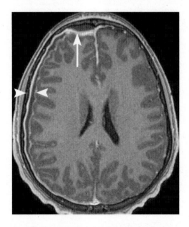

Axial T1 postcontrast image shows the epidural collection is superficial to the enhancing dura (*arrow*) while the subdural collection has enhancement in the dura and leptomeninges (*arrowheads*).

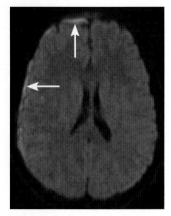

Axial DWI ADC map shows decreased diffusion of the epidural and subdural collections (*arrows*).

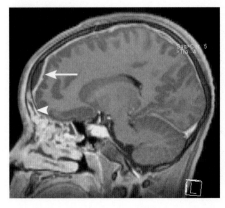

Sagittal T1 postcontrast shows the epidural empyema (*arrow*) associated with sinusitis (*arrowhead*).

Answers

1. The differential for extraaxial fluid collections includes subdural hematomas, hygromas, and effusions. Thick enhancement should suggest empyema or dural metastasis.

2. Restricted diffusion is typical of subdural empyema and is the most sensitive modality.

3. Paranasal sinusitis or mastoiditis accounts for 75% of the cases of empyema in adults and older children. Paranasal sinusitis is the cause in 2/3 of cases leading to supratentorial empyema while mastoiditis occurs in 20% with infratentorial empyema.

4. Bacterial meningitis is the most common etiology of empyema in infants.

5. Lumbar puncture has been associated with rapid decline and death in patients with empyema.

Pearls

- Empyema is a collection of pyogenic material in the subdural or epidural space, with subdural being more common.
- Majority of cases are from paranasal sinus disease (supratentorial) or mastoiditis (infratentorial)
- Empyema in infants is more common from bacterial meningitis.
- Complications such as cerebritis, abscess, hydrocephalus, and sinus thrombosis are more likely with subdural than with epidural empyema.
- Imaging typically shows peripherally enhancing extraaxial fluid collection without FLAIR suppression (hyperintense).
- Restricted diffusion is typical.
- Empyema is an emergency necessitating neurosurgical drainage.
- Lumbar puncture can be fatal.

Suggested Readings

Han KT, Choi DS, Ryoo JW, et al. Diffusion-weighted MR imaging of pyogenic intraventricular empyema. *Neuroradiology*. 2007 Oct;49(10):813-818.

Nickerson JP, Richner B, Santy K, et al. Neuroimaging of pediatric intracranial infection—part 1: techniques and bacterial infections. *J Neuroimaging*. 2012 Apr;22(2):e42-e51.

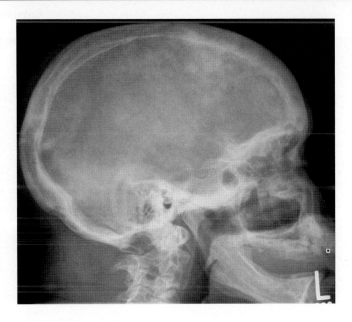

1. Where is the abnormality located?

2. What are the classic imaging findings for this entity?

3. What is the differential diagnosis?

4. What are presenting symptoms for this lesion?

5. What is the treatment for this entity?

Case ranking/difficulty:

Category: Meninges, skull, and scalp

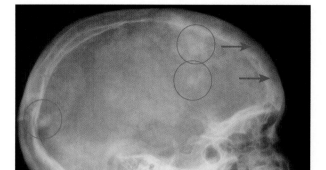

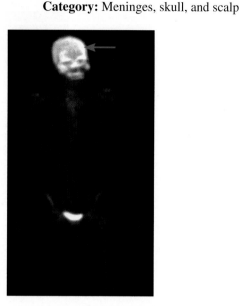

Lateral skull radiograph shows areas of patchy increased density involving the skull both anteriorly and posteriorly (*circles*). Note that the diploic space is widened with increased density (*arrow*). Increased density is also noted involving the skull base and floor of the anterior cranial fossa.

Technetium 99m MDP bone scan shows marked radiotracer uptake involving the skull (*arrow*).

Answers

1. Areas of patchy increased density are seen involving the skull both anteriorly within the frontal bone and posteriorly within occipital bone.

2. The skull in the early phase of Paget disease demonstrates focal areas of lucency involving the frontal and occipital bones termed osteoporosis circumscripta. Later, osteoblastic activity dominates and focal, patchy opacities are seen termed "cotton wool" skull. Marked thickening of the diploic space with thickening of the inner table and resultant enlargement may also be seen called "tam-o-shanter" skull. Platybasia with basilar invagination may be seen.

3. The differential diagnosis includes Paget disease, metastasis, and renal osteodystrophy.

4. Patient symptoms include pain, increased bone size, bowing deformities, cranial nerve deficits (from compression), and decreased range of motion. Patients will have elevated serum alkaline phosphatase during the mixed phase. Secondary osteoarthritis, gout, CPPD, and rheumatoid are all associated with Paget disease. Sarcomatous transformation is rare (most commonly osteosarcoma).

5. The goal of treatment is pain control and is achieved via the inhibition of bone resorption. The medications used include calcitonin, bisphosphonates, mithramycin, and gallium nitrate.

Pearls

- Paget disease has three phases: lytic phase (bone resorption), mixed phase (gradual return of yellow marrow), and blastic phase (sclerosis).
- Paget disease is most common in the axial skeleton and polyostotic.
- The skull is involved in 25%-65% of cases.
- Osteoporosis circumscripta is seen early in the lytic phase.
- Later in disease "cotton wool" skull is seen.
- Sarcomatous transformation rare especially in skull (<1%).
- Sarcomatous degeneration hallmarks include cortical destruction and soft tissue mass.
- Giant cell tumor transformation shows a lytic lesion with marrow replacement without periosteal reaction or soft tissue mass.

Suggested Readings

Love C, Din AS, Tomas MB, Kalapparambath TP, Palestro CJ. Radionuclide bone imaging: an illustrative review. *Radiographics*. 2007 Oct;23(2):341-358.

Smith SE, Murphey MD, Motamedi K, Mulligan ME, Resnik CS, Gannon FH. From the archives of the AFIP. Radiologic spectrum of Paget disease of bone and its complications with pathologic correlation. *Radiographics*. 2007 Oct;22(5):1191-1216.

Tjon-A-Tham RT, Bloem JL, Falke TH, et al. Magnetic resonance imaging in Paget disease of the skull. *AJNR Am J Neuroradiol*. 2008 Jan;6(6):879-881.

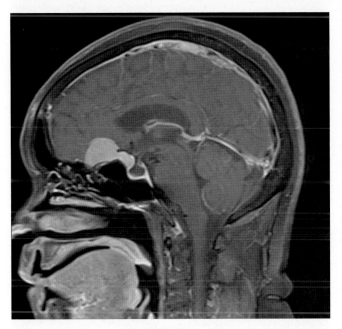
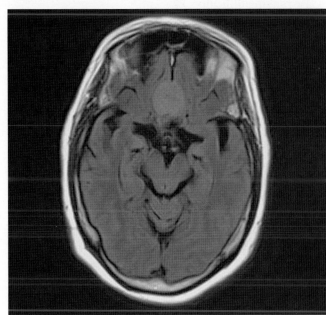

1. Where is the abnormality?

2. What is the differential diagnosis?

3. In which diseases can focal hyperostosis also be seen?

4. What percentage of these lesions are symptomatic?

5. With which syndromes or history is an increased incidence of meningiomas associated?

Case ranking/difficulty: 🌑

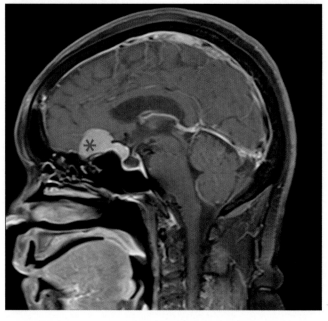

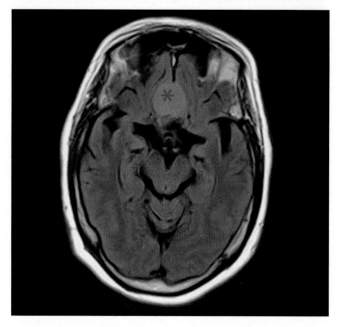

Sagittal T1 postcontrast image shows a homogeneously enhancing extraaxial lesion above the planum sphenoidale and extends posteriorly into the sella turcica (*asterisk*). This lesion causes mass effect on the diaphragma sellae and there is an associated empty sella.

Axial FLAIR image shows the interhemispheric lesion with iso- to slightly hyperintense signal to gray matter (*asterisk*).

Answers

1. This is an extraaxial lesion with mass effect on the optic chiasm sitting on the planum sphenoidale. There is extension into the sella turcica.

2. The differential includes dural metastasis, hemangiopericytoma, and meningioma.

3. Focal hyperostosis is present with meningioma, fibrous dysplasia, Paget disease, Dyke-Davidoff-Mason syndrome, and hyperostosis frontalis interna. Generalized skull thickness occurs with chronic severe anemia, acromegaly, osteopetrosis, Camurati-Engelmann disease, and hyperparathyroidism.

4. Less than 10% of all meningiomas are symptomatic.

5. Neurofibromatosis 2, basal cell nevus syndrome, and prior radiation therapy are associated with increased incidence of meningiomas.

Pearls

- Meningiomas are neoplasms that arise from the meningeal arachnoid cells.
- Meningioma may grow very large and can demonstrate dural venous sinus invasion as well as intraosseous extension.
- Most common extraaxial CNS tumor.
- Key imaging findings include extraaxial lesion with associated hyperostosis of adjacent inner table, bright/homogenous enhancement, and occasional calcifications.
- Consider NF2 when a young patient presents with a meningioma.
- Meningiomas may grow during pregnancy.

Suggested Readings

Buetow MP, Buetow PC, Smirniotopoulos JG. Typical, atypical, and misleading features in meningioma. *Radiographics*. 1991 Nov;11(6):1087-1106.

Wang CW, Li YY, Zhu SG, et al. Surgical management and evaluation of prognostic factors influencing postoperative visual outcome of suprasellar meningiomas. *World Neurosurg*. 2011 Feb;75(2):294-302.

Wong RH, Wong AK, Vick N, Farhat HI. Natural history of multiple meningiomas. *Surg Neurol Int*. 2013 Nov;4(4):71.

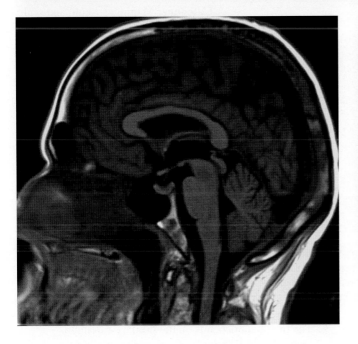 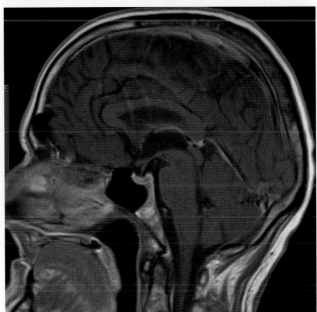

1. Where is the abnormality located?

2. What are the classic imaging findings for this entity?

3. What is the differential diagnosis?

4. What are common etiologies for this finding?

5. What is the treatment for this entity?

Case ranking/difficulty:

Category: Meninges, skull, and scalp

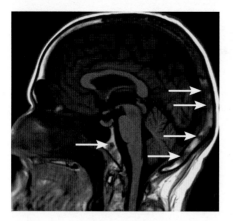

Sagittal T1 noncontrast image shows multiple, irregular, low T1 signal lesions within the clivus and occipital bone (*arrows*).

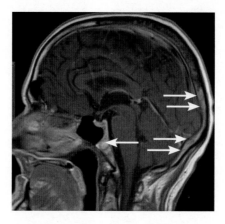

Sagittal T1 postcontrast image shows the multiple low T1 signal lesions within the calvarium on precontrast imaging demonstrate contrast enhancement (*arrows*).

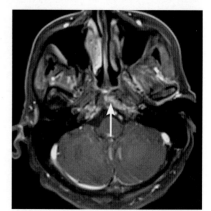

Axial T1 postcontrast shows the clivus lesion with more obvious contrast enhancement with fat saturation (*arrow*).

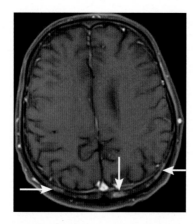

Axial T1 postcontrast image shows the posterior skull lesions with more obvious contrast enhancement with fat saturation (*arrows*).

Answers

1. The abnormality is located within the clivus and posterior skull (occipital and parietal bones).

2. On MR, the classic findings of osseous metastasis are focal low T1 signal that is lower than skeletal muscle and demonstrates enhancement. The enhancement is variable. There is also variable T2 signal depending on the primary neoplasm.

3. The differential diagnosis includes metastasis, red marrow expansion in anemia, sarcoidosis, and renal osteodystrophy.

4. Skull metastases are commonly seen in adults with primary cancers including breast, lung, prostate, renal cell, follicular thyroid, melanoma, and multiple myeloma.

5. The treatment depends on the primary carcinoma and if the skull metastases are symptomatic. A combination of radiotherapy (usually for single lesions) and chemotherapy (typically aimed at systemic or widespread disease) is typically utilized.

Pearls

- The most common skull metastases in adults include breast, lung, prostate, renal cell, follicular thyroid, melanoma, and multiple myeloma.
- Direct spread from head and neck carcinomas into the skull base may be seen (squamous cell, lymphoma, and adenoid cystic carcinoma).
- Postcontrast fat saturation images increase sensitivity.
- Lytic metastasis is more common.
- If a low T1 signal bone lesion is detected without a primary carcinoma history, then further evaluation must be performed in order to find the primary tumor.
- Consider whole-body bone scan to assess the extent of osseous involvement.
- High T1 signal bone lesions are likely benign.

Suggested Readings

Abdel Khalek Abdel Razek A, King A. MRI and CT of nasopharyngeal carcinoma. *AJR Am J Roentgenol.* 2012 Jan;198(1):11-18.

Barakos JA, Dillon WP, Chew WM. Orbit, skull base, and pharynx: contrast-enhanced fat suppression MR imaging. *Radiology.* 1991 Apr;179(1):191-198.

Lauenstein TC, Goehde SC, Herborn CU, et al. Whole-body MR imaging: evaluation of patients for metastases. *Radiology.* 2004 Oct;233(1):139-148.

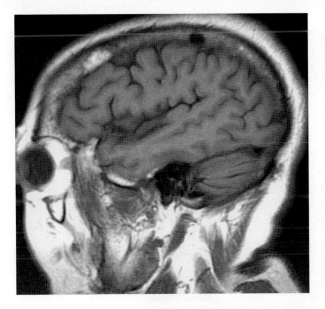
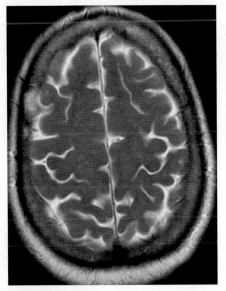
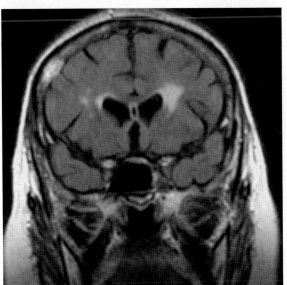

1. Where is the abnormality located?

2. What are the classic imaging findings for this entity?

3. What is the differential diagnosis?

4. What are presenting symptoms for this lesion?

5. What is the typical treatment for this entity?

Case ranking/difficulty:

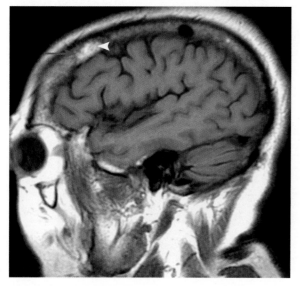

Axial T1 noncontrast image shows a well-marginated right frontal bone lesion with high T1 signal (*arrow*). Note the internal punctate areas of thickened trabeculation (*arrowhead*).

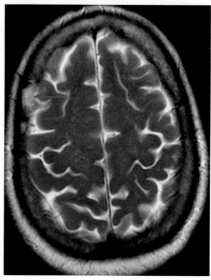

Axial T2 image shows the lesion to be mildly expansile and with high T2 signal (*arrow*).

3. The differential diagnosis includes metastasis, hemangioma, dermoid/epidermoid, hemangioendothelioma, and Paget disease.

4. Hemangiomas are benign vascular lesions. Typically the lesions are asymptomatic. Rarely, larger lesions may cause extraaxial intracranial hemorrhage.

5. Usually no treatment is needed. Larger lesions may require surgical resection due to mass effect, hemorrhage, or cosmesis.

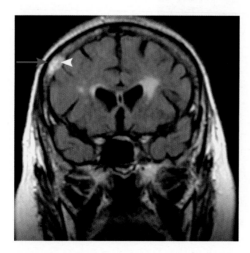

Coronal FLAIR image shows the lesion is mildly expansile and thins the inner table (*arrow*). Note the punctate thickened trabeculae within the lesion (*arrowhead*) suggesting hemangioma.

Pearls

- Hemangiomas are benign vascular lesions.
- The most common locations are frontal and parietal bones.
- Hemangiomas are usually located in the medullary space of the skull.
- Bright T1 bone lesions are almost always benign.
- Well circumscribed.
- May demonstrate enhancement on postcontrast imaging.
- Inner and outer table typically intact.
- Look for thickened trabecula on CT.

Answers

1. The abnormality is located within the frontal bone.

2. On CT, the hemangiomas classically have thickened trabeculae. On MR, the tumors may have iso- to hyperintense T1 and T2 bright signal. Interosseous hemangiomas may demonstrate enhancement on postcontrast imaging. Stages of blood products can occur within the lesion.

Suggested Reading

Bastug D, Ortiz O, Schochet SS. Hemangiomas in the calvaria: imaging findings. *AJR Am J Roentgenol.* 1995 Mar;164(3):683-687.

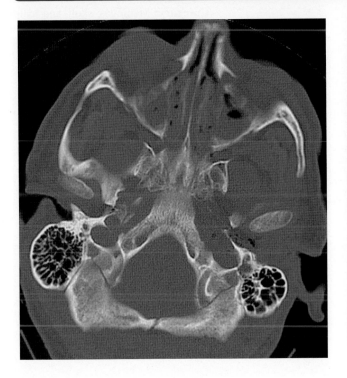 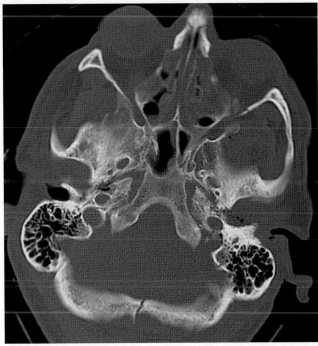

1. Where is the abnormality located?

2. What are the classic imaging findings for this entity?

3. What imaging modality is useful for evaluation of possible arterial injury?

4. What is the etiology of this finding?

5. What are common sequelae of this entity?

Case ranking/difficulty:

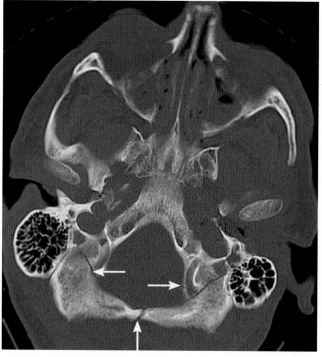

Axial CT bone window image shows fracture lines involving the occiput (*arrows*).

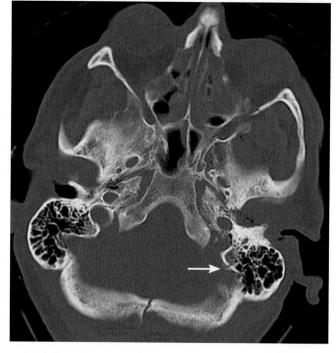

Axial CT bone window image shows a fracture extending from the left occiput into the left temporal bone (*arrow*).

Answers

1. The abnormality is located within the occipital bone.

2. The classic imaging findings for this entity are comminuted or depressed fractures of the skull base involving the basiocciput, basisphenoid, and/or temporal bones.

3. Basilar skull fractures that have suspected vascular injury can be studied with CTA. The gold standard remains catheter angiogram, but this is minimally invasive.

4. Most commonly a direct blow to the back of the head or a fall on the back of the head can cause basilar skull fractures.

5. Basilar skull fractures may have depressed fragments resulting in brain parenchymal contusion. These fractures may also extend into the temporal bones or vascular canals/cranial nerve foramen resulting in hearing loss, arterial dissection, thrombosis, or pseudoaneurysm.

Pearls

- Basilar skull fractures may have comminution or depressed fragments.

- Depressed fragments may result in intracranial hemorrhage or brain injury (parenchymal contusion).
- Evaluate brain for parenchymal contusions and extraaxial hemorrhage.
- Follow fracture lines for involvement of foramina.
- CTA needed if fracture traverses vascular foramen to exclude arterial dissection, thrombosis, or pseudoaneurysm.
- Pneumocephalus is a clue for fracture.
- Venous epidural hematoma may occur with disruption of venous sinus.

Suggested Readings

Aiken AH, Gean AD. Imaging of head trauma. *Semin Roentgenol.* 2010 Apr;45(2):63-79.

York G, Barboriak D, Petrella J, DeLong D, Provenzale JM. Association of internal carotid artery injury with carotid canal fractures in patients with head trauma. *AJR Am J Roentgenol.* 2005 May;184(5):1672-1678.

Zayas JO, Feliciano YZ, Hadley CR, Gomez AA, Vidal JA. Temporal bone trauma and the role of multidetector CT in the emergency department. *Radiographics.* 2011 Oct;31(6):1741-1755.

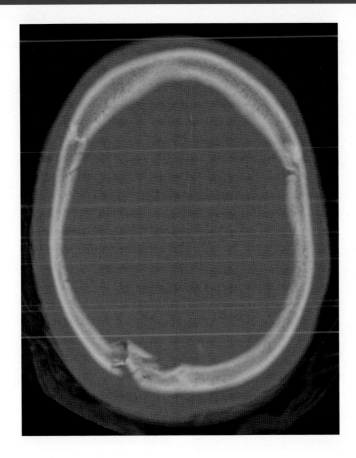

1. Where is the abnormality located?

2. What are the imaging findings for this entity?

3. What is the differential diagnosis?

4. What is the etiology of this finding?

5. What is the treatment for this entity?

Case ranking/difficulty:

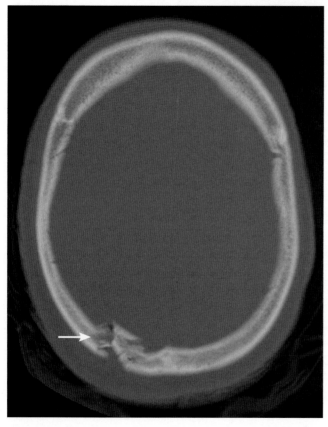

Axial CT bone window image shows a depressed, comminuted fracture posteriorly involving the right parietal bone (*arrow*).

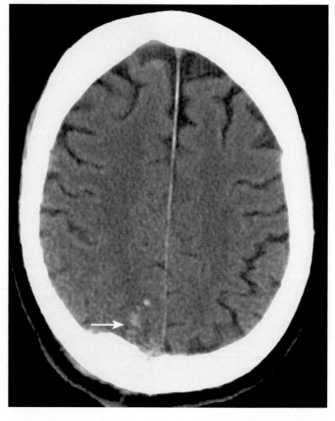

Axial CT brain window image shows multiple punctate foci of hemorrhage from brain contusion (*arrow*).

Answers

1. The abnormality involves the right parietal bone.

2. The imaging findings for depressed skull fracture include displacement of the inner table into the skull with fragments.

3. The differential diagnosis includes suture diastasis, arachnoid granulation, and depressed fracture.

4. Depressed skull fractures are caused by high-energy blunt trauma to a small area of the skull.

5. Depressed fractures also are at risk for infection and injury to venous sinuses. Therefore, these fractures are typically explored surgically and fracture fragments are elevated and/or removed.

Pearls

- There are three main types of skull fracture: basilar, linear, and depressed.
- Evaluate brain for parenchymal contusion and extraaxial hemorrhage.
- Skull fracture may disrupt venous sinuses.
- Depressed fractures also are at risk for infection.
- Pneumocephalus is a clue for fracture.

Suggested Reading

Aiken AH, Gean AD. Imaging of head trauma. *Semin Roentgenol*. 2010 Apr;45(2):63-79.

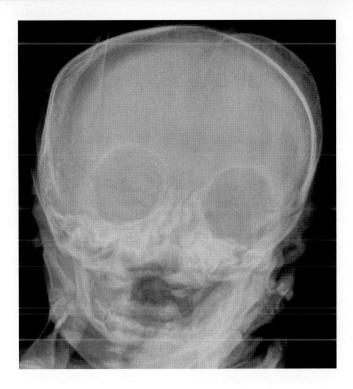

1. Where is the abnormality located?

2. What are the classic imaging findings for this entity?

3. What is the differential diagnosis?

4. What is the etiology of this entity?

5. What is the treatment for this entity?

Case ranking/difficulty: 🦞

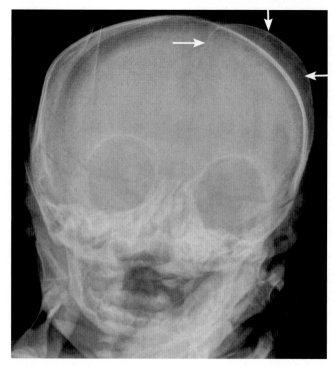

AP view of the skull shows a well-circumscribed oval-shaped structure over the left parietal bone. Notice that it does not cross midline and has peripheral calcification (*arrows*).

Pearls

- Cephalohematoma is a subperiosteal hematoma that is bound by sutures.
- If hematoma crosses midline, consider caput succedaneum or subgaleal hematoma.
- Cephalohematoma may peripherally calcify, then ossify and be incorporated in the skull over time.
- Cephalohematoma most commonly involves the parietal bone followed by the occipital bone.
- Do not mistake for fibrous dysplasia, which does not typically present in the neonatal period.

Suggested Readings

Nabavizadeh SA, Bilaniuk LT, Feygin T, Shekdar KV, Zimmerman RA, Vossough A. CT and MRI of pediatric skull lesions with fluid-fluid levels. *AJNR Am J Neuroradiol.* 2014;35(3):604-608.

Winter TC, Mack LA, Cyr DR. Prenatal sonographic diagnosis of scalp edema/cephalohematoma mimicking an encephalocele. *AJR Am J Roentgenol.* 1993 Dec;161(6):1247-1248.

Answers

1. The abnormality is located along the left parietal bone.

2. A cephalohematoma typically appears as a well-circumscribed scalp mass that is bound by cranial sutures.

3. The differential diagnosis includes cephalohematoma, subgaleal hematoma, caput succedaneum, and cephalocele.

4. Cephalohematoma is typically from trauma and commonly seen in newborns with instrument delivery. There can be associated skull fracture.

5. No treatment is needed for this entity. Cephalohematomas can eventually ossify and be remodeled with the calvarium.

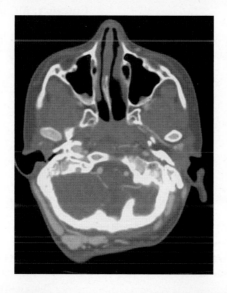
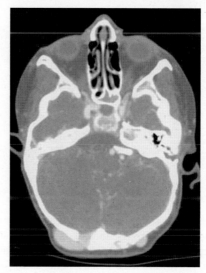
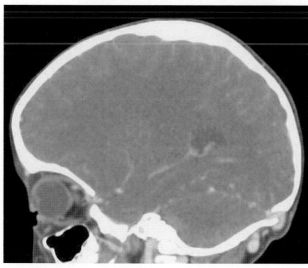
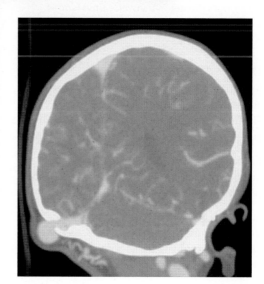

1. What is the differential diagnosis?

2. What intracranial vascular structures communicate with the mass?

3. What imaging should be performed prior to possible surgical resection?

4. What imaging findings can be seen in the extracranial component?

5. What are the causes of this lesion?

Case ranking/difficulty: **Category:** Meninges, skull, and scalp

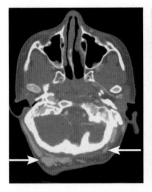 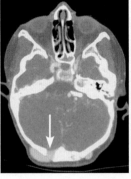 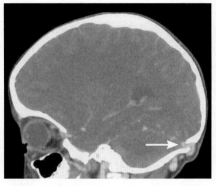 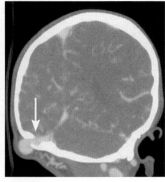

Axial CT image with contrast in the venous phase shows serpentine vascular structures in the occipital scalp (*arrows*), right greater than left.	Axial CT postcontrast image delayed phase shows bony defect connecting the scalp vascular mass with the right transverse sinus (*arrow*).	Sagittal CT postcontrast delayed phase image shows the bony defect with communication with the right transverse sinus (*arrow*).	Oblique reformat of CT with contrast delayed phase shows the right bony defect (*arrow*) with communication of scalp vascular mass and right transverse sinus.

Answers

1. Differentials for vascular masses of the scalp include sinus pericranii, venous and arteriovenous malformations. Infantile hemangiomas may also be considered, although this appearance is not typical.

2. Sinus pericranii typically communicate with dural venous sinuses or cortical veins and rarely developmental venous anomalies.

3. Venography, CT, MR, or catheter is essential for evaluating the associated venous structures in sinus pericranii and evaluate for adequate venous drainage of the brain to prevent venous infarcts after ligation.

4. Extracranial component of sinus pericranii typically involves a scalp venous varix that may be dilated and serpentine or a vascular malformation with cysts, septations, and phleboliths.

5. The majority of sinus pericranii are thought to be congenital, possibly associated with other venous malformations and variations, or from sinus thrombosis. Posttraumatic laceration of emissary veins is also an etiology.

Pearls

- Sinus pericranii represents a variant communication between intracranial and extracranial venous circulation.
- Typically seen as a scalp venous varix communicating with a dural venous sinus through a transcalvarial emissary vein.
- Etiology can be congenital or traumatic.
- The extracranial venous structure may also present as a venous malformation with septations, cysts, and phleboliths.
- Intracranial communications are typically a dural venous sinus, cortical vein, or less commonly, a developmental venous anomaly.
- CT or MR venography is helpful to identify all associated venous vascular components.
- Assessment of appropriate pathways of venous drainage is necessary to prevent venous infarcts, prior to surgical ligation.

Suggested Readings

Gandolfo C, Krings T, Alvarez H, et al. Sinus pericranii: diagnostic and therapeutic considerations in 15 patients. *Neuroradiology*. 2007 Jun;49(6):505-514.

Kim YJ, Kim IO, Cheon JE, Lim YJ, Kim WS, Yeon KM. Sonographic features of sinus pericranii in 4 pediatric patients. *J Ultrasound Med*. 2011 Mar;30(3):411-417.

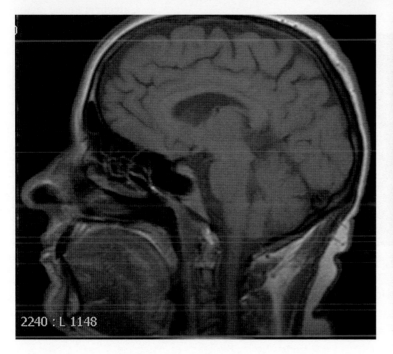

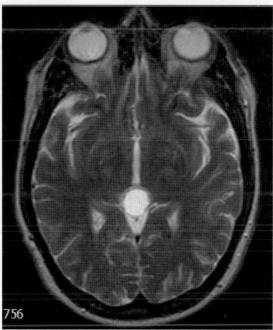

1. Where is the abnormality located?

2. What are the imaging findings for this entity?

3. What is the differential diagnosis?

4. What is a complication of this entity?

5. What is the treatment for this entity?

Case ranking/difficulty: 　　　　　　　　　　　　**Category:** Pineal region

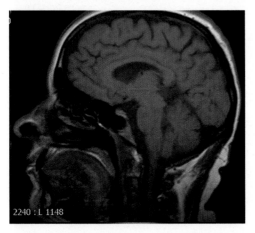

Sagittal T1 image shows a lesion within the pineal gland that is hypointense but has more T1 shortening than CSF (*arrow*).

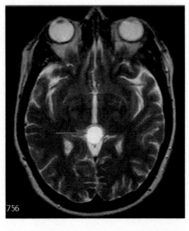

Axial T2 image shows a cystic lesion in the pineal gland that is hyperintense and follows CSF signal (*arrow*).

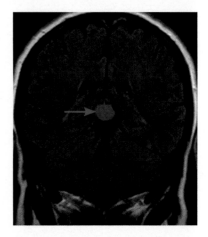

Coronal FLAIR shows that the lesion in the pineal gland is hyperintense to CSF (*arrow*).

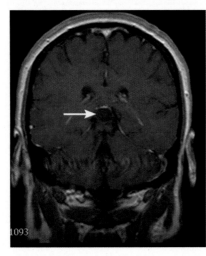

Coronal postcontrast image shows that the lesion in the pineal gland does not enhance (*arrow*).

Pearls

- Pineal cysts (PC) have an outer fibrous connective tissue layer with pineal parenchyma with or without hemorrhagic products internally.
- Key to diagnosis is noting a fluid signal lesion within the pineal gland.
- PC larger than 1.5 cm may compress the aqueduct resulting in hydrocephalus.
- Check lateral ventricle size.
- Check aqueduct for compression.
- Consider pineocytoma when solid components are seen.

Suggested Reading

Osborn AG, Preece MT. Intracranial cysts: radiologic-pathologic correlation and imaging approach. *Radiology*. 2006 Jun;239(3):650-664.

Answers

1. The abnormality is located in the pineal gland.

2. The imaging findings for this entity include intermediate and slightly brighter than CSF on T1, follow CSF on T2, and have peripheral or rim contrast enhancement.

3. The differential diagnosis includes arachnoid cyst, pineal cyst, and pineocytoma.

4. This entity may result in obstructive hydrocephalus when lesions are larger than 1.5 cm in size.

5. Usually no treatment is needed unless it gets large enough to cause obstructive hydrocephalus.

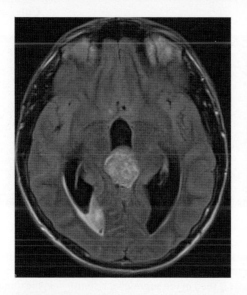
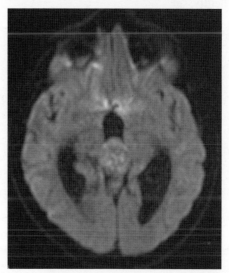
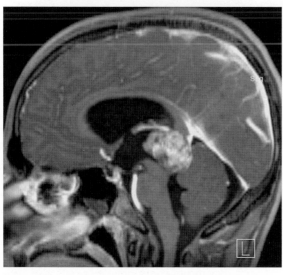
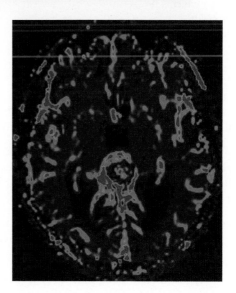

1. What is the differential diagnosis?

2. What are the most common locations for this tumor?

3. What is the most common location of these tumors in males and females?

4. What are the typical imaging characteristics of this tumor?

5. What is the prognosis for this disease?

Case ranking/difficulty:

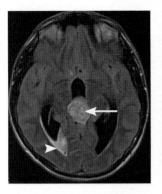

Axial FLAIR image shows a lobular mass in the pineal region, which is slightly hyperintense to gray matter (*arrow*), which causes hydrocephalus and transependymal CSF (*arrowhead*).

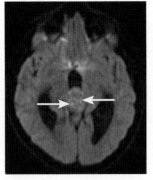

Axial DWI b = 1000 image shows areas of decreased diffusion (*arrows*) due to hypercellularity.

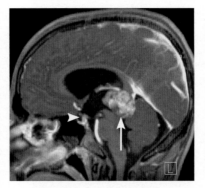

Sagittal T1 postcontrast shows intense enhancement of the pineal mass with possible invasion of the tectal plate (*arrow*). A second smaller enhancing mass is seen in the suprasellar cistern (*arrowhead*).

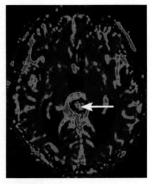

Axial color CBV map from dynamic susceptibility contrast perfusion imaging shows areas of hyperperfusion in the tumor (*arrow*).

Answers

1. A pineal region mass should include the differentials of germ cell tumor, pineoblastoma, and tectal plate glioma.

2. The most common locations for germ cell tumors are the pineal region and suprasellar locations. Pineal region germ cell tumors are more common than suprasellar with a ratio of 2:1.

3. Pineal germinomas are 10× more likely to occur in males than females while 75% of germ cell tumors in females are in the suprasellar location.

4. Germinomas typically show homogeneous enhancement with restricted diffusion due to hypercellularity. Tumor cysts and necrosis, along with adjacent structure invasion, can be seen as the tumor increases in size. CSF dissemination is not uncommon at presentation.

5. Pure germinomas have good prognosis despite the hypercellular nature due to sensitivity to radiation and platinum-based chemotherapy. Greater than 90% 5-year survival is seen with radiation alone. By contrast, nongerminomatous germ cell tumors typically have poorer prognosis due to relative insensitivity to treatment.

Pearls

- Germinomas are a subclassification of germinomatous germ cell tumors while nongerminomatous germ cell tumors include yolk sac tumors and teratomas.
- CNS germ cell tumors commonly occur in the midline at the pineal and suprasellar locations.
- CNS germinoma in the pineal region have a 10:1 predilection for boys while those in the suprasellar location have a 75% predilection for girls.
- Imaging shows lobular-enhancing tumors engulfing the pineal gland or infundibulum. Pituitary calcifications are engulfed rather than exploded as in pineoblastomas.
- Germinomas can show restricted diffusion due to high cellularity. On CT, this shows hyperdensity.
- Larger tumors can invade adjacent brain parenchyma.
- Pure germinomas are highly responsive to radiation and chemotherapy, with favorable prognosis.

Suggested Readings

Dumrongpisutikul N, Intrapiromkul J, Yousem DM. Distinguishing between germinomas and pineal cell tumors on MR imaging. *AJNR Am J Neuroradiol.* 2012 Mar;33(3):550-555.

Mathews VP, Broome DR, Smith RR, Bognanno JR, Einhorn LH, Edwards MK. Neuroimaging of disseminated germ cell neoplasms. *AJNR Am J Neuroradiol.* 2003 Jan;11(2):319-324.

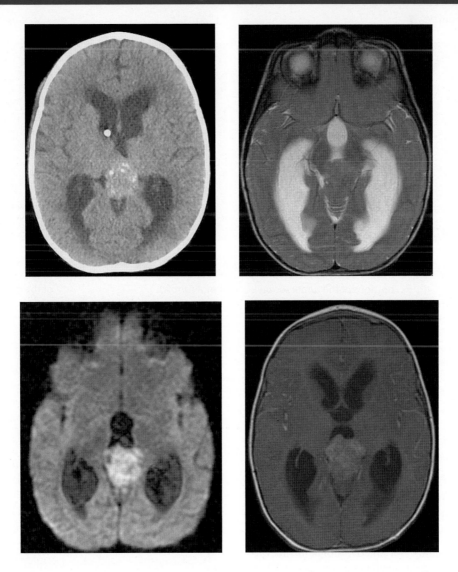

1. What is the differential diagnosis of this tumor?

2. How does diffusion imaging help in differentiating these tumors?

3. What are typical imaging findings in this entity?

4. What hereditary conditions are associated with this tumor?

5. What is the prognosis of these pineal tumors?

Case ranking/difficulty: **Category:** Pineal region

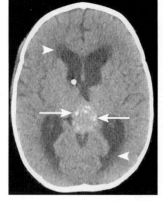

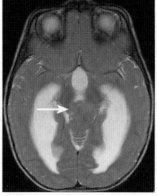

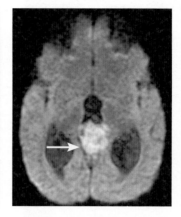

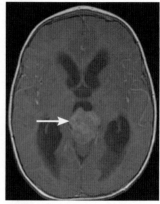

Axial CT image shows a pineal region tumor with "exploded" peripheral calcifications (*arrows*). There is obstructive hydrocephalus with transependymal CSF (*arrowheads*). A shunt catheter is noted in the right lateral ventricle.

Axial T2 image shows hypointensity of the solid portions of the tumor (*arrow*).

Axial DWI b = 1000 image shows restricted diffusion of the pineal tumor (*arrow*).

Axial postcontrast image shows heterogeneous enhancement of the pineal tumor (*arrow*).

Answers

1. Pineal parenchymal tumors, germ cell tumors, and tectal plate glial tumors should be considered in tumors of the pineal region.

2. Pineal tumors with decreased diffusion suggest high-grade lesions such as pineoblastoma and poorly differentiated germ cell tumors.

3. Typical imaging findings for pineoblastoma include an "exploded" peripheral calcification, decreased T2 and diffusion of the solid components, heterogeneous enhancement, and invasion of adjacent structures.

4. Pineoblastomas and the related pineal region primitive neuroectodermal tumors have well-known associations with familial retinoblastoma (adding bilateral retinoblastomas forms the "trilateral retinoblastoma"). Also, pineoblastomas have also been reported with Turcot syndrome, a subset of familial adenomatous polyposis.

5. Two major tumor types occur in the pineal region, pineal parenchymal tumors and germ cell tumors. As a whole, pineal parenchymal tumors have worse survival than germ cell tumors. This is likely reflected in that 45% of pineal parenchymal tumors are pineoblastomas. Pineoblastomas have 1- to 2-year median survival after presentation despite treatment.

Pearls

- Pineoblastomas are poorly differentiated, embryonal WHO grade IV tumors originating from the pineal gland.
- There is significant histological overlap with PNET, with pineal region PNETs and pineoblastomas considered as related entities.
- Known association with sporadic and hereditary retinoblastoma, forming the "trilateral retinoblastoma" in the mutations of RB1 gene.
- Imaging shows a large lobular and heterogeneous tumor in the pineal region with frequent invasion of adjacent structures.
- CT can show "exploded" peripheral calcification rather than central engulfed calcification as seen with germ cell tumors.
- Solid components show T2 hypointensity and restricted diffusion due to hypercellularity.
- Heterogeneous enhancement, necrosis, and hemorrhage can be common.
- The typical clinical profile is a toddler with increased intracranial pressure and possible Parinaud syndrome.

Suggested Readings

Kakigi T, Okada T, Kanagaki M, et al. Quantitative imaging values of CT, MR, and FDG-PET to differentiate pineal parenchymal tumors and germinomas: are they useful? *Neuroradiology*. 2014;56(4):297-303.

Rodjan F, de Graaf P, Moll AC, et al. Brain abnormalities on MR imaging in patients with retinoblastoma. *AJNR Am J Neuroradiol*. 2010 Sep;31(8):1385-1389.

21-year-old female with headache

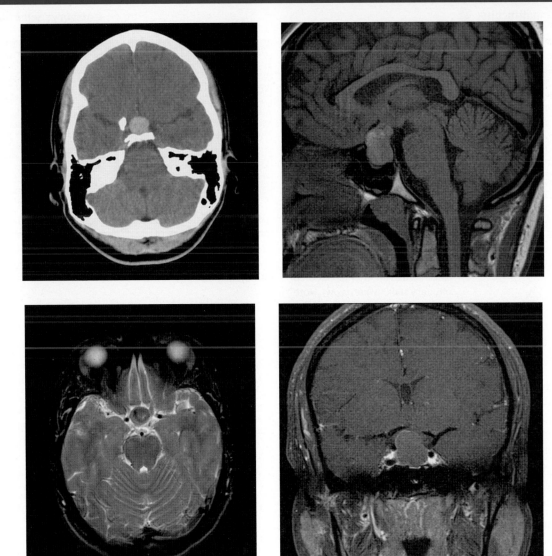

1. What is the differential diagnosis?

2. What imaging sign is specific for this disease?

3. What is the most common clinical symptom in this diagnosis?

4. What are the characteristic radiographic features?

5. What is the primary treatment option for this disease?

Case ranking/difficulty:

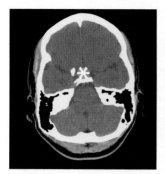 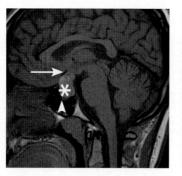 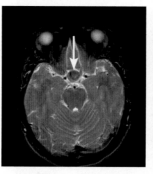 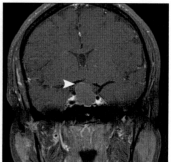

Noncontrast CT brain demonstrates a round hyperdense mass in the sellar/suprasellar region (*asterisk*).

Sagittal T1 image demonstrates a large T1 slightly hyperintense mass in the sella extending to the suprasellar region (*asterisk*), causing mild anterior deviation of pituitary stalk (*white arrow*). Note a pituitary gland in the floor of pituitary fossa (*white arrowhead*).

Axial T2 image demonstrates mixed signal intensity of a sellar/suprasellar mass. There is a T2 hypointense intracystic nodule (*arrow*).

Postcontrast coronal T1 image demonstrates mild peripheral enhancement of a sellar/suprasellar mass (*white arrowhead*).

Answers

1. Craniopharyngioma, pituitary macroadenoma, Rathke cleft cyst, thrombosed aneurysm, and dermoid/epidermoid cyst can all occur in the same location, usually suprasellar in origin, and should be considered in the differential diagnosis.

2. Specific imaging findings of Rathke cleft cyst include the "claw" sign of a peripheral enhancing pituitary gland and an intracystic T2 hypointense nodule.

3. Most Rathke cleft cysts are incidentally discovered and asymptomatic. When present, headaches are usually the most common symptom, and can be accompanied by symptoms referable to compression on the optic chiasm, pituitary, and hypothalamus.

4. A nonenhancing, midline cystic lesion in the sellar/suprasellar region arising from the anterior lobe and pars intermedia of the pituitary gland are characteristic radiographic features. However, wall calcification and enhancement may be present in some cases (10%-15%) Internal calcification and enhancement are not seen.

5. When symptomatic, Rathke cleft cysts are typically treated by surgical resection.

- Usually incidentally found and asymptomatic, 1 in 10 autopsies.
- Radiographic features seen as well-defined, nonenhancing midline cyst within the sella arising between the anterior lobes and pars intermedia.
- 60% suprasellar extension.
- Varying signal characteristics due to cystic protein concentration.
- T2 hypointense intracystic nodule in the majority of cases.
- Top three differential diagnoses include craniopharyngioma, cystic microadenoma, and aneurysm.
- Transsphenoidal resection is a treatment option in the symptomatic patient.

Suggested Readings

Bonneville F, Cattin F, Marsot-Dupuch K, Dormont D, Bonneville JF, Chiras J. T1 signal hyperintensity in the sellar region: spectrum of findings. *Radiographics*. 2006 May;26(1):93-113.

Sumida M, Uozumi T, Mukada K, Arita K, Kurisu K, Eguchi K. Rathke cleft cysts: correlation of enhanced MR and surgical findings. *AJNR Am J Neuroradiol*. 1994 Mar;15(3):525-532.

Takanashi J, Tada H, Barkovich AJ, Saeki N, Kohno Y. Pituitary cysts in childhood evaluated by MR imaging. *AJNR Am J Neuroradiol*. 2005 Sep;26(8):2144-2147.

Pearls

- Benign, sellar/suprasellar epithelium-lined cystic lesion arising from the remnants of Rathke pouch.
- Female predominance.

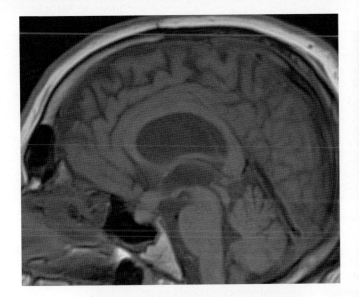
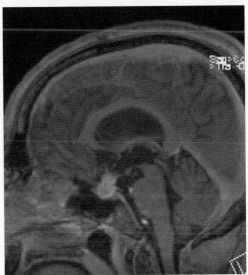
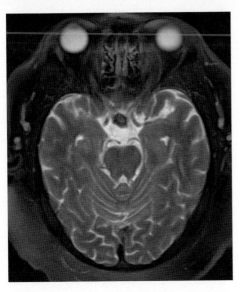
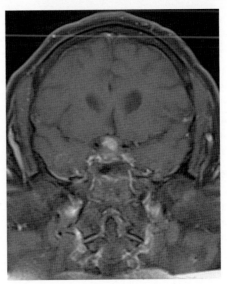

1. What is the differential diagnosis?

2. What imaging feature can help separate the top 2 differential considerations?

3. What is the pathophysiology of the disease?

4. What percentage of patients will have other autoimmune diseases?

5. What is the treatment for this disease?

Case ranking/difficulty:

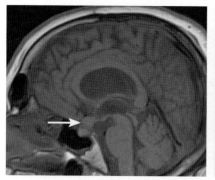

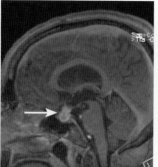

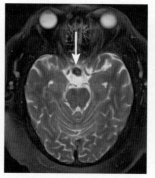

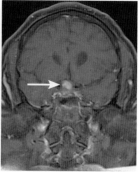

Sagittal T1 postcontrast at midline shows an isointense mass centered at the pituitary stalk (*arrow*). There is loss of the posterior pituitary bright spot.

Sagittal postcontrast image at midline shows solid enhancement of the pituitary stalk, which also involves predominantly the anterior pituitary gland (*arrow*).

Axial T2 of the suprasellar cistern shows T2 hypointensity of the infundibular mass (*arrow*). This is specific for lymphocytic hypophysitis over pituitary adenoma.

Coronal T1 postcontrast again shows the infundibular mass with extension into the sella (*arrow*).

Answers

1. Likely differentials of a homogeneous enhancing mass involving the infundibulum and extending into the anterior pituitary gland include lymphocytic hypophysitis and pituitary adenoma. While germinoma and hypothalamic glioma are considered, invasion into the pituitary is rare.

2. The main differential for a sellar and suprasellar homogeneous enhancing mass is lymphocytic hypophysitis and pituitary macroadenoma. Both can have homogeneous enhancement, but lymphocytic hypophysitis has not been described with cystic change. Loss of posterior pituitary bright spot is seen in 3/4 of lymphocytic hypophysitis, but if the pituitary adenoma is large enough, the neurohypophysis can be obliterated. T2 hypointensity of lymphocytic hypophysitis is a specific sign, not seen with adenomas.

3. Lymphocytic hypophysitis is an autoimmune-mediated inflammation of the adenohypophysis and stalk.

4. Nearly a quarter of patients with lymphocytic hypophysitis will have other autoimmune diseases.

5. Lymphocytic hypophysitis is treated with immunosuppression such as corticosteroids with hormone replacement as needed.

Pearls

- Lymphocytic hypophysitis (LH) is an autoimmune inflammation of the anterior pituitary gland and the pituitary stalk.
- While there is an association with peripartum women, LH can affect both men and women from adolescence through old age.
- Males are eight times less likely to have LH than females and tend to present a decade later with mean age of 45 years.
- MRI imaging shows homogeneous enhancement with thickening of the pituitary stalk with or without enlargement of the pituitary gland.
- 75% of LH have loss of the posterior pituitary bright spot on T1.
- T2 hypointensity is a characteristic sign of LH and may help differentiate from pituitary adenoma.

Suggested Readings

Bellastella A, Bizzaro A, Coronella C, Bellastella G, Sinisi AA, De Bellis A. Lymphocytic hypophysitis: a rare or underestimated disease? *Eur J Endocrinol.* 2003 Nov;149(5):363-376.

Nakata Y, Sato N, Masumoto T, et al. Parasellar T2 dark sign on MR imaging in patients with lymphocytic hypophysitis. *AJNR Am J Neuroradiol.* 2010 Nov;31(10):1944-1950.

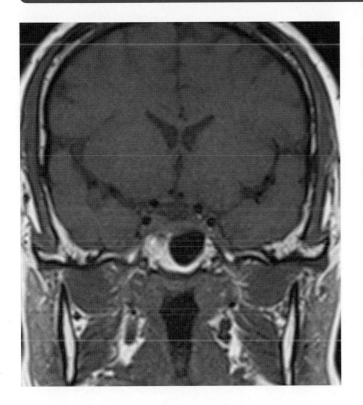
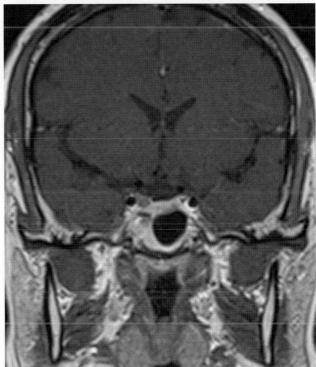

1. Where is the abnormality located?

2. What are the classic imaging findings for this entity?

3. What is the differential diagnosis?

4. What are possible presenting symptoms for this lesion?

5. What is the treatment for this entity?

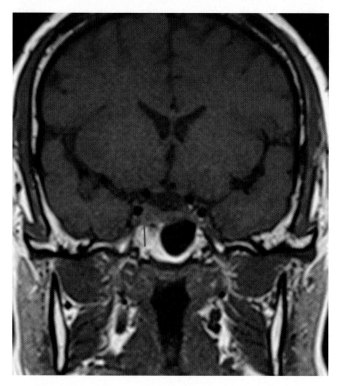

Coronal T1 of the sella without contrast shows fullness along the right parasagittal pituitary gland (*arrow*).

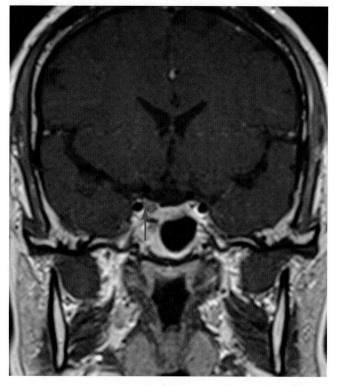

Coronal T1 of the sella postcontrast shows an area of diminished contrast enhancement relative to the remainder of the gland (*arrow*).

Answers

1. The abnormality is located in the right aspect of the pituitary gland.

2. Classically pituitary microadenomas are isointense to gray matter on T1- and T2-weighted images and demonstrate diminished contrast enhancement, which appears as a "filling defect" in the pituitary gland.

3. The differential diagnosis includes microadenoma, craniopharyngioma, and Rathke cleft cyst.

4. Prolactinomas are the most common type of hormonally active microadenomas. This usually results in galactorrhea in females and decreased libido in male patients.

5. The treatment for this entity includes medical treatment for hormonally active lesions versus surgical resection. Most microadenomas can be treated conservatively if nonfunctioning.

Pearls

- Pituitary adenomas are benign tumors of the pituitary gland.
- Pituitary microadenomas < 1 cm.
- Microadenomas typically are hormonally active in contrast to macroadenomas, which usually are not.
- The most common microadenoma is the prolactinoma.
- Adenomas usually enhance more slowly than rest of the gland; 10%-30% can be seen only with dynamic sella imaging.
- Consider Rathke cleft cyst with a nonenhancing midline pituitary lesion.
- If heterogeneous sellar lesion with calcifications, consider craniopharyngioma.

Suggested Reading

Johnsen DE, Woodruff WW, Allen IS, Cera PJ, Funkhouser GR, Coleman LL. MR imaging of the sellar and juxtasellar regions. *Radiographics*. 1991 Sep;11(5):727-758.

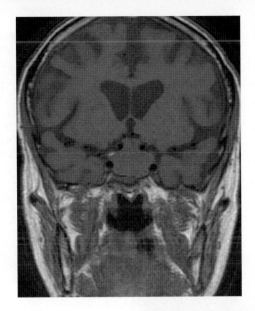
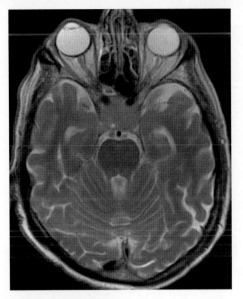
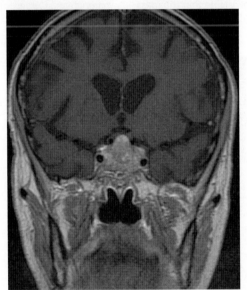

1. Where is the abnormality located?

2. What are the classic imaging findings for this entity?

3. What is the differential diagnosis?

4. What are presenting symptoms for this lesion?

5. What is the treatment for this entity?

Case ranking/difficulty: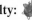

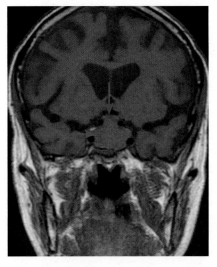

Coronal T1 noncontrast image shows a large sellar mass that is isointense to brain parenchyma (*green arrow*). Note that the mass is extending into the suprasellar cistern and impressing upon the optic chiasm (*red arrow*).

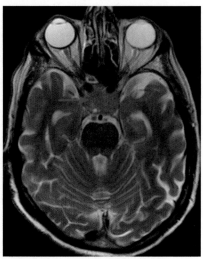

Axial T2 image shows a large sellar mass that is isointense to brain parenchyma (*arrow*).

5. The treatment for this entity is medical (when tumors are hormonally active) or surgical removal if symptomatic compression occurs.

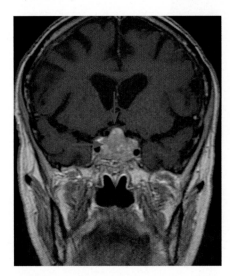

Coronal T1 postcontrast image shows enhancement of the sellar mass (*green arrow*). Note that the mass is impressing upon the optic chiasm (*red arrow*).

Answers

1. The abnormality is located within the pituitary gland.

2. These lesions classically are isointense to gray matter on T1- and T2-weighted images. There is associated enhancement of the tumor.

3. The differential diagnosis includes pituitary macroadenoma, meningioma, and aneurysm.

4. Patients usually present with bitemporal hemianopsia from compression of the optic chiasm.

Pearls

- Pituitary adenomas are benign tumors of the pituitary gland.
- Macroadenoma has a classic "snowman or figure 8" shape and is greater than 1 cm.
- Macroadenomas may invade the cavernous sinus or sphenoid sinus.
- If flow voids are seen consider aneurysm.
- If a lesion is seen that is isointense to brain and does not involve the pituitary consider a diaphragmatic meningioma.
- Total encasement of the cavernous ICA is a highly specific but not sensitive sign for cavernous sinus invasion.
- CTA or MRA for exclusion of aneurysm.

Suggested Readings

Douglas-Akinwande AC, Hattab EM. AJR teaching file: central skull base mass. *AJR Am J Roentgenol*. 2010 Sep;195(3 suppl):S22-S24.

Johnsen DE, Woodruff WW, Allen IS, Cera PJ, Funkhouser GR, Coleman LL. MR imaging of the sellar and juxtasellar regions. *Radiographics*. 1991 Sep;11(5):727-758.

86-day-old male with enlarging head circumference

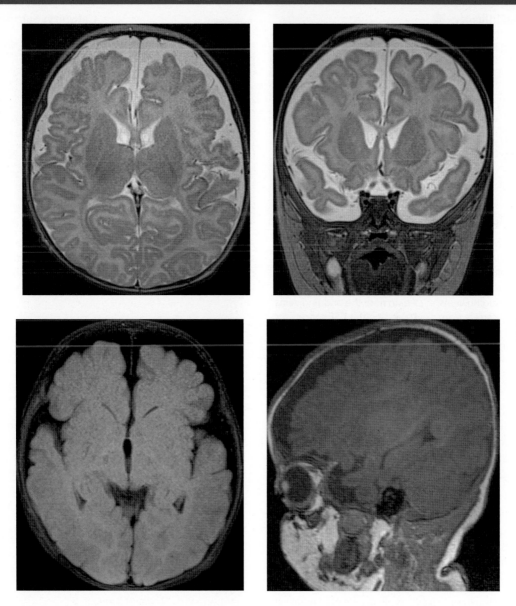

1. What is the differential diagnosis?

2. What are typical imaging findings for this entity?

3. What is the gender predilection for this entity?

4. What is the natural history of this entity?

5. What must be excluded with subdural hematomas?

Case ranking/difficulty:

Category: Subarachnoid spaces

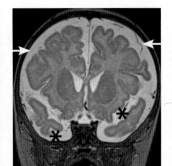

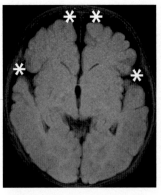

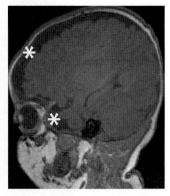

Axial T2 image shows enlarged CSF spaces overlying the frontal lobes (*asterisks*). Note the lack of mass effect with prominence of the sulci and bridging veins, which traverse this space from the cortex to the inner table of the skull (*arrows*).

Coronal T2 shows increased subarachnoid spaces associated with the frontal and temporal lobes (*asterisks*). Again note the bridging veins traversing this CSF space (*arrows*).

Axial FLAIR shows complete suppression of the symmetric prominent frontal and temporal subarachnoid spaces (*asterisks*).

Sagittal T1 image off midline shows the frontal and temporal enlarged subarachnoid spaces following CSF signal (*asterisks*).

Answers

1. The differential diagnosis for prominent extra-axial spaces in an infant includes enlarged subarachnoid spaces, subdural hematoma, communicating hydrocephalus (extraventricular obstructive hydrocephalus), and brain atrophy.

2. In enlarged subarachnoid spaces, the frontal and anterior temporal symmetric fluid collections follow CSF on all imaging sequences. A key finding is the visualization of bridging veins that travel through this space from the cortex to inner table. No mass effect on the parenchyma is seen.

3. Enlarged subarachnoid spaces typically involve males at a 4 to 1 ratio.

4. Likely due to maturation of arachnoid villi, almost all cases resolve without any intervention by 2 years of age, with resolution of enlarged subarachnoid spaces and any associated mild motor delays. Persistent macrocephaly is common.

5. Enlarged subarachnoid spaces have been suggested to be a risk factor for small subdural hematomas with minimal head trauma. However, a good clinical history must be obtained to exclude nonaccidental trauma.

Pearls

- Accumulation of increased CSF in the subarachnoid spaces due to immaturity of the arachnoid villi.
- No mass effect on brain parenchyma with bridging veins traversing through subarachnoid space.
- MRI is the most sensitive and specific for the evaluation of bridging veins through the enlarged subarachnoid spaces.
- CT with contrast may be helpful to distinguish the bridging veins.
- Ultrasound with Doppler may be useful with persistence of the anterior fontanelle.
- Follows CSF on all sequences.
- Difficult to exclude chronic subdural hematomas on CT, raising the possibility of nonaccidental trauma.
- Possible increased risk of small subdural hematomas with minimal head trauma with enlarged subarachnoid spaces—clinical history very important!

Suggested Readings

Greiner MV, Richards TJ, Care MM, Leach JL. Prevalence of subdural collections in children with macrocrania. *AJNR Am J Neuroradiol*. 2013 Dec;34(12):2373-2378.

Kendall B, Holland I. Benign communicating hydrocephalus in children. *Neuroradiology*. 1981 Mar;21(2):93-96.

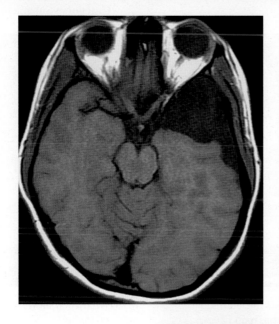
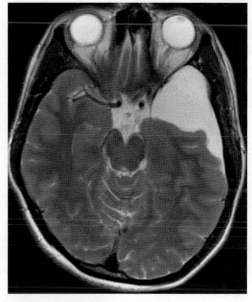
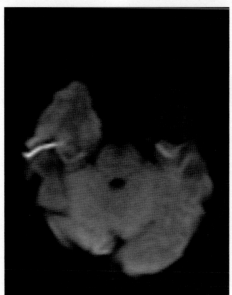

1. Where is the abnormality located?

2. What are the classic imaging findings?

3. What is the differential diagnosis?

4. What is the etiology of this entity?

5. What is the treatment for this entity?

Case ranking/difficulty: 🌑

Category: Subarachnoid spaces

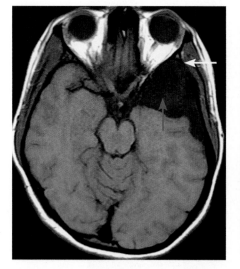

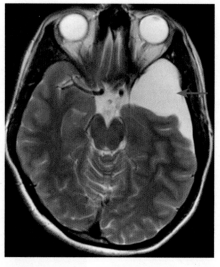

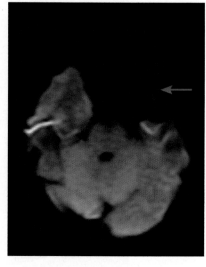

Axial T1 image shows a hypointense CSF signal lesion (*green arrow*) in the extraaxial space within the left middle cranial fossa. Note the bony remodeling (*white arrow*) suggesting a long-standing lesion.

Axial T2 image shows the left middle cranial fossa lesion has high T2 signal following CSF (*arrow*). There is displacement of the brain parenchyma.

Axial DWI b-1000 shows no restricted diffusion (*arrow*).

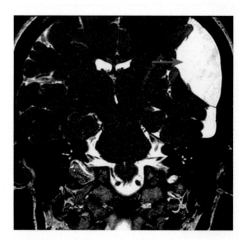

Coronal FIESTA image shows extension of cystic lesion to involve the sylvian fissure (*arrow*).

5. Arachnoid cysts are benign, and the majority of cases do not require treatment. However, a small number of cases can cause symptoms that can be relieved by surgical resection, fenestration, or shunting.

Pearls

- Arachnoid cysts are the most common congenital cystic lesion
- The most common location is the middle cranial fossa (60%).
- Follows CSF on all MRI pulse sequences.
- No contrast enhancement.
- If DWI shows restriction, then consider epidermoid/dermoid cyst and neurenteric cyst.

Answers

1. The abnormality is within the left middle cranial fossa.

2. These lesions will follow CSF on CT and all MRI sequences. Therefore, T1 prolongation (low signal) and T2 prolongation (high signal).

3. The differential diagnosis includes dermoid cyst, epidermoid cyst, and arachnoid cyst.

4. Arachnoid cysts are primarily congenital, although rarely they are associated with surgery or infection.

Suggested Reading

Osborn AG, Preece MT. Intracranial cysts: radiologic-pathologic correlation and imaging approach. *Radiology*. 2006 Jun;239(3):650-664.

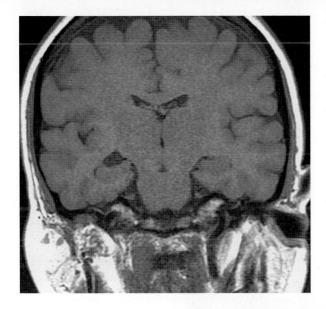
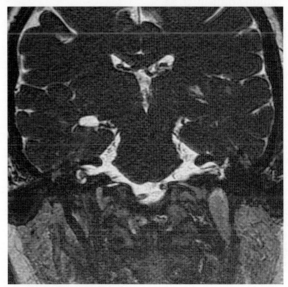

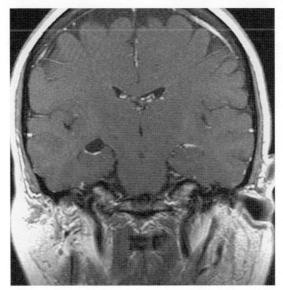

1. Where is the abnormality located?

2. What are the classic imaging findings for this entity?

3. What is the differential diagnosis?

4. What is the etiology of this entity?

5. What is the treatment for this entity?

Choroidal fissure cyst

Case 71 (3548)

Case ranking/difficulty: 🌰

Category: Subarachnoid spaces

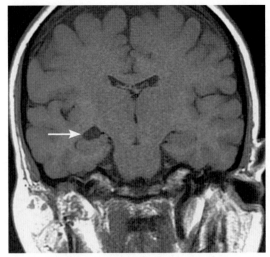

Coronal T1 image shows a well-circumscribed low signal lesion within the right choroidal fissure (*arrow*).

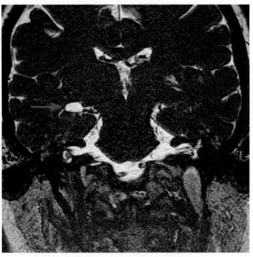

Coronal FIESTA image shows the right choroidal fissure cystic lesion with high signal following CSF (*arrow*).

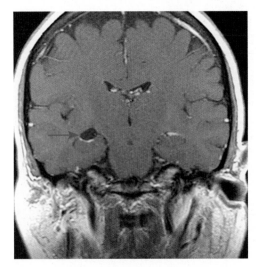

Coronal T1 postcontrast image demonstrates no contrast enhancement of the cystic lesion (*arrow*). The enhancement inferior to the lesion is from choroid plexus.

4. Choroidal fissure cysts are extraaxial neuroepithelial or arachnoid cysts, which are likely congenital in nature.

5. No treatment is typically necessary for this entity. Some authors advocate surgical resection in the setting of medically refractory seizures.

Pearls

- A benign extraaxial cyst located within the choroidal fissure.
- The choroidal fissure is a cleft located along the wall of the lateral ventricle where the choroid plexus attaches.
- May be associated with seizures and may be secondary to compression of the hippocampus.
- Follows CSF on all sequences without contrast enhancement.
- If contrast enhancement is seen, consider neoplasm.
- If gyral enhancement is seen, consider infarct.

Answers

1. The abnormality is within the right choroidal fissure.

2. On CT and MRI, the key to diagnosis is the location within the choroidal fissure and that the lesion follows CSF signal on all sequences. After the administration of contrast, no enhancement is seen.

3. The differential diagnosis includes hippocampal sulcus remnant, choroidal fissure cyst, and mesial temporal sclerosis.

Suggested Readings

de Jong L, Thewissen L, van Loon J, Van Calenbergh F. Choroidal fissure cerebrospinal fluid-containing cysts: case series, anatomical consideration, and review of the literature. *World Neurosurg*. 2011 Dec;75(5-6):704-708.

Osborn AG, Preece MT. Intracranial cysts: radiologic-pathologic correlation and imaging approach. *Radiology*. 2006 Jun;239(3):650-664.

Sherman JL, Camponovo E, Citrin CM. MR imaging of CSF-like choroidal fissure and parenchymal cysts of the brain. *AJR Am J Roentgenol*. 1990 Nov;155(5):1069-1075.

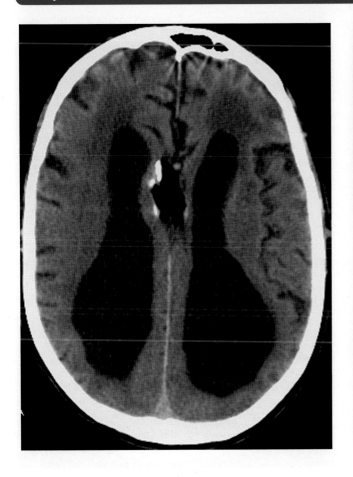 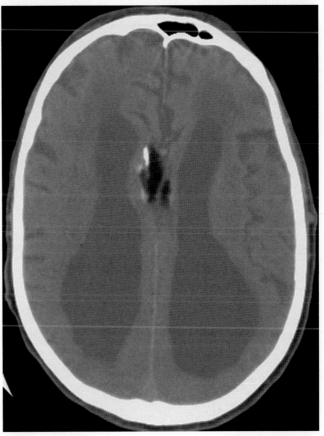

1. Where is the abnormality located?

2. What are the classic imaging findings for this entity?

3. What is the differential diagnosis?

4. What is the etiology of this entity?

5. What is the treatment for this entity?

Case ranking/difficulty:

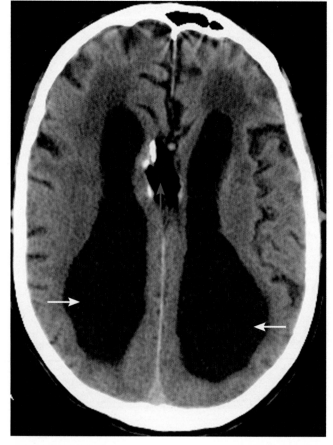

Axial CT image shows a low attenuating lesion consistent with fat within the midline with associated calcifications (*green arrow*). Also note that there is colpocephaly (*white arrows*) with associated agenesis of the corpus callosum.

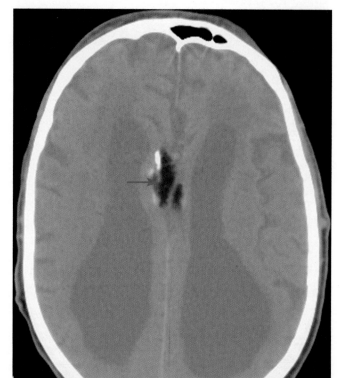

Axial CT demonstrates the midline lipoma that is easier to visualize utilizing a wide window, demonstrating decreased attenuation compared to fluid (*arrow*).

Answers

1. The abnormality is located within the interhemispheric fissure.

2. The classic imaging findings are low attenuation, fat density within the lesion.

3. The differential diagnosis includes lipoma, dermoid, and teratoma.

4. Intracranial lipomas are a product of maldifferentiation of the meninx primitiva (meninges precursor). The most common location for intracranial lipomas is within the pericallosal region. Lipomas will follow fat on CT and MRI. Calcifications are commonly seen. There is an association with corpus callosum dysgenesis.

5. No treatment needed.

Pearls

- Intracranial lipomas are a product of maldifferentiation of the meninx primitiva (meninges precursor).
- The most common location for intracranial lipomas is within the pericallosal region.
- Will follow fat on all MRI pulse sequences.
- Loss of signal on MRI fat saturation sequences is confirmatory.
- No enhancement.
- Hounsfield units less than −30.

Suggested Readings

Ginat DT, Meyers SP. Intracranial lesions with high signal intensity on T1-weighted MR images: differential diagnosis. *Radiographics*. 2012;32(2):499-516.

Ho ML, Moonis G, Ginat DT, Eisenberg RL. Lesions of the corpus callosum. *AJR Am J Roentgenol*. 2013 Jan;200(1):W1-W16.

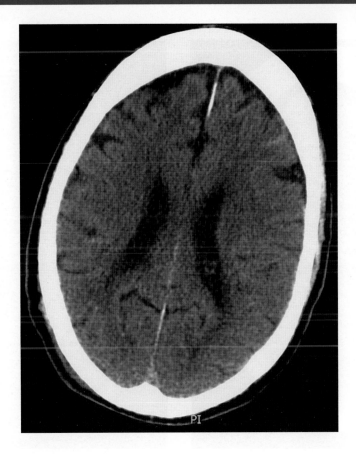

1. Where is the abnormality located?

2. What is the differential diagnosis for high attenuation within a sulcus?

3. What is the most common cause of the high attenuation?

4. What other common etiologies can cause this appearance?

5. Which routine MRI sequences are highly sensitive to this sequence?

Case ranking/difficulty: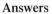

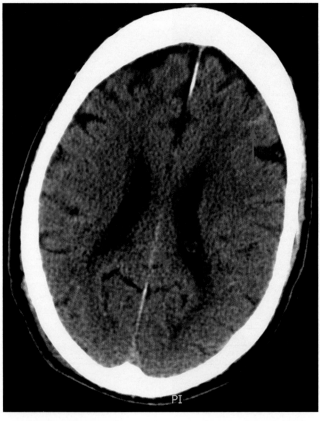

Axial CT shows linear high attenuation within one of the left frontal lobe sulcus (*arrow*).

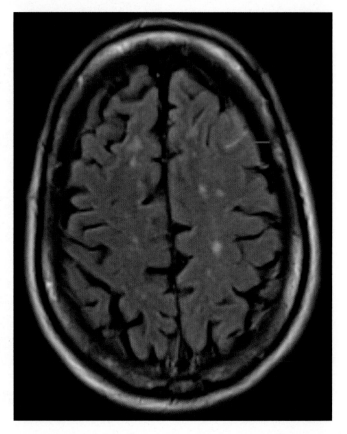

Axial FLAIR shows linear high signal within one of the left frontal lobe sulci (*arrow*). The remaining sulci all have dark or nulled signal, which is normal on this fluid attenuated inversion recovery image.

Answers

1. Subarachnoid hemorrhage (SAH) is blood within the subarachnoid space and may fill sulci and/or cisterns.

2. The differential diagnosis for high attenuation within a sulcus includes subarachnoid hemorrhage, metastatic disease (leptomeningeal spread), and an infectious process.

3. SAH is usually the result of injury to pial or arachnoidal cortical vessels from trauma.

4. SAH is also associated with aneurysms of the circle of Willis. Trauma is the most common cause, with vascular malformations and amyloid angiopathy as other potential causes. Perimesencephalic nonaneurysmal subarachnoid hemorrhage is an uncommon clinically benign entity that is likely venous in origin.

5. Of the "routine" MRI sequences, SAH is easiest to diagnose on FLAIR images from lack of CSF suppression.

Pearls

- Subarachnoid hemorrhage (SAH) fills sulci and cisterns.
- CT noncontrast, check for high attenuation within sulci and/or cisterns.
- Check dependent sylvian fissures and interpeduncular cistern.
- Nontraumatic SAH needs to be followed with vascular imaging in order to exclude an aneurysm or AVM.
- With infection history, consider pus from meningitis.
- With cancer history, consider carcinomatosis.

Suggested Reading

Aiken AH, Gean AD. Imaging of head trauma. *Semin Roentgenol.* 2010 Apr;45(2):63-79.

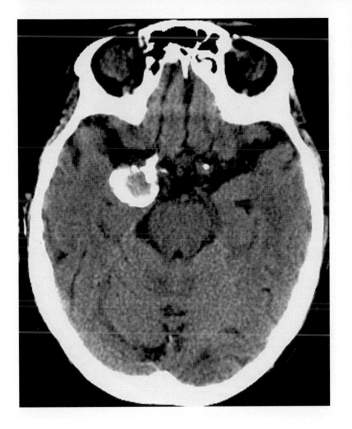 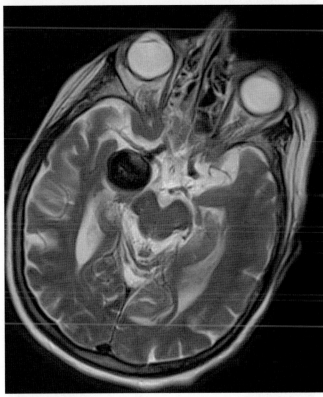

1. Where is the abnormality located?

2. What are the classic imaging findings for this entity?

3. What is the differential diagnosis?

4. What are acute presenting symptoms for this lesion?

5. What is the treatment for this entity?

Case ranking/difficulty:

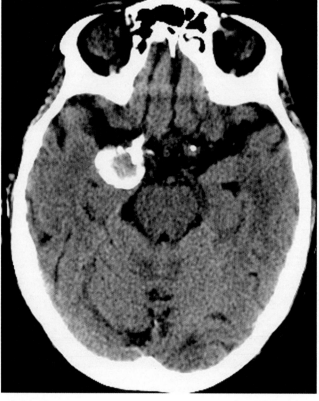

Axial CT image shows high-density structure with associated peripheral calcification adjacent to the right ICA bifurcation (*arrow*).

Axial T2 image shows spherical low signal structure (*arrow*) that appears to arise from the right ICA bifurcation.

Answers

1. The abnormality is located in the extraaxial space adjacent to the circle of Willis.

2. Key to the diagnosis is to confirm aneurysm connection to its arterial origin. Commonly, giant aneurysms will exhibit peripheral calcification. Heterogeneous contrast enhancement and flow characteristics may be seen due to partial aneurysm thrombosis.

3. The differential diagnosis includes aneurysm, meningioma, and metastasis.

4. In the acute setting, patients may present with the "worst headache of my life" secondary to subarachnoid hemorrhage, loss of consciousness, nausea, and vomiting.

5. The treatment for this entity depends on multiple factors, some of which include neck dimensions, shape (saccular vs fusiform), and the presence of collateral circulation. Endovascular coiling vs surgical clipping are typical options for saccular aneurysms. Fusiform aneurysms can be treated endovascularly with covered or pipeline stents.

Pearls

- Giant aneurysms are defined as aneurysms larger than 25 mm.
- Most of these are saccular type.
- On CT, peripheral calcifications may be helpful for diagnosis.
- Key to the diagnosis is to confirm aneurysm connection to its arterial origin (utilize MRA and CTA).
- Angiography reserved for treatment.
- If no vascular connection, consider meningioma.

Suggested Reading

Mehta RI, Salamon N, Zipser BD, Mehta RI. Best cases from the AFIP: giant intracranial aneurysm. *Radiographics.* 2010;30(4):1133-1138.

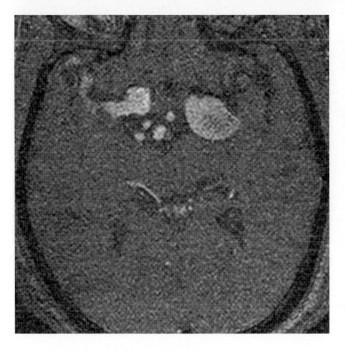
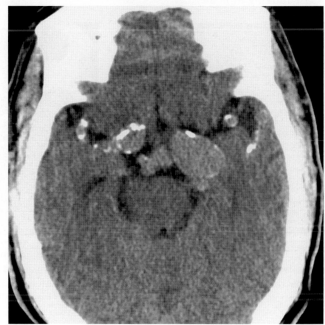

1. What is the abnormality?

2. What are the classic imaging findings for this entity?

3. What is the differential diagnosis?

4. What are associated risk factors for this entity?

5. What is the treatment for this entity?

Case ranking/difficulty: 🦴

Category: Subarachnoid spaces

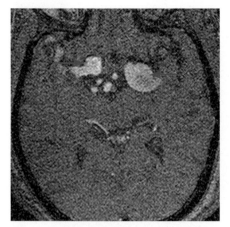

Axial 3D time of flight image demonstrates circumferential enlargement of both internal carotid arteries involving their supraclinoid portions (*arrows*).

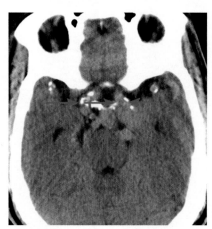

Axial CT image shows the bilateral circumferential enlargement to originate from the internal carotid arteries (*green arrows*). Also, note the dolichoectasia of the basilar artery (*red arrow*).

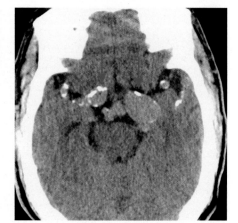

Axial CT image shows circumferential enlargement of both supraclinoid portions of the internal carotid arteries. Note the peripheral calcifications in these vessels indicating atherosclerotic disease (*arrows*).

Answers

1. The internal carotid arteries are abnormally dilated.

2. Fusiform aneurysms typically demonstrate abnormal enlargement that does not protrude away from the lumen (saccular aneurysm) but involves the whole lumen. Peripheral calcification is common, with no contrast filling of the intraluminal thrombus. MRI demonstrates mixed signal due to thrombus and flow characteristics.

3. The differential diagnosis includes aneurysm, meningioma, and vascular malformation. The key to the diagnosis is noting focal dilation involving the whole vessel circumferentially. This excludes meningioma and a vascular malformation.

4. Fusiform aneurysms involve the whole vessel circumferentially. These are also called dolichoectatic aneurysms and are often associated with atherosclerotic disease. Risk factors include family history of aneurysms, hypertension, hyperlipidemia, tobacco use, vasculopathies, connective tissue disorders, trauma, and vascular malformations.

5. The treatment for this entity includes endovascular therapy (stenting).

Pearls

- Fusiform aneurysms are typically related to atherosclerotic disease.
- More common in vertebrobasilar arteries.
- Calcification common.
- Intraluminal clot and flow turbulence cause heterogeneous signal on MR.
- CTA provides better spatial resolution than MRA.
- Aneurysms less than 7 mm have a rupture rate of 0.1%.
- In general the larger the aneurysms, the more likely it is to rupture.
- Reformatted images including maximum intensity projection images and 3D volume-rendered images may also be helpful.
- Utilize noncontrast CT in order to exclude subarachnoid hemorrhage.

Suggested Readings

Hacein-Bey L, Provenzale JM. Current imaging assessment and treatment of intracranial aneurysms. *AJR Am J Roentgenol.* 2011 Jan;196(1):32-44.

Kemmling A, Noelte I, Gerigk L, Singer S, Groden C, Scharf J. A diagnostic pitfall for intracranial aneurysms in time-of-flight MR angiography: small intracranial lipomas. *AJR Am J Roentgenol.* 2008 Jan;190(1):W62-W67.

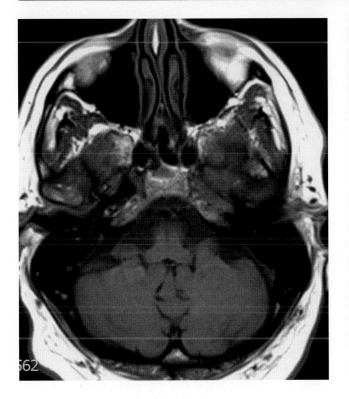 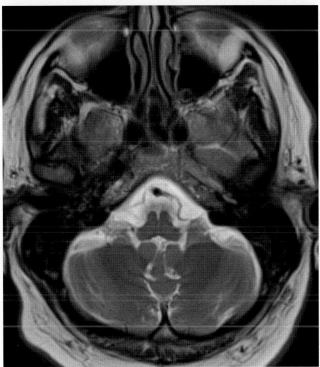

1. Where is the abnormality?

2. What are the classic imaging findings for this entity?

3. What is the differential diagnosis?

4. What is the most common etiology of this finding?

5. What is the treatment for this entity?

Case ranking/difficulty: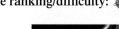

Category: Subarachnoid spaces

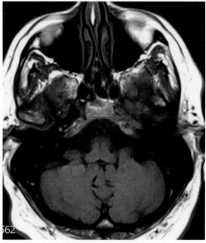

Axial T1 noncontrast image shows loss of the normal "flow void" of the left petrous internal carotid artery (*arrow*).

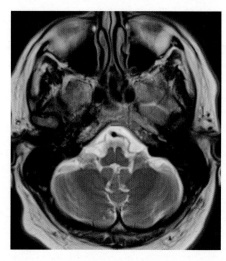

Axial T2 image shows increased signal and loss of the normal "flow void" of the left petrous internal carotid artery (*arrow*).

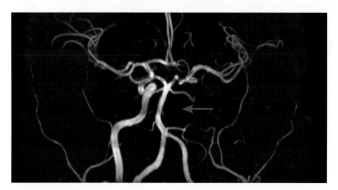

Maximum intensity projection image from time of flight imaging again shows nonvisualization of the left internal carotid artery (*arrow*).

Answers

1. The abnormality involves the left internal carotid artery.

2. On imaging, nonvisualization of the vessel is the classic appearance.

3. The differential diagnosis includes vasculitis, dissection, and atherosclerotic occlusive disease.

4. Arterial occlusion is usually the manifestation of atherosclerotic disease, which is an acquired process.

5. The treatment for occlusive disease is supportive care. Endarterectomy and endovascular therapy are classically reserved for symptomatic nonocclusive stenosis over 70% at the internal carotid bulb.

Pearls

- Arterial occlusion is usually the manifestation of atherosclerotic disease.
- Cerebral infarction occurs in greater than two-thirds of patients with carotid occlusion.
- Consider CTA or US (neck) to confirm occlusion on time of flight MRA, as this technique overestimates stenosis.
- Catheter angiogram remains gold standard.
- T1 and T2 demonstrate "flow void" loss with increased signal.
- 2D time of flight useful for detecting flow direction and is instrumental in diagnosing "subclavian steal" (no flow in vertebral artery on time of flight MRA, normal contrast opacification with contrast-enhanced MRA, CTA, or DSA).

Suggested Readings

Huang BY, Castillo M. Radiological reasoning: extracranial causes of unilateral decreased brain perfusion. *AJR Am J Roentgenol*. 2007 Dec;189(6 suppl):S49-S54.

Kerwin WS, Hatsukami T, Yuan C, Zhao XQ. MRI of carotid atherosclerosis. *AJR Am J Roentgenol*. 2013 Mar;200(3):W304-W313.

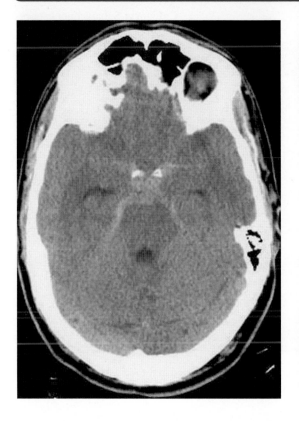

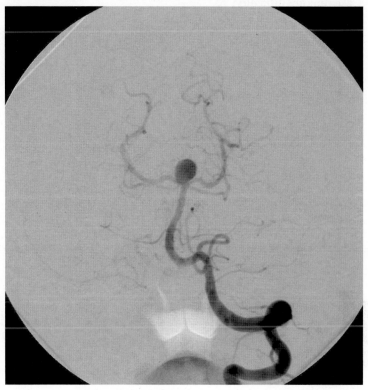

1. What can be seen on MRI imaging within the sulci diffusely in this entity?

2. What percentage of patients with this lesion have more than one?

3. What is the most common location of these lesions?

4. What are relative contraindications to endovascular coiling?

5. What is the lifetime risk of aneurysm rupture?

Case ranking/difficulty: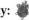

Axial CT image shows hyperdensity within the suprasellar cistern consistent with subarachnoid blood (*arrowheads*). There is prominence in the prepontine cistern at the location of the basilar tip (*arrow*).

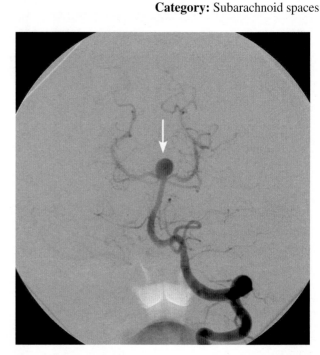

Frontal angiogram with injection in the left vertebral artery shows a basilar tip saccular aneurysm (*arrow*).

Answers

1. Subarachnoid hemorrhage from aneurysm rupture can demonstrate increased susceptibility on gradient echo or susceptibility-weighted imaging and incomplete suppression (bright signal) on FLAIR.

2. Approximately 20% of patients with an aneurysm will have multiple.

3. 85%-90% of intracranial aneurysms present in the anterior circulation. Intracranial saccular aneurysms are thought to be more common due to lack of the internal elastic lamina.

4. Relative contraindications to endovascular coiling of intracranial aneurysms include a wide neck, existence of branch vessels arising from the aneurysm, and MCA aneurysms.

5. The risk of aneurysm rupture is correlated with size; however, there is a lifetime risk of 1%-2% per year, cumulative regardless of size.

Pearls

- Only 10%-15% of intracranial aneurysms arise from the posterior circulation with a majority of them being basilar tip aneurysms.
- 20% of patients with aneurysms are multiple.
- 80%-90% of nontraumatic subarachnoid hemorrhage is due to aneurysm rupture with a "thunderclap" severe headache.
- Vasospasm occurs in 5-10 days after subarachnoid hemorrhage in up to 70% of patients and is a significant contributor to morbidity and mortality from brain ischemia.
- CT angiography is >95% sensitive for aneurysms >2 mm and 3D time of flight MRA is >90% sensitive for aneurysms >3 mm.
- Digital subtraction angiography remains the gold standard as a workup for treatment.

Suggested Readings

Sforza DM, Putman CM, Scrivano E, Lylyk P, Cebral JR. Blood-flow characteristics in a terminal basilar tip aneurysm prior to its fatal rupture. *AJNR Am J Neuroradiol.* 2010 Jun;31(6):1127-1131.

Tsurumi A, Tsurumi Y, Negoro M, et al. Delayed rupture of a basilar artery aneurysm treated with coils: case report and review of the literature. *J Neuroradiol.* 2013 Mar;40(1):54-61.

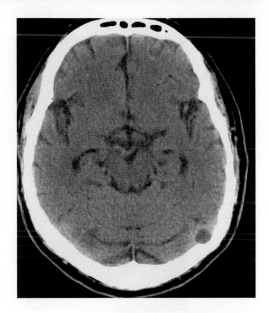
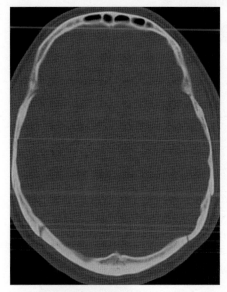
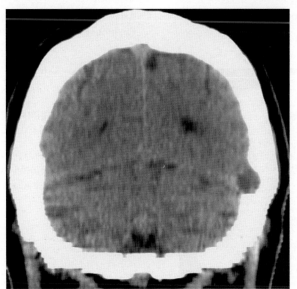

1. Where is the abnormality located?

2. What are the classic imaging findings for this entity?

3. What is the differential diagnosis?

4. What is the etiology of this entity?

5. What is the treatment for this entity?

Case ranking/difficulty: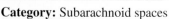

Category: Subarachnoid spaces

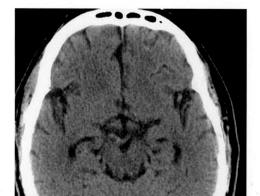

Axial CT image shows a low attenuation lesion within the left transverse sinus (*arrow*).

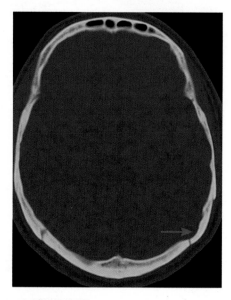

Axial CT bone window image demonstrates smooth erosion of the inner table of calvarium (*arrow*)

3. The differential diagnosis includes arachnoid granulation, thrombus, and skull metastasis.

4. Arachnoid granulations may be a normal variant, or developmental from CSF pulsations.

5. No treatment is typically needed for this entity. Aberrant AGs do not communicate with the dural venous sinus and can rarely cause CSF leaks, requiring surgical repair.

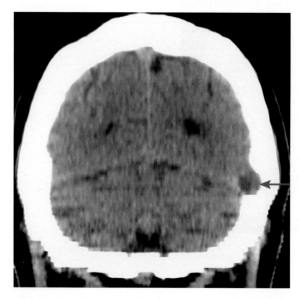

Coronal CT reformat shows the low-density lesion with smooth inner table erosion (*arrow*).

Pearls

- Arachnoid granulation (AG) is an enlarged arachnoid villus that is macroscopic.
- Smooth inner table erosion.
- The most common location for AG is the transverse sinus (left greater than right).
- Follows CSF on MR.
- AG can mimic thrombus in dural venous sinus but is usually round or oval.
- Sinus thrombus is typically long, cylinder shape.

Answers

1. The abnormality is located within the transverse sinus.

2. An arachnoid granulation (AG) on imaging classically follows CSF on CT and MRI. Therefore on MR imaging, they have high T2 signal and low T1 signal. On CT, they will be hypodense and show inner table smooth calvarial erosion. AGs do not show enhancement.

Suggested Reading

Kan P, Stevens EA, Couldwell WT. Incidental giant arachnoid granulation. *AJNR Am J Neuroradiol.* 2006 Aug;27(7):1491-1492.

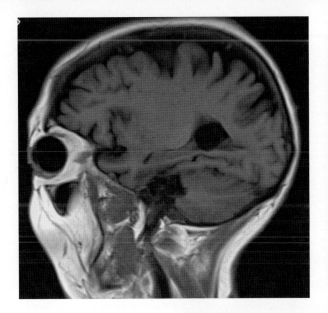
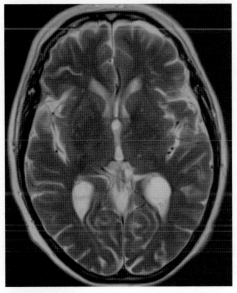
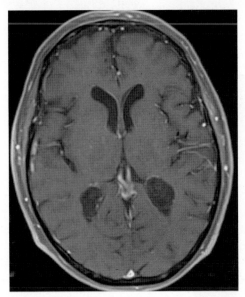

1. Where is the abnormality located?

2. What are enhancement characteristics of this entity?

3. What is the differential diagnosis?

4. What material is within this entity?

5. What is the treatment for this entity?

Case ranking/difficulty: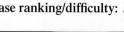

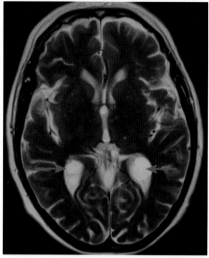

Axial T2 image shows within the choroid plexus are bilateral high signal lesions (*arrows*).

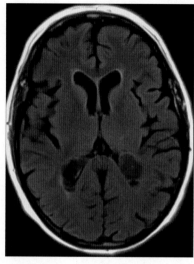

Axial T2 inversion recovery image demonstrates the choroid plexus bilateral lesions have low signal that is higher than CSF.

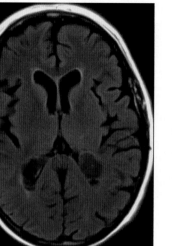

Axial T1 shows nonenhancement of the mass-like well-circumscribed cystic lesions involving the atria of the bilateral lateral ventricles (*arrows*).

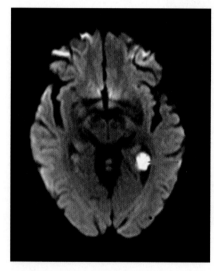

Axial DWI shows restriction within the choroid plexus on the left (*arrow*).

Answers

1. The abnormality is located within the lateral ventricles, involving the choroid plexus.

2. Enhancement is variable from none to ring or solid.

3. The differential diagnosis includes arachnoid cyst, choroid plexus cyst, and ependymal cyst.

4. Choroid plexus cysts (CPC) are lipid filled (lipid-laden histiocytes) and/or with desquamating choroid epithelium.

5. No treatment is needed for this entity.

Pearls

- Choroid plexus cysts (CPC) are the most common of all neuroepithelial cysts.
- CPC are usually bilateral.
- On MRI, CPC can be slightly hyperintense on T1 and T2 compared to CSF.
- Enhancement is variable from none to ring to solid.
- 60%-80% will show diffusion restriction.

Suggested Reading

Osborn AG, Preece MT. Intracranial cysts: radiologic-pathologic correlation and imaging approach. *Radiology*. 2006 Jun;239(3):650-664.

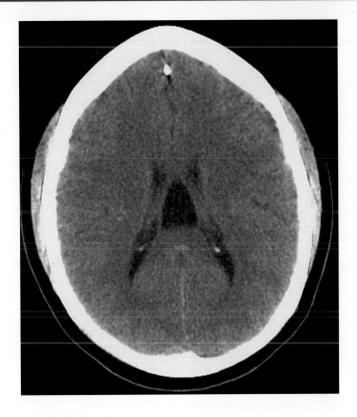

1. Where is the abnormality located?

2. What are the classic imaging findings?

3. What is the differential diagnosis?

4. What is the etiology for this finding?

5. What is the treatment for this entity?

Case ranking/difficulty:

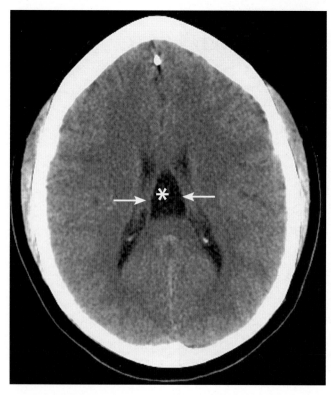

Axial CT image shows triangular CSF collection between both lateral ventricles (*asterisk*). The collection splays the columns of the fornix (*arrows*).

Pearls

- Cavum velum interpositum (CVI) is a normal variant of the ventricular system that occurs when the tela choroidea fails to fuse in fetal life.
- CVI is also called cavum velum triangulare and cyst of the velum interpositum.
- Triangle-shaped CSF space between lateral ventricles.
- Splays and elevates the fornix.
- Consider epidermoid if peripheral contrast enhancement and diffusion restriction.
- On imaging, CVI will follow CSF signal and attenuation.
- CVI does not enhance.

Suggested Readings

Ciołkowski MK. Cavum velum interpositum, cavum septum pellucidum and cavum Vergae: a review. *Childs Nerv Syst.* 2011 Dec;27(12):2027-2028; author reply 2029.

Tubbs RS, Krishnamurthy S, Verma K, et al. Cavum velum interpositum, cavum septum pellucidum, and cavum vergae: a review. *Childs Nerv Syst.* 2011 Nov;27(11):1927-1930.

Answers

1. The abnormality is located between the lateral ventricles.

2. On imaging, the cavum velum interpositum will follow CSF on CT and all pulse sequences on MRI. Therefore, high signal on T2 and low signal on T1.

3. The differential diagnosis includes arachnoid cyst, cavum velum interpositum, and cavum vergae.

4. Cavum velum interpositum is a normal variant of the ventricular system, with congenital failure of fusion of the double layers of the tela choroidea.

5. No treatment is usually needed for this normal variant. Cysts of the velum interpositum may be large enough to cause hydrocephalus, for which shunting may be necessary.

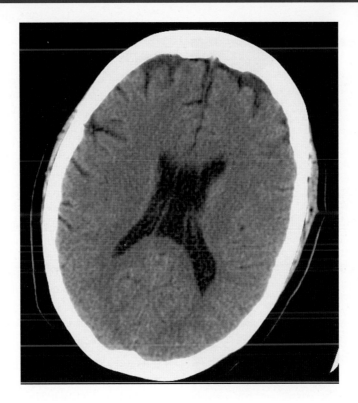

1. Where is the abnormality located?

2. What are the classic imaging findings for this entity?

3. What is the differential diagnosis?

4. What is the etiology of this entity?

5. What is the treatment for this entity?

Case ranking/difficulty:

Category: Ventricles and cisterns

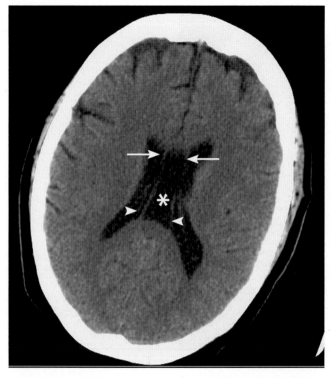

Axial CT image shows rectangular CSF collection located between lateral ventricles extending from the genu of the corpus callosum to the splenium (*asterisk*), bound by the septi pellucidi leaflets anteriorly (*arrows*), and fornices posteriorly (*arrowheads*).

Pearls

- Cavum vergae (CV) is a normal variant of the ventricular system (also called Verga ventricle, sixth ventricle, and cavum psalterii).
- Rectangular-shaped CSF space between lateral ventricles.
- CV typically never occurs without cavum septum pellucidum (CSP).
- 100% of fetal age of 6 months have CV, 30% at term, and <1 % of adults.
- 100% of premature infants have CSP, with 85% at term, typically with normal progressive fusion and residual 1%-20% in adults.
- On imaging, the CV will follow CSF on CT and all pulse sequences on MRI.

Suggested Readings

Ciołkowski MK. Cavum velum interpositum, cavum septum pellucidum and cavum Vergae: a review. *Childs Nerv Syst.* 2011 Dec;27(12):2027-2028; author reply 2029.

Tubbs RS, Krishnamurthy S, Verma K, et al. Cavum velum interpositum, cavum septum pellucidum, and cavum vergae: a review. *Childs Nerv Syst.* 2011 Nov;27(11):1927-1930.

Answers

1. The abnormality is located between the lateral ventricles.

2. On imaging, the cavum septi pellucidi (CSP) with cavum vergae (CV) will follow CSF on CT and all pulse sequences on MRI. It will not enhance after administration of contrast. CSP is only between the frontal horns of the lateral ventricle while the addition of CV will extend back to the splenium between the fornices.

3. The differential diagnosis includes cavum septum pellucidum et vergae, arachnoid cyst, and cavum velum interpositum.

4. Cavum septum pellucidum with cavum vergae is a congenital normal variant of the ventricular system, due to failure of fusion.

5. There is no treatment needed for this entity. Rarely cystic enlargement may cause mass effect.

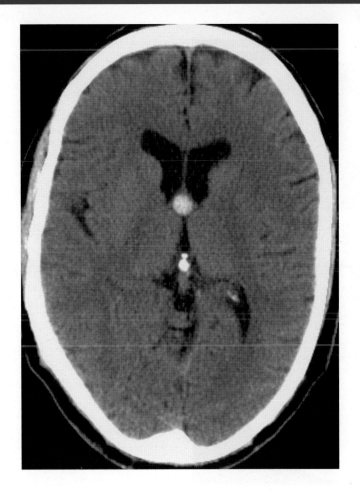

1. Where is the abnormality located?

2. What are the classic imaging findings for this entity?

3. What is the differential diagnosis?

4. What are presenting symptoms for this lesion?

5. What is the treatment for this entity?

Case ranking/difficulty: 🦷

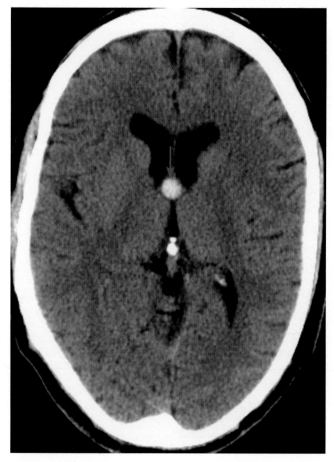

Axial CT noncontrast image shows a spherical focal high attenuated structure in the anterior third ventricle at the foramen of Monro (*arrow*).

Pearls

- Colloid cysts (CC) are benign cysts derived from endoderm and lined by a pseudostratified epithelium with scattered cilia which are filled with a viscous gel (a combination of mucin, blood products, and cholesterol crystals).
- 99% of CC are within the foramen of Monro/anterior third ventricle.
- This can result in sudden death of the patient from rapid hydrocephalus.
- Always check for hydrocephalus or lateral ventricle asymmetry.
- CC can be differentiated from other lesions with contrast, showing no or mild rim enhancement.

Suggested Readings

Armao D, Castillo M, Chen H, Kwock L. Colloid cyst of the third ventricle: imaging-pathologic correlation. *AJNR Am J Neuroradiol*. 2000 Sep;21(8):1470-1477.

Osborn AG, Preece MT. Intracranial cysts: radiologic-pathologic correlation and imaging approach. *Radiology*. 2006 Jun;239(3):650-664.

Wilms G. MR imaging of colloid cysts of the third ventricle. *AJNR Am J Neuroradiol*. 2001 Sep;22(8):1632.

Answers

1. The abnormality is located at the anterior third ventricle roof at the foramen of Monro.

2. The classic imaging findings for this entity are a high-density lesion on CT within the anterior third ventricle at the foramen of Monro.

3. A nonenhancing cystic lesion at this site is characteristic for colloid cyst. Other cystic differentials can include a choroid plexus cyst or subependymoma (cyst-like mass). CSF flow artifacts on MRI also occur at this location.

4. More than half of patients may present with headaches, which may be positional.

5. These patients are followed and only surgically resected when symptomatic.

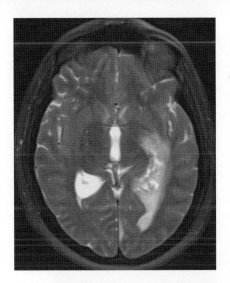
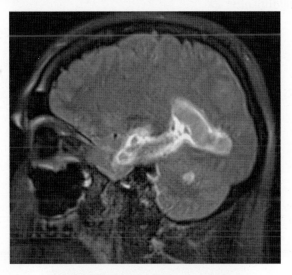
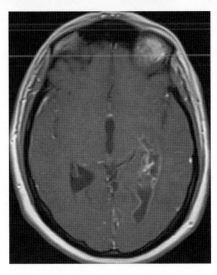
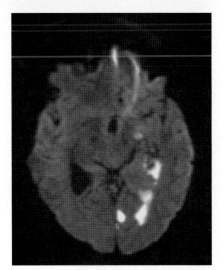

1. What is the differential diagnosis?

2. What imaging sequences are sensitive for layering pyogenic debris?

3. What is the most common class of pathogens in immunocompetent patients?

4. What is a common iatrogenic cause of this disease?

5. What age group has a high association of this disease with meningitis?

Case ranking/difficulty: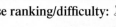

Category: Ventricles and cisterns

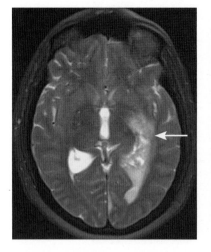

Axial T2 image shows heterogeneous material within the left lateral ventricle with adjacent T2 hyperintense edema (*arrow*).

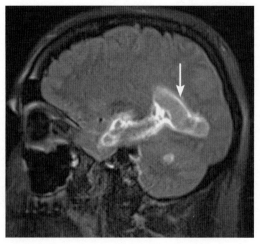

Sagittal FLAIR image demonstrates incomplete suppression of the left lateral ventricle fluid with adjacent T2 hyperintensity (*arrow*).

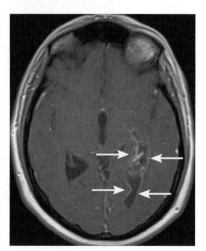

Axial T1 postcontrast image demonstrates ependymal enhancement of the left lateral ventricle (*arrows*).

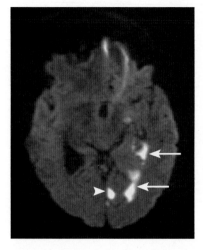

Axial DWI b = 1000 image shows restricted diffusion within the left lateral ventricle from pyogenic material (*arrows*). There is also a left occipital parafalcine focal subdural empyema (*arrowhead*).

Answers

1. The differential for ependymal enhancement of the ventricular walls includes ventriculitis, ependymal carcinomatosis, and CNS lymphoma.

2. DWI and FLAIR are sensitive for dependent layering pyogenic debris and can show restricted diffusion and hyperintensity on FLAIR.

3. Fungal and viral ventriculitis are commonly seen in immunocompromised patients with bacterial ventriculitis more common in the immunocompetent.

4. Intraventricular catheters are a common cause of ventriculitis and can be seen in up to 20% of ventricular catheters. These patients may have little initial clinical symptoms.

5. 80%-90% of bacterial meningitis in infants less than 6 months are associated with ventriculitis.

Pearls

- Ventriculitis is an ependymal ventricular infection that may be an extension of cerebral abscess or meningitis, or a complication of neurosurgical procedure, typically involving an intraventricular catheter
- Etiology is most commonly bacterial, with fungal or viral ventriculitis occurring mostly in immunosuppressed patients.
- The dependent debris within the ventricles may be hyperdense on CT, hyperintense on T1, hypointense on T2, hyperintense on FLAIR, with restricted diffusion.
- Postcontrast imaging may show enhancing ventricular ependymal margins with associated T2 hyperintense edema.
- Ventriculitis may carry a high mortality rate especially when associated with extension of CNS infection.

Suggested Readings

Mohan S, Jain KK, Arabi M, Shah GV. Imaging of meningitis and ventriculitis. *Neuroimaging Clin N Am.* 2012 Nov;22(4):557-583.

Vandesteen L, Drier A, Galanaud D, et al. Imaging findings of intraventricular and ependymal lesions. *J Neuroradiol.* 2013 Oct;40(4):229-244.

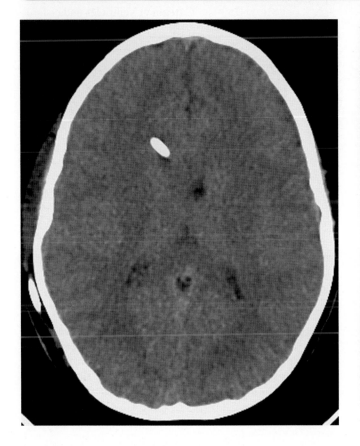 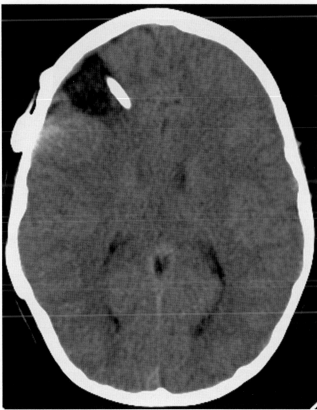

1. What is the differential diagnosis?

2. What is the clinical presentation?

3. What are complications of shunt placement?

4. What are initial imaging modalities to evaluate shunt malfunction?

5. What percentage of patients will need multiple shunt revisions?

Case ranking/difficulty: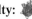

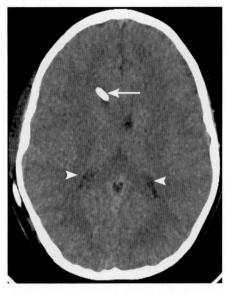

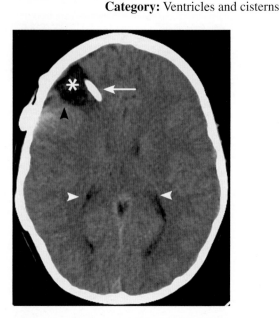

CT image 1 month ago demonstrates right frontal ventriculostomy catheter (*white arrow*) with slit-like appearance of the lateral ventricles (*white arrowheads*).

CT image demonstrates a hypodense cystic collection (*white asterisk*) along the right frontal ventriculostomy catheter (*white arrow*) with mass effect on the adjacent brain parenchyma (*black arrowhead*), suggestive of CSF pseudocyst. There is slight increase in the size of the lateral ventricles bilaterally (*white arrowheads*).

Answers

1. A CSF density collection along the ventriculostomy catheter in conjunction with increased size of the ventricle is highly suggestive of VP shunt malfunction with a CSF pseudocyst. Abscess may be considered but is unlikely given lack of parenchymal edema. Arachnoid cyst does not typically grow rapidly.

2. Clinical presentations of shunt malfunction include headache, vomiting, lethargy, irritability, increasing head size, and seizure.

3. Complications of VP shunt placement include infection, mechanical complications (occlusion, disconnection and fracture, migration), improper placement, and overdrainage.

4. CT brain and shunt series radiographs can evaluate for change in ventricular size and continuity of the shunt. Nuclear medicine shunt study can evaluate the function and patency of the shunt.

5. 50% of patients will need multiple shunt revisions, with progressively shorter intervals to next shunt failure.

- Clinical presentations of shunt malfunction include headache, vomiting, neuropsychologic, cognitive, and behavioral impairment.
- CT is usually an initial imaging modality to evaluate shunt malfunction by evaluation of ventricular size compared to the prior study.
- Tc-99m sulfur colloid or DTPA is an available option to evaluate shunt function. However, it takes more time and needs a gamma camera to obtain images.
- Shunt series radiographs are useful to evaluate shunt disconnections or fractures.
- Disconnection usually occurs at the connector while shunt fracture usually occurs in the area of greater mobility.
- Chronic overdrainage can cause noncompliance of the ventricle, which do not significantly enlarge even with shunt obstruction.
- Acute overdrainage can present with subdural hematomas.

Pearls

- Ventriculoperitoneal shunt is the most commonly used shunt to bypass obstruction of the CSF.
- Complications include shunt obstruction, malfunction, fractures, infections, or overdrainage.

Suggested Reading

Goeser CD, McLeary MS, Young LW. Diagnostic imaging of ventriculoperitoneal shunt malfunctions and complications. *Radiographics*. 2000 Oct;18(3):635-651.

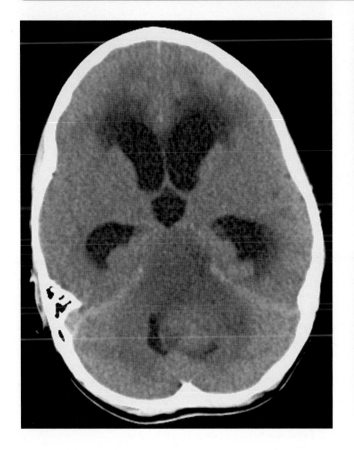 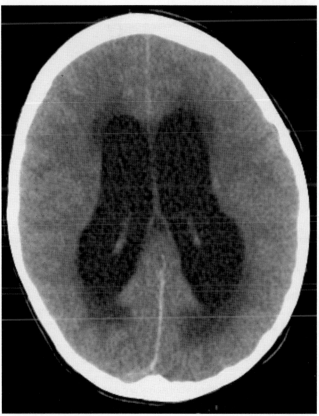

1. Where is the abnormality located?

2. What are the classic imaging findings for this entity?

3. What is the differential diagnosis?

4. What is the significance of periventricular low attenuation in this entity?

5. What is the treatment for this entity?

Case ranking/difficulty:

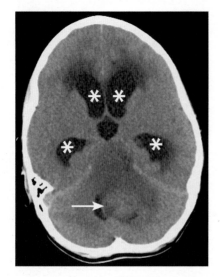

CT axial image shows the fourth ventricle effaced by a mass (*arrow*). This results in dilation of the frontal horns and temporal horns of the lateral ventricles (*asterisks*) and third ventricle.

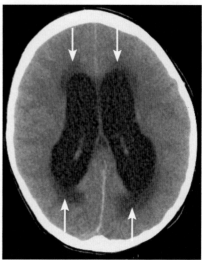

CT axial image shows enlargement of the lateral ventricles with periventricular hypodensity (*arrows*). This indicates interstitial CSF, seen in an acute, uncompensated obstructive process.

Answers

1. The lateral and third ventricles are abnormal in size with associated periventricular edema due to obstruction by a mass in the fourth ventricle.

2. On imaging, at least the lateral ventricular size will be enlarged with both intraventricular and extraventricular hydrocephalus. With intraventricular obstruction, depending upon where the obstruction is located, the ventricles downstream will be effaced or normal in size. In extraventricular obstruction, all the ventricles are enlarged.

3. The differential diagnosis includes obstructive hydrocephalus, normal-pressure hydrocephalus, and atrophy.

4. The significance of periventricular low attenuation, which appears as a "halo" of water signal or low attenuation, is the flow of CSF retrograde through the ependymal lining of the ventricle. This indicates an acute, uncompensated process.

5. The treatment for hydrocephalus is CSF diversion typically with an intraventricular shunt or ventriculostomy to relieve the acute obstruction. If possible, the cause of obstruction should be addressed.

Pearls

- Intraventricular obstructive hydrocephalus = "noncommunicating," obstruction proximal to the foramina of Luschka and Magendie.
- Extraventricular hydrocephalus = "communicating," typically due to decreased CSF absorption at the arachnoid granulations.
- CSF signal around the ventricular horns signifies an uncompensated, acute process.
- Chronic hydrocephalus will typically not have periventricular interstitial CSF due to compensation over time.
- Size of ventricles does not correlate with intracranial pressure.

Suggested Readings

Glastonbury CM, Osborn AG, Salzman KL. Masses and malformations of the third ventricle: normal anatomic relationships and differential diagnoses. *Radiographics*. 2011;31(7):1889-1905.

Siddiqui A, Chew NS, Miszkiel K. Vertebrobasilar dolichoectasia: a rare cause of obstructive hydrocephalus: case report. *Br J Radiol*. 2008 Apr;81(964):e123-e126.

Uluğ AM, Truong TN, Filippi CG, et al. Diffusion imaging in obstructive hydrocephalus. *AJNR Am J Neuroradiol*. 2003 Aug;24(6):1171-1176.

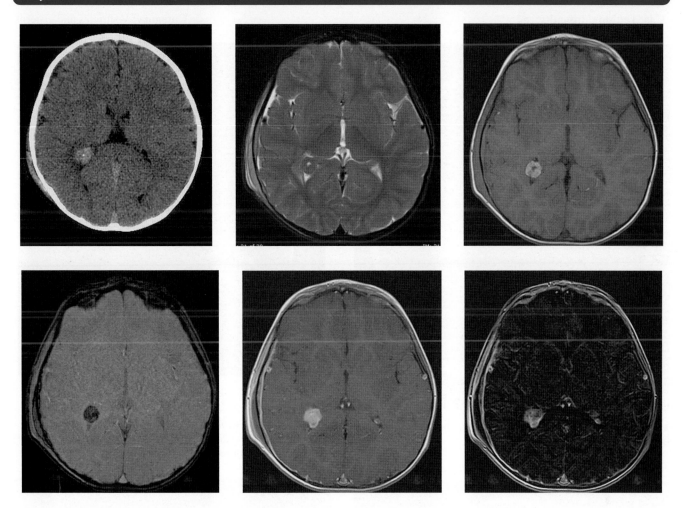

1. What is the differential diagnosis for this finding in a young child?

2. What location is the most common for these tumors?

3. What are typical MRI findings for this tumor?

4. In which patient age group is this tumor the most common?

5. What syndromes are associated with this tumor?

Case ranking/difficulty: 🌰

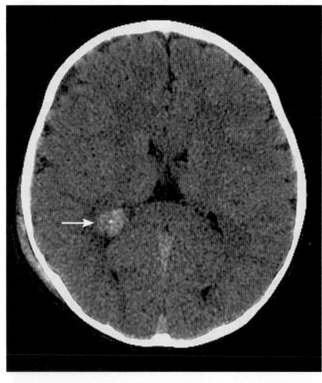

Axial CT image shows a hyperdense right intraventricular mass at the atria (*arrow*).

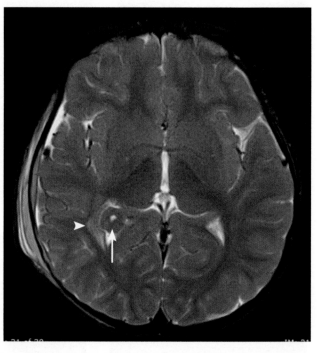

Axial T2 image shows the well-circumscribed, lobular right intraventricular mass, which is predominantly T2 hypointense likely due to calcification (*white arrow*). There is adjacent periventricular T2 hyperintensity (*white arrowhead*). There is an unrelated epidural hematoma from a history of trauma (*red arrow*).

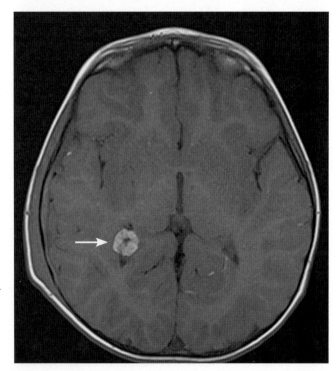

Axial T1 image shows increased T1 signal of the lobular intraventricular mass (*arrow*).

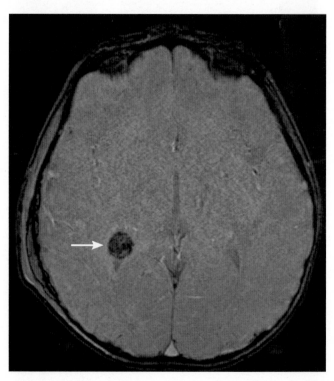

Axial susceptibility-weighted image shows significant hypointensity without blooming, consistent with calcification (*arrow*).

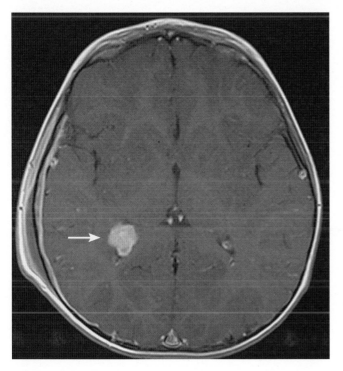

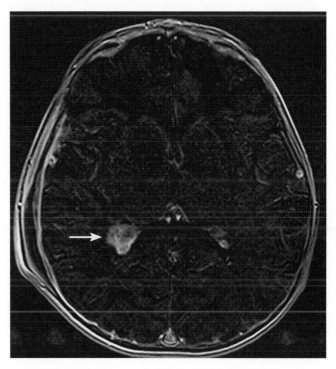

Axial T1 postcontrast image shows intense enhancement of the tumor (*arrow*).

Axial pre- and postcontrast subtraction image shows the enhancement beyond precontrast T1 shortening (*arrow*).

Answers

1. Choroid plexus papillomas and carcinomas are not reliably distinguishable on imaging, but are the most likely diagnoses for this well-circumscribed intraventricular tumor in a young child. Supratentorial ependymoma occur in children but tend to be periventricular. Intraventricular meningiomas can appear similar but is primarily a tumor occurring in adults.

2. The commonest occurrence of choroid plexus tumors also coincides with the amount of choroid tissue by location. In decreasing order of frequency, choroid plexus tumors occur in the trigone of the lateral ventricle, fourth ventricle, and third ventricle.

3. Intense enhancement is typical for choroid plexus papillomas. Calcification is seen in 25% of tumors that demonstrate decreased T2 and increased T1 signal. Periventricular edema and invasion are not reliable differentiators between papillomas, atypical papillomas, and carcinomas.

4. Choroid plexus tumors occur most commonly in younger children and are the most common brain tumor under 1 year of age. Choroid plexus tumors have been described in fetal imaging, also making it a common congenital CNS tumor.

5. Increased incidence of choroid plexus tumors are seen in Li-Fraumeni and Aicardi syndromes.

Pearls

- Choroid plexus tumors can appear in all ages but are most common in young children.
- Choroid plexus papillomas are the most common tumor in a child less than 1 year of age.
- They are typically lobulated, well-circumscribed intraventricular tumors with intense enhancement.
- Calcification is seen in 25% with increased T1 and decreased T2 signal on MR imaging.
- The atrium is the most common location followed by fourth and third ventricles.
- No neuroimaging criteria currently exist to differentiate papillomas from carcinomas.

Suggested Readings

Naeini RM, Yoo JH, Hunter JV. Spectrum of choroid plexus lesions in children. *AJR Am J Roentgenol*. 2009 Jan;192(1):32-40.

Pereira DB, Gasparetto EL, Marcondes de Souza J, Chimelli L. Choroid plexus papilloma with osseous metaplasia as a differential diagnosis of calcifying pseudoneoplasms of the neuraxis. *AJNR Am J Neuroradiol*. 2010 Jun;31(6):E51-E52; author reply E53.

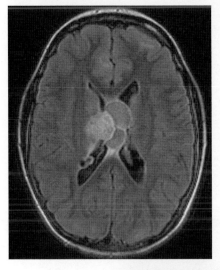
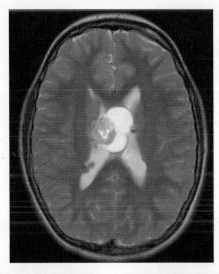
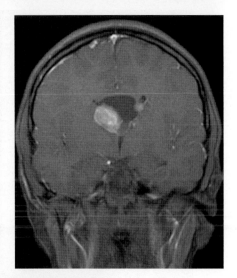
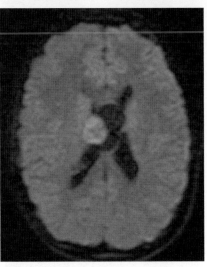
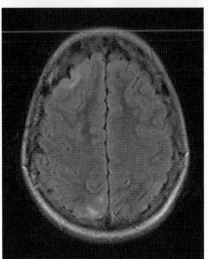

1. What is the differential diagnosis?

2. What other lesional findings narrow the differential diagnosis for the intraventricular tumor?

3. What are typical neuroimaging characteristics of this tumor?

4. What is the prognosis for this tumor?

5. What is the WHO grade for this neoplasm?

Case ranking/difficulty:

Category: Ventricles and cisterns

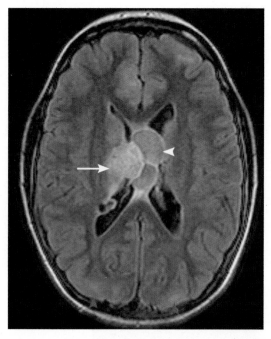

Axial FLAIR image shows a heterogeneous mass in the right lateral ventricle arising near the foramen of Monro with T2 hyperintensity of the solid component (*white arrow*). There are associated cysts (*white arrowhead*). Multiple T2 hyperintense lesions are also noted in the cortical and subcortical areas in the frontal and parietal lobes (*red arrowheads*).

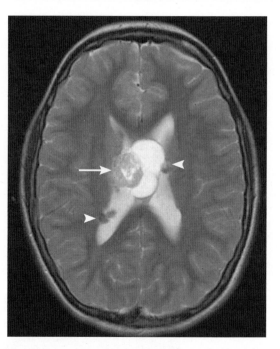

Axial T2 image shows iso- to hypointense signal of the solid nodule (*arrow*). There are multiple hypointense subependymal nodules, which are calcified (*arrowheads*).

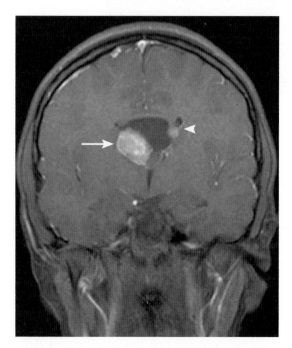

Coronal T1 postcontrast image shows the enhancing mass near the right foramen of Monro (*arrow*). There is a second contralateral smaller enhancing mass (*arrowhead*).

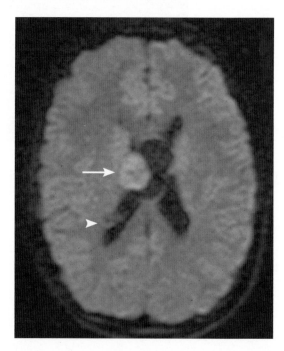

Axial DWI b = 1000 image shows the right ventricular mass has increased signal (*arrow*) representing decreased diffusion relative to the other subependymal nodules (*arrowhead*).

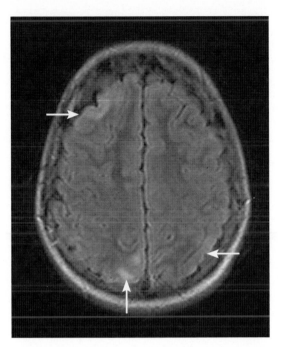

Axial FLAIR image near the vertex shows multiple cortical and subcortical areas of T2 hyperintensity associated with gyral thickening (*arrows*) consistent with cortical tubers.

Answers

1. Intraventricular tumors should include subependymal giant cell astrocytoma, choroid plexus tumor, and central neurocytoma in the differential.

2. Location of the tumor at the foramen of Monro, findings of other subependymal nodules, and cortical tubers narrow the differential to subependymal giant cell astrocytoma in a tuberous sclerosis patient.

3. Subependymal giant cell astrocytomas are greater than 1 cm, located exclusively at the foramen of Monro, typically lobular and well circumscribed with intense enhancement of the solid components.

4. Surgical resection is usually curative for subependymal giant cell astrocytoma. Recurrence is uncommon. Chemotherapy and radiation are usually not indicated.

5. Subependymal giant cell astrocytomas are low-grade, WHO grade I tumors. While case reports of atypia have been described, these may not have significant impact on prognosis, which is usually excellent in regard to the tumor.

Pearls

- Subependymal giant cell astrocytomas (SEGA) are low-grade neoplasms and are almost always associated with tuberous sclerosis.
- Up to 15% of tuberous sclerosis patients will have SEGAs, which is also the most common CNS tumor in tuberous sclerosis.
- SEGAs always occur at the foramen of Monro, demonstrate slow growth, and are larger than 1 cm.
- These tumors are usually lobular and well marginated.
- They can have heterogeneous signal intensity with calcification and cysts.
- Intense enhancement of solid components is typical.
- SEGAs may show decreased diffusion relative to other subependymal nodules.
- Obstructive hydrocephalus is a common presenting symptom.
- Spontaneous or intraoperative hemorrhage is a significant risk factor.

Suggested Readings

Jelinek J, Smirniotopoulos JG, Parisi JE, Kanzer M. Lateral ventricular neoplasms of the brain: differential diagnosis based on clinical, CT, and MR findings. *AJR Am J Roentgenol*. 1990 Aug;155(2):365-372.

Roth J, Roach ES, Bartels U, et al. Subependymal giant cell astrocytoma: diagnosis, screening, and treatment. Recommendations from the International Tuberous Sclerosis Complex Consensus Conference 2012. *Pediatr Neurol*. 2013 Dec;49(6):439-444.

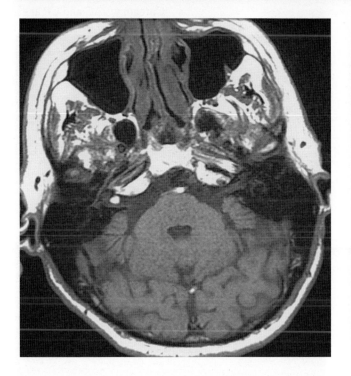 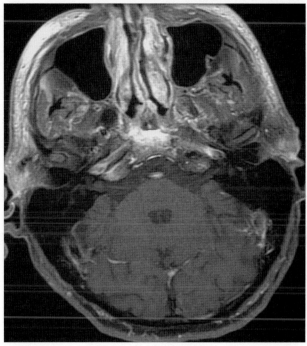

1. Where is the abnormality located?

2. What are the classic imaging findings for this entity?

3. What is the differential diagnosis?

4. What are possible presenting symptoms?

5. What is the treatment for this entity?

Case ranking/difficulty:

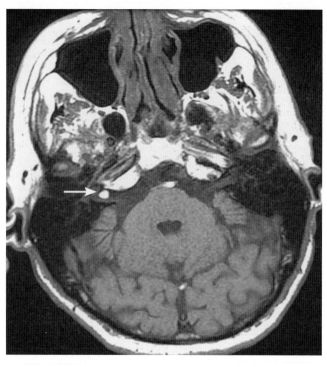

Axial T1 noncontrast image shows a bright subcentimeter lesion centered at the right internal auditory canal (*arrow*).

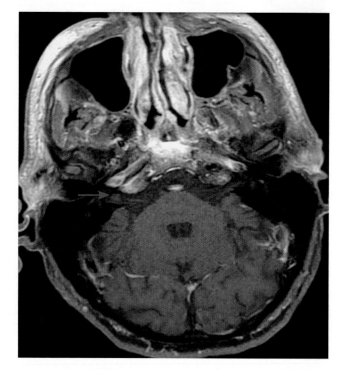

Axial T1 postcontrast with fat saturation shows that the subcentimeter lesion demonstrates loss of signal on fat saturation images (*arrow*). Note there is no enhancement of the lesion.

Answers

1. The abnormality is located within the internal auditory canal.

2. The classic imaging findings for this entity include a classic homogeneous fatty appearance. Lipomas will follow fat on all MR pulse sequences and have high signal on T1 and fast spin echo T2. Fat saturation is confirmatory and shows loss of signal. Typically, no contrast enhancement is seen.

3. The differential diagnosis includes schwannoma, dermoid cyst, and lipoma.

4. Patients with a mass in the internal auditory canal may present with sensorineural hearing loss, vertigo, headache, or facial muscle weakness.

5. Surgical removal is needed if the lesion is symptomatic.

Pearls

- Cerebellar pontine angle (CPA) lipomas are uncommon lesions but they can mimic schwannomas.
- These lesions are no different than other lipomas within the skull at other locations and are from maldevelopment of the meninx primitiva.
- Fat sat images are confirmatory and show loss of signal.
- If the CPA lesion enhances, consider schwannoma.
- If the CPA lesion restricts diffusion, consider epidermoid cyst.

Suggested Reading

Bonneville F, Sarrazin JL, Marsot-Dupuch K, et al. Unusual lesions of the cerebellopontine angle: a segmental approach. *Radiographics.* 2001;21(2):419-438.

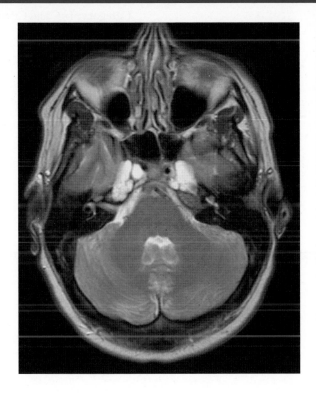 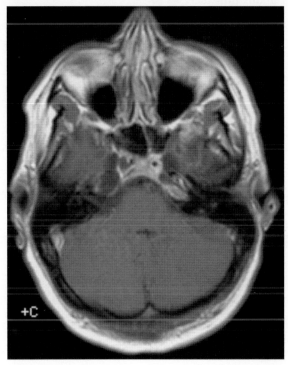

1. Where is the abnormality located?

2. What are the classic imaging findings for this entity?

3. What is the differential diagnosis?

4. What is the etiology of this finding?

5. What is the treatment for this entity?

Case ranking/difficulty: **Category:** IAC and CP angle

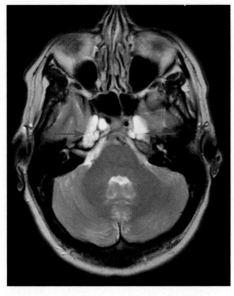

Axial T2 image shows multiloculated fluid signal lesion connecting the right Meckel cave and the petrous apex. A similar lesion is seen on the left (*arrows*).

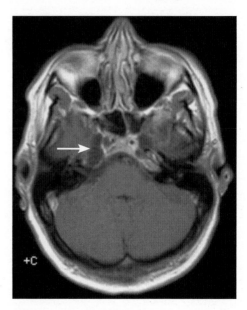

Axial T1 postcontrast shows no enhancement of the fluid-filled lesion connecting the right Meckel cave and the petrous apex. A similar lesion is seen on the left (*arrow*).

Answers

1. The abnormality is located within the trigeminal (Meckel) cave.

2. On MRI, petrous apex cephalocele will follow CSF with corresponding low T1 and high T2 signal. These lesions do not enhance. The key to diagnosis is noting the connection between the trigeminal cave and the petrous apex cyst.

3. The differential diagnosis includes petrous apex cephalocele, mucocele, cholesterol granuloma, and cholesteatoma.

4. Petrous apex cephalocele (PAC) are either acquired or congenital herniation of the trigeminal cave contents into the petrous apex.

5. No treatment is usually needed for this entity. On occasion, if complicated by infection or CSF leak, then surgery may be necessary.

- PAC is contiguous with the trigeminal cave.
- Identifying the epicenter of the cyst outside of the petrous apex makes mucocele and cholesteatoma unlikely.
- On imaging, PAC will follow CSF signal and attenuation.
- PAC lesions do not enhance.
- The key to diagnosis is noting the connection between the trigeminal cave and the PA.
- PAC may be associated with idiopathic intracranial hypertension.

Suggested Readings

Bialer OY, Rueda MP, Bruce BB, Newman NJ, Biousse V, Saindane AM. Meningoceles in idiopathic intracranial hypertension. *AJR Am J Roentgenol*. 2014 Mar;202(3):608-613.

Lin BM, Aygun N, Agrawal Y. Imaging case of the month: cystic lesions of the petrous apex: identification based on magnetic resonance imaging characteristics. *Otol Neurotol*. 2012 Dec;33(9):e75-e76.

Moore KR, Fischbein NJ, Harnsberger HR, et al. Petrous apex cephaloceles. *AJNR Am J Neuroradiol*. 2009 Feb;22(10):1867-1871.

Pearls

- Petrous apex cephalocele (PAC) are cystic structures that occur in the trigeminal (Meckel) cave representing arachnoid cysts or meningoceles that erode into the petrous apex (PA)
- PAC is a "don't touch lesion."

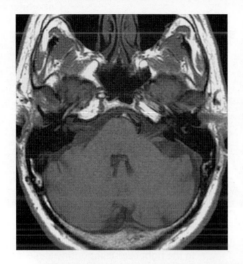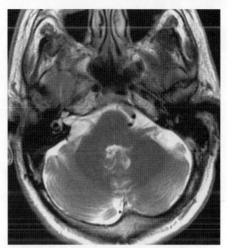

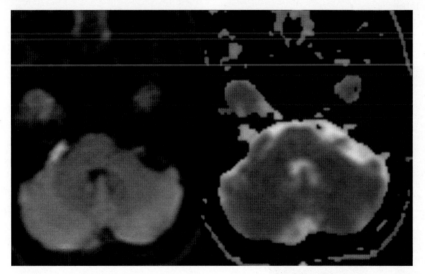

1. Where is the abnormality located?

2. This entity is best diagnosed on MRI with which sequence?

3. What is the differential diagnosis for a cystic extraaxial lesion in this location?

4. This entity can have what effect on adjacent nerves?

5. Where are the most common intracranial locations of this entity?

Case ranking/difficulty:

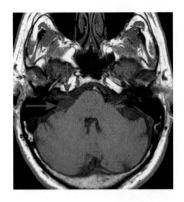

Axial T1 image demonstrates anterior displacement of the seventh or eighth cranial nerve (*red arrow*) by a CSF isointense mass (*green arrow*) in the right cerebellopontine angle.

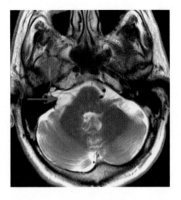

Axial T2 image demonstrates CSF isointensity of the mass (*arrow*) in the right cerebellopontine angle.

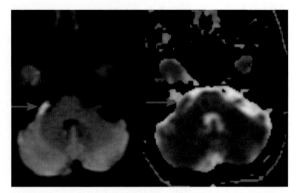

Axial DWI b-1000 and ADC images demonstrate restricted diffusion (increased DWI signal and dark ADC) of the mass in the right cerebellopontine angle (*arrows*).

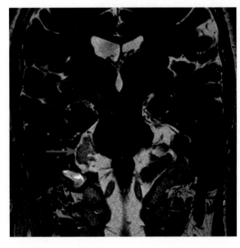

Coronal FIESTA image demonstrates an obvious mass that is of intermediate signal in the right cerebellopontine angle (*arrow*).

Answers

1. The abnormality is located in the cerebellopontine angle.

2. Epidermoid cysts (EC) are readily seen on diffusion-weighted imaging, and demonstrate incomplete suppression on FLAIR. They usually follow CSF signal on standard T2 and T1 imaging and are difficult to visualize.

3. The differential diagnosis includes arachnoid cyst, epidermoid cyst, and dermoid.

4. EC can encase adjacent nerves, compared to arachnoid cyst that displaces the nerves.

5. EC are most commonly located in the cerebellopontine angle. The second most common location is the fourth ventricle followed by the sella.

Pearls

- Epidermoid cysts (EC) are due to an accumulation of keratin and cholesterol with a stratified squamous epithelial lining.
- EC are the third most common CPA tumors.
- Use FLAIR and DWI to differentiate EC from arachnoid cyst.
- Use T1 to differentiate EC from dermoid.
- EC encase nerves and vessels.

Suggested Readings

Bonneville F, Sarrazin JL, Marsot-Dupuch K, et al. Unusual lesions of the cerebellopontine angle: a segmental approach. *Radiographics*. 2009 Nov;21(2):419-438.

Kallmes DF, Provenzale JM, Cloft HJ, McClendon RE. Typical and atypical MR imaging features of intracranial epidermoid tumors. *AJR Am J Roentgenol*. 1997 Sep;169(3):883-887.

Osborn AG, Preece MT. Intracranial cysts: radiologic-pathologic correlation and imaging approach. *Radiology*. 2006 Jun;239(3):650-664.

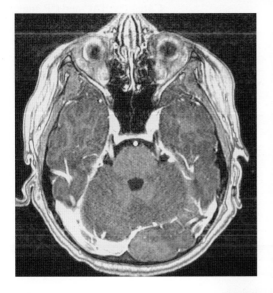
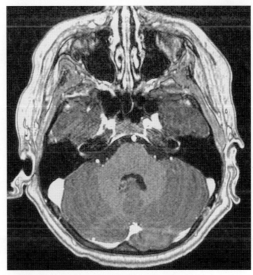
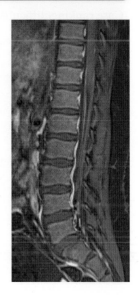
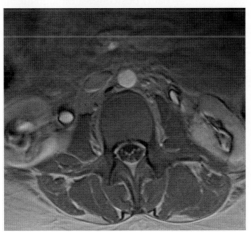

1. What is the differential diagnosis?

2. What is the typical clinical presentation?

3. How often are cranial nerves involved in this disease process?

4. What is the pathophysiology of this disease?

5. What is the prognosis for the disease?

Case ranking/difficulty:

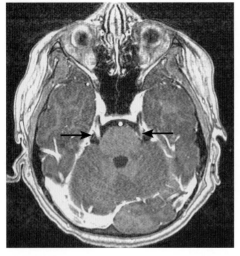

Axial T1 postcontrast through the pons shows thickened and enhancing bilateral trigeminal nerves (*black arrows*). This is a case of Guillain-Barre syndrome.

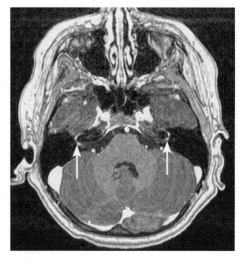

Axial T1 postcontrast through the internal auditory canals shows bilateral enhancement of the labyrinthine segments of the facial nerves (*white arrows*).

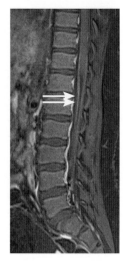

Sagittal T1 postcontrast of the lumbar spine shows diffuse enhancement of the ventral nerve roots of the cauda equina (*white arrows*).

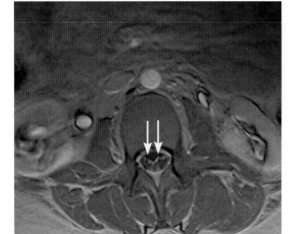

Axial T1 postcontrast through the L1 vertebral body level shows enhancement of the ventral nerve roots of the cauda equina (*white arrows*).

Answers

1. The differential for diffuse cranial nerve and peripheral nerve enhancement includes both acute and chronic inflammatory demyelinating polyneuropathy, carcinomatous neural invasion, and radiation neuritis.

2. The classic presentation of Guillain-Barre is a rapidly progressive paralysis after a bacterial or viral infection.

3. Cranial nerve involvement is common in Guillain-Barre, in 45%-75% of cases.

4. Guillain-Barre is an immune-mediated inflammation of the myelin sheath of peripheral nerves induced from prior exposure to a foreign antigen.

5. In Guillain-Barre, 75%-80% of patient fully recover within a year. Mortality is at 2%-6% with severe disability in 5% of patients.

Pearls

- Symmetric bilateral cranial nerve enhancement is likely to be inflammatory.
- With a history of ascending paralysis, acute inflammatory demyelinating polyneuropath (AIDP) should be considered.
- Cranial nerves are involved in 45%-75% of AIDP (Guillain-Barre).
- Classic findings of AIDP include diffuse enhancement of the ventral nerve roots.
- Clinical history of a recent prior infection is typical.

Suggested Readings

Li HF, Ji XJ. The diagnostic, prognostic, and differential value of enhanced MR imaging in Guillain-Barre syndrome. *AJNR Am J Neuroradiol.* 2011 Aug;32(7):E140; author reply E141.

Zuccoli G, Panigrahy A, Bailey A, Fitz C. Redefining the Guillain-Barré spectrum in children: neuroimaging findings of cranial nerve involvement. *AJNR Am J Neuroradiol.* 2011 Apr;32(4):639-642.

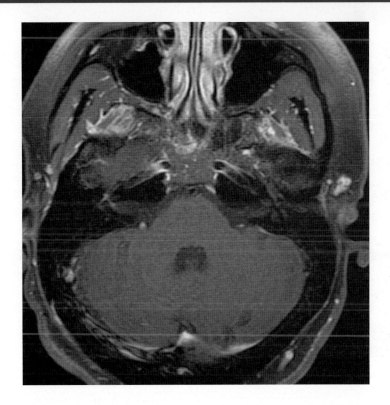

1. Where is the abnormality located?

2. What are the classic imaging findings for this entity?

3. What is the differential diagnosis?

4. What is the etiology of this entity?

5. What is the treatment for this entity?

Case ranking/difficulty:

Category: IAC and CP angle

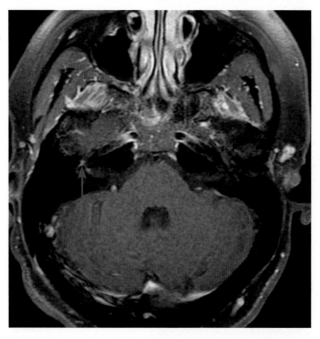

Axial T1 postcontrast with fat saturation image through the internal auditory canal shows asymmetric enhancement involving the seventh cranial nerve. Specifically, enhancement is seen involving the distal intracanalicular segment, labyrinthine segment, geniculate ganglion (*red arrow*), and proximal tympanic segment.

Answers

1. The abnormality involves the seventh cranial nerve.

2. On MRI, the facial nerve will demonstrate asymmetric linear contrast enhancement from the intracanalicular segment through the temporal bone. CT is typically not useful as the findings of neuritis are not seen.

3. The differential diagnosis includes Bell palsy, hemangioma, and schwannoma.

4. Bell palsy is a latent herpes simplex infection particularly of the geniculate ganglion with inflammatory spread to other segments of the facial nerve.

5. The treatment for this entity includes a corticosteroid taper with possible surgical decompression reserved for profound denervation.

Pearls

- Bell palsy is an inflammatory process involving the seventh cranial nerve (facial nerve) characterized by the acute onset of unilateral facial paralysis.
- Labyrinthine and intracanalicular segment enhancement of the seventh cranial nerve should be considered abnormal.
- Mild enhancement of the geniculate ganglion, tympanic, and mastoid segments is normal (use contralateral nerve for comparison).
- Assess the facial nerve for a focal mass.
- Labyrinth, seventh, and eighth cranial nerve enhancement consider Ramsay Hunt syndrome.
- Both facial nerves may enhance but typically the symptomatic side enhances more intensely.
- Facial nerve enhancement may also be seen with a temporal bone fracture.

Suggested Readings

Al-Noury K, Lotfy A. Normal and pathological findings for the facial nerve on magnetic resonance imaging. *Clin Radiol*. 2011 Aug;66(8):701-707.

Tien R, Dillon WP, Jackler RK. Contrast-enhanced MR imaging of the facial nerve in 11 patients with Bell's palsy. *AJR Am J Roentgenol*. 1990 Sep;155(3):573-579.

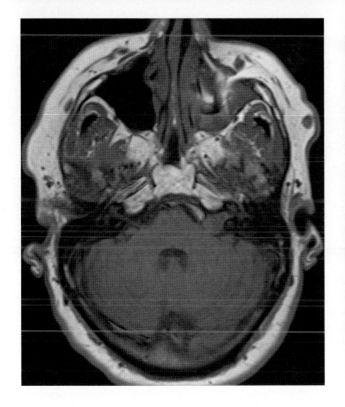 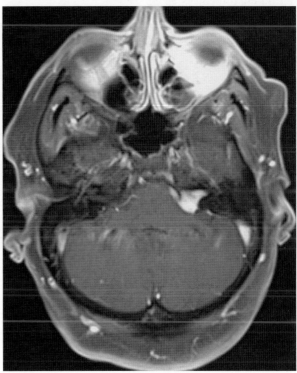

1. Where is the abnormality located?

2. What are the classic imaging findings for this entity?

3. What is the differential diagnosis for a mass at the cerebellopontine angle?

4. What symptoms are associated with this entity?

5. What is the treatment for this entity?

Case ranking/difficulty:

Category: IAC and CP angle

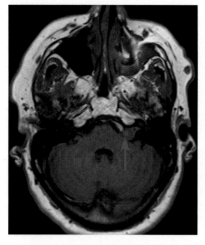

Axial T1 image shows a left cerebellopontine angle "ice-cream cone" shaped mass (*arrow*) which is isointense to the cerebellum.

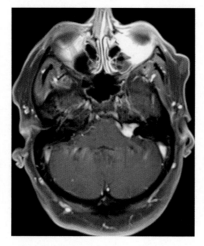

Axial T1 postcontrast with fat saturation shows the lesion within the left cerebellopontine angle is a contrast-enhancing mass with extension into the internal auditory canal (*arrow*).

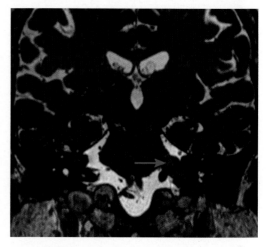

Coronal FIESTA image again shows the left cerebellopontine angle mass (*arrow*) which fills the internal auditory canal.

Answers

1. The abnormality is located within the cerebellopontine angle and internal auditory canal (IAC).

2. Vestibular schwannomas (VS) have a classic "ice-cream cone" shaped mass at the cerebellopontine angle and IAC. Smaller lesions may only be in the IAC while larger lesions extrude into the CP angle.

3. The differential diagnosis for a mass at the cerebellopontine angle includes meningioma, epidermoid cyst, and schwannoma. Vestibular schwannomas (VS) are the most common cerebellopontine angle (CPA) mass.

4. Patients with VS usually present with sensorineural hearing loss, vertigo, or tinnitus.

5. Surgical removal vs gamma knife is very successful with minimal recurrence.

Pearls

- Vestibular schwannomas (VS) are the most common cerebellopontine angle (CPA) mass.
- Classic appearance is "ice-cream cone" shaped.
- On CT beware of a widened internal auditory canal as VS may not be visible.
- VS are the most common CPA mass.
- VS may show cystic degeneration.
- Bilateral vestibular schwannomas are diagnostic for neurofibromatosis II.
- CT may be helpful to distinguish meningioma (hyperostosis and hyperdense) from VS.

Suggested Readings

Babu R, Sharma R, Bagley JH, et al. Vestibular schwannomas in the modern era: epidemiology, treatment trends, and disparities in management. *J Neurosurg*. 2013 Jul;119(1):121-130.

Bonneville F, Sarrazin JL, Marsot-Dupuch K, et al. Unusual lesions of the cerebellopontine angle: a segmental approach. Radiographics. 2009 Nov;21(2):419-438.

Silk PS, Lane JI, Driscoll CL. Surgical approaches to vestibular schwannomas: what the radiologist needs to know. *Radiographics*. 2009 Nov;29(7):1955-1970.

1-day-old female with a posterior head mass

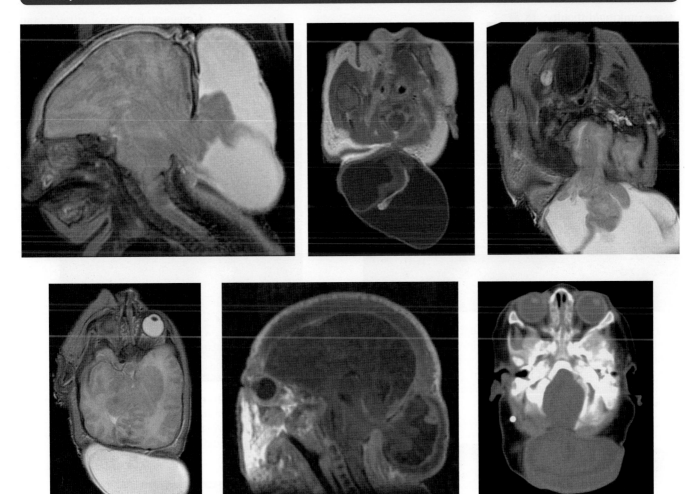

1. According to some authors what bony structure should be defective to make this diagnosis?

2. What can be included in the sac contents?

3. What are the intracranial findings in this malformation?

4. What is the treatment for this disease?

5. What are relative risk factors for this disease?

Case ranking/difficulty:

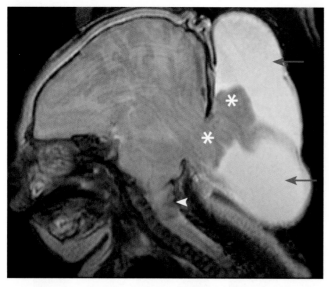

Sagittal T2 image at midline shows a large encephalocele herniating through the low occipital bone involving defects of the opisthion and C1. There is primarily dysplastic occipital lobe (*asterisks*) with bilateral CSF collections (*red arrows*). Note brainstem and tonsillar descent into the spinal canal (*white arrowhead*).

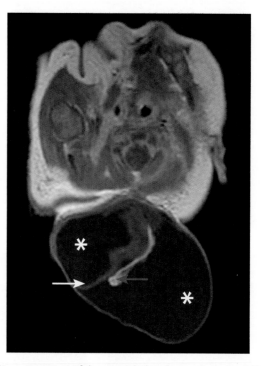

Axial T1 postcontrast of the encephalocele sac shows a midline structure, likely falx (*white arrow*), with bilateral fluid from herniated occipital horns of the lateral ventricles (*asterisks*). Note the enhancing choroid plexus (*red arrow*).

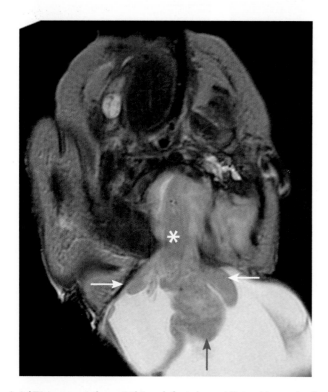

Axial T2 image at the opisthion defect shows bilateral hypoplastic cerebellar hemispheres (*white arrows*), a severely elongated and distorted midbrain and tectum (*asterisk*), and dysplastic occipital lobe (*red arrow*).

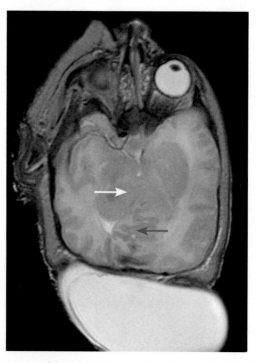

Axial T2 image of the brain shows enlarged massa intermedia (*white arrow*), and gyral interdigitation (*red arrow*).

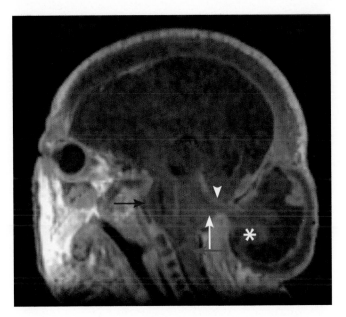

Sagittal T1 postcontrast image of midline after encephalocele repair shows persistent herniation of occipital lobes (*asterisk*), enhancing choroid (*arrowhead*), severe beaking of the midbrain (*white arrow*), tonsillar descent (*red arrow*), and herniation of the temporal lobe into the prepontine cistern (*blue arrow*). Note the lack of corpus callosum.

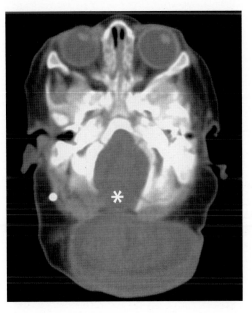

Axial CT of the skull base shows the opisthion defect (*asterisk*).

Answers

1. Some authors suggest that the opisthion must be involved in the low occipital/high cervical encephalocele to diagnose a Chiari III. Chiari III was first described as essentially a high cervical myelocystocele through dysraphic C1-C2 levels.

2. The encephalocele sac typically includes dysplastic cerebellum and cerebral elements, and may also include brainstem/upper cervical cord, lateral ventricles including choroid plexus, and dural venous sinuses.

3. The intracranial findings of Chiari III are similar to Chiari II, including brainstem descent, tectal beaking, callosal dysgenesis, and falcine fenestration with gyral interdigitation.

4. Folate supplementation before and during embryo organogenesis may help reduce the incidence of neural tube defects associated with Chiari malformations. Surgical repair or resection of the encephalocele is indicated as long as there is more CNS tissue in the cranium than in the sac. CSF diversion of hydrocephalus is also indicated.

5. Increased risks of neural tube defects such as folate deficiency, through diet or genetic mutation of methylene tetrahydrofolate reductase, are associated with increased incidence of Chiari malformations. Toxins such as arsenic and tripterygium wilfordii (a Chinese herb) have also been shown to cause neural tube defects.

Pearls

- Chiari III includes a low occipital and high cervical encephalocele in addition to other Chiari II morphologic findings in the brain.
- Some authors suggest that Chiari III encephaloceles must always involve the opisthion of the foramen magnum.
- Herniated contents may include cerebellum, cerebrum, brainstem, and cord, or even lateral ventricles and dural venous sinuses.
- Chiari II changes of the brain include tectal beaking, enlarged massa intermedia, callosal dysgenesis, falcine fenestration and gyral interdigitation, stenogyria and periventricular nodular heterotopia.

Suggested Readings

Aribal ME, Gürcan F, Aslan B. Chiari III malformation: MRI. *Neuroradiology*. 1996 May;38 (suppl 1):S184-S186.

Castillo M, Quencer RM, Dominguez R. Chiari III malformation: imaging features. *AJNR Am J Neuroradiol*. 1996 May;13(1):107-113.

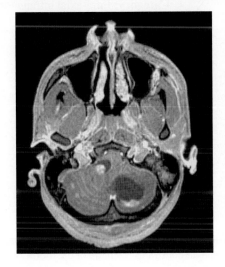
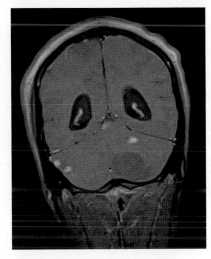
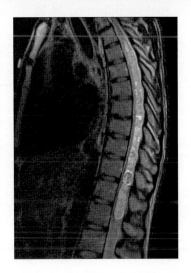
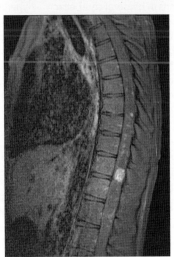

1. What chromosome is associated with von Hippel-Lindau disease?

2. What is the most common location of CNS hemangioblastomas?

3. What is the classic radiographic finding in intracranial hemangioblastoma?

4. What is the radiographic finding of spinal hemangioblastoma?

5. What is the most common cause of hearing loss in these patients?

Case ranking/difficulty:

Category: Intra-axial infratentorial

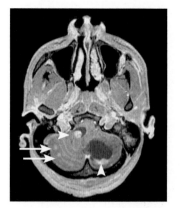 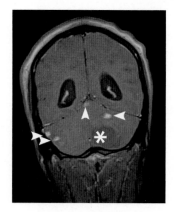 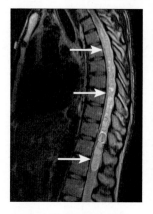 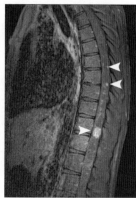

Axial T1 postcontrast image demonstrates cystic lesions with mural nodular enhancement (*white arrowheads*) in the left cerebellum and right-sided pons. Also noted are few nodular-enhancing foci in the right cerebellar hemisphere (*white arrows*).

Coronal T1 postcontrast image demonstrates multiple nodular-enhancing lesions in bilateral cerebellar hemispheres (*white arrowheads*), with cystic lesion in the left cerebellum (*asterisk*) and obstructive hydrocephalus. Note that the enhancing nodules are close to a pial surface, which is typical of hemangioblastomas due to the vascular nature of these tumors.

Sagittal STIR image of the thoracic spine demonstrates hyperintensity involving the entire spinal cord and central spinal canal, suggestive of combination of cord edema and syringohydromyelia (*arrows*).

Sagittal T1 postcontrast image of the thoracic spine demonstrates several enhancing lesions in the spinal cord (*white arrowheads*). The associated edema is usually out of proportion to the enhancing nodules.

Answers

1. von Hippel-Lindau disease is a rare, autosomal dominant inherited multisystemic disorder associated with inactivation of a tumor suppressor gene (VHL gene) located on Chromosome 3. Sporadic mutation is found in 20% of cases.

2. The most common location of CNS hemangioblastoma is the cerebellum (40%-70%), followed by the spinal cord (10%-60%) and medulla (5%). Supratentorial lesions are less common.

3. Classic radiographic finding is a cystic lesion with mural nodular enhancement, typically in the cerebellum.

4. Intramedullary enhancing nodule typically on the pial surface with edema out of proportion to the size of the nodule, associated with syringohydromyelia, is a characteristic finding of spinal hemangioblastoma.

5. The most common cause of hearing loss in VHL disease is due to an increased risk of developing endolymphatic sac tumors, with a tendency for bilateral lesions.

- endolymphatic sac tumors, renal cysts and tumors, pancreatic cysts and tumors, pheochromocytomas, epididymal cystadenomas.
- CNS hemangioblastoma is one of the most common manifestations following pancreatic cysts.
- Typical location for CNS hemangioblastoma is cerebellum (40%-70%), spinal cord (10%-60%), and medulla (5%).
- Classic radiographic findings of CNS hemangioblastoma include cystic lesion with solid-enhancing mural nodules, usually near a pial surface.
- Spinal cord lesions may be associated with syringohydromyelia, with greater than expected edema.
- Renal cell carcinoma and neurological complications are common causes of death.
- Combination of clinical and radiographic screening substantially decreases complications, morbidity, and mortality.

Pearls

- Rare, autosomal dominant, inherited multisystemic disorder.
- Broad clinical manifestations involving retinal and central nervous system (CNS) hemangioblastomas,

Suggested Readings

Leung RS, Biswas SV, Duncan M, Rankin S. Imaging features of von Hippel-Lindau disease. *Radiographics.* 2009 Apr;28(1):65-79; quiz 323.

Slater A, Moore NR, Huson SM. The natural history of cerebellar hemangioblastomas in von Hippel-Lindau disease. *AJNR Am J Neuroradiol.* 2003 Sep;24(8):1570-1574.

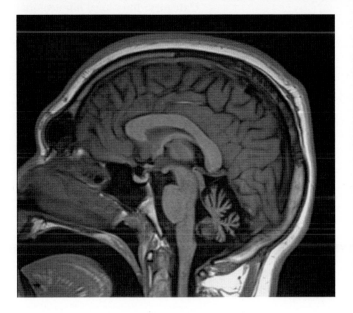
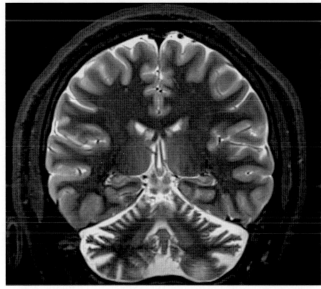

1. What is the clinical presentation of this disease?

2. What is the differential diagnosis of this finding?

3. What are typical neuroimaging findings in this disease?

4. What radiographic exams are relatively contraindicated in this disease?

5. What is the clinical course and prognosis of this disease?

Case ranking/difficulty: **Category:** Intra-axial infratentorial

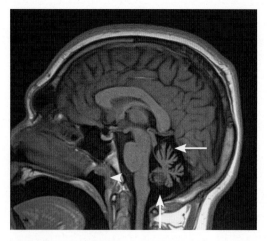

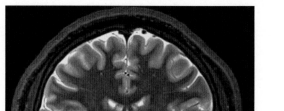

Sagittal T1 image demonstrates severe atrophy of the cerebellar hemisphere with widening of the cerebellar folia and CSF space (*white arrows*). Note the hypoplastic adenoid tissue for this age (*arrowhead*).

Coronal T2 image demonstrates cerebellar brain volume loss with enlargement of extra axial CSF space (*white arrows*).

Answers

1. Main clinical characteristics of ataxia telangiectasia include progressive cerebellar ataxia, oculomucocutaneous telangiectasias, and recurrent sinopulmonary infection.

2. Cerebellar atrophy can be caused by multiple etiologies, from inherited degeneration, the most common being Friedreich ataxia, to damage to the Purkinje cells from hyperthermia, autoimmune paraneoplastic process, and seizure medications. This case is from ataxia telangiectasia, which is considered a neurocutaneous disorder.

3. Neuroimaging findings in ataxia telangiectasia include progressive cerebellar atrophy, beginning in the vermis, and hypoplastic or absent pharyngeal lymphoid tissue from immunodeficiency. CNS angiomas and associated hemorrhage can be seen in adults with the disease.

4. Patients with ataxia telangiectasia have increased sensitivity to the DNA breakage effects of ionizing radiation. Benefits from the modality of diagnostic imaging should be carefully considered.

5. Ataxia is usually a presenting symptom in patients with ataxia telangiectasia becoming apparent when child begins to walk. Ataxia telangiectasia patients usually have recurrent sinopulmonary infections, which is the most common cause of death. Median age at death is approximately 20 years.

Pearls

- Ataxia telangiectasia is an autosomal recessive, complex multisystemic disorder with cerebellar degeneration, telangiectasia formation, immunodeficiency, tumor formation, and progeria.
- Clinical features include cerebellar ataxia, oculocutaneous telangiectasia, and recurrent bronchopulmonary infections.
- Ataxia is usually an initial presenting symptom and becoming apparent when the child begins to walk.
- Most common cause of death is recurrent sinopulmonary infection.
- MRI is a modality of choice due to nonionizing radiation.
- Radiographic findings include diffuse cerebellar volume loss with compensatory enlargement of the fourth ventricle, cerebral white matter dysmyelination/demyelination, microhemorrhages, or telangiectasias, as well as decreased or absent adenoid gland, thymus, and mediastinal lymphoid tissue.

Suggested Readings

Farina L, Uggetti C, Ottolini A, et al. Ataxia-telangiectasia: MR and CT findings. *J Comput Assist Tomogr.* 1994;18(5):724-727.

Lin DD, Barker PB, Lederman HM, Crawford TO. Cerebral abnormalities in adults with ataxia-telangiectasia. *AJNR Am J Neuroradiol.* 2014 Jan;35(1):119-123.

Wallis LI, Griffiths PD, Ritchie SJ, Romanowski CA, Darwent G, Wilkinson ID. Proton spectroscopy and imaging at 3T in ataxia-telangiectasia. *AJNR Am J Neuroradiol.* 2007 Jan;28(1):79-83.

12-month-old male with ataxia, nystagmus, alternating apnea, and hyperpnea

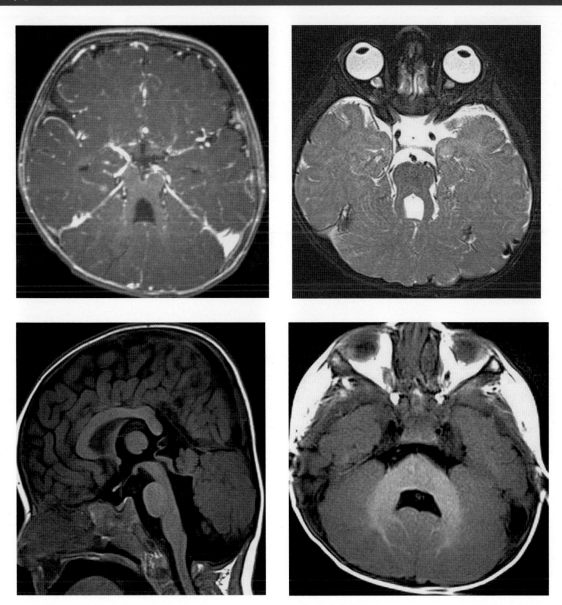

1. What is the differential diagnosis?

2. What are the classic imaging findings for this entity?

3. What is the classic clinical presentation?

4. What are the subtypes of this entity?

5. What is the prognosis for this disease?

Case ranking/difficulty:

Category: Intra-axial infratentorial

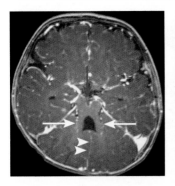

Axial T1 postcontrast image shows the "molar tooth sign" with deep interpeduncular cistern (*red arrow*) and thickened superior cerebellar peduncles (*white arrows*). Note the leptomeningeal vessels within a midline vermian cleft (*arrowheads*).

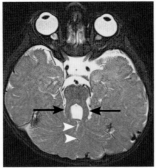

Axial T2 image shows the thickened cerebellar peduncles (*arrows*) and midline vermian cleft (*arrowheads*).

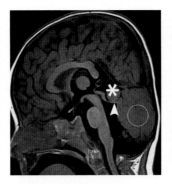

Sagittal T1 image shows hypoplastic superiorly displaced vermis (*asterisk*) with dysmorphic fourth ventricular roof (*arrowhead*). The cerebellar hemispheres are apposed (*circle*).

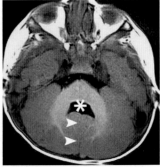

Axial T1 noncontrast image shows the "bat-wing fourth ventricle (*asterisk*) and vermian cleft (*arrowheads*).

Answers

1. The differential for vermian hypoplasia/clefting includes Joubert syndrome–related disorders (JSRD), Dandy-Walker, pontocerebellar hypoplasia, and vermian atrophy from heterogeneous insult.

2. Joubert syndrome–related disorders all have the obligatory "molar tooth" midbrain malformation with deep interpeduncular cleft and elevated and thickened superior cerebellar peduncles. Additional findings include vermian clefting, and "bat wing" fourth ventricle.

3. Neurologic cardinal features of hypotonia, ataxia, developmental delay, alternating apnea and tachypnea, nystagmus, and intellectual disability are seen in all JSRD.

4. JSRD includes syndromes previously considered separate entities such as Dekaban-Arima, COACH, Senior-Loken, Varadi-Papp, and Joubert-polymicrogyria syndromes. However, recent classification starts with pure Joubert syndrome (JS) with the cardinal neurologic features and molar tooth malformation. Related disorders include JS with ocular defect (retinal dystrophy), JS with renal defect, JS with oculorenal defects, JS with hepatic defect, and JS with orofaciodigital defects.

5. Treatment is supportive, with early death in patients not well supported for episodes of prolonged apneas. In most cases these respiratory abnormalities will resolve spontaneously with renal and hepatic complications representing major causes of death in older children.

Pearls

- Joubert syndrome (JS)–related disorders (JSRD) all have the midbrain-hindbrain malformation of "molar tooth" sign and vermian clefting.
- Multiple genes have been implicated that encode for proteins of primary cilia.
- Eye abnormalities, renal, liver, and orofaciodigital defects are associated with the cardinal neurologic findings of JS and help classify JSRD into subsets.
- Other neuroimaging findings includes "bat-wing" fourth ventricle, prominent CSF spaces, migrational anomalies, and abnormal myelination.

Suggested Readings

Poretti A, Huisman TA, Scheer I, Boltshauser E. Joubert syndrome and related disorders: spectrum of neuroimaging findings in 75 patients. *AJNR Am J Neuroradiol.* 2011 Sep;32(8):1459-1463.

Saleem SN, Zaki MS. Role of MR imaging in prenatal diagnosis of pregnancies at risk for Joubert syndrome and related cerebellar disorders. *AJNR Am J Neuroradiol.* 2010 Mar;31(3):424-429.

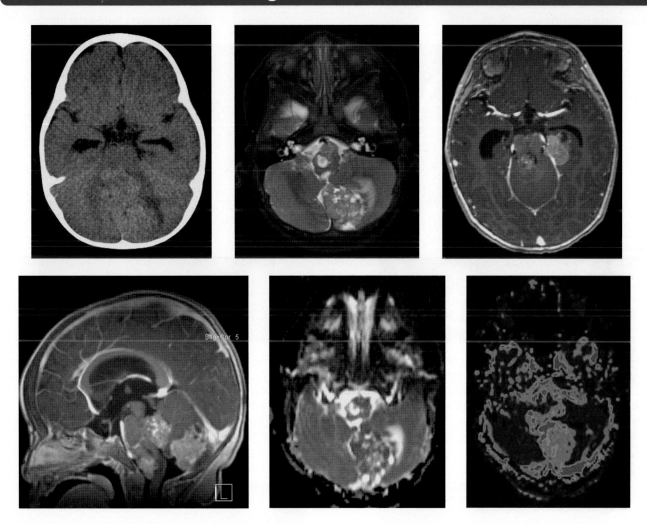

1. What is the differential diagnosis?

2. What are typical MRI findings for this entity?

3. What is the prognosis of this disease?

4. Which other tumors have similar histological features from which the name is derived?

5. What is the most common location for this tumor?

Case ranking/difficulty:

Category: Intra-axial infratentorial

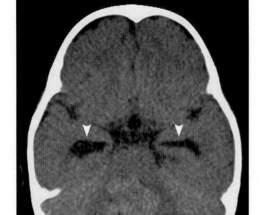

Axial CT image of the posterior fossa shows a hyperdense mass (typically seen with high grade tumors) filling the fourth ventricle and extending to the left cerebellar hemisphere (*arrow*) causing obstructive hydrocephalus as demonstrated by dilated temporal horns (*arrowheads*).

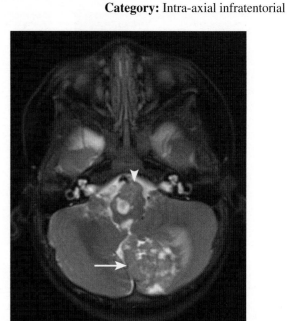

Axial T2 image of the posterior fossa shows separate heterogeneous tumors in the left cerebellar hemisphere (*arrow*) with a mild amount of adjacent peritumoral T2 hyperintensity, as well as a mass anterior to the medulla (*arrowhead*). Note areas of tumor which show decreased signal on T2, corresponding with hypercellular regions of tumor seen with high grade malignancies.

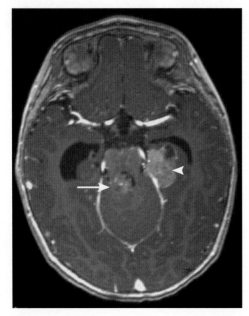

Axial T1 post contrast of the same patient shows multiple heterogenously enhancing tumors in the superior fourth ventricle (*arrow*) and adjacent to the left tentorial incisura involving the left temporal lobe (*arrowhead*).

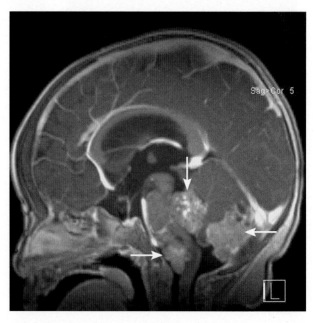

Sagittal postcontrast image at midline shows three of the four separate heterogeneously enhancing masses (*arrows*).

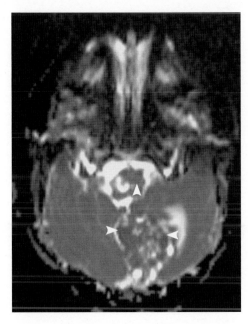

Axial ADC map shows that these masses have areas of decreased diffusion corresponding likely corresponding with hypercellularity (*arrowheads*).

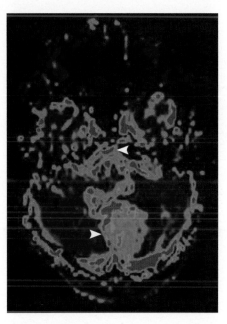

Axial relative cerebral blood volume map from dynamic susceptibility contrast perfusion technique shows increased CBV of these masses (*arrowheads*) favoring a high grade malignancy.

Answers

1. This tumor demonstrates decreased ADC, and increased perfusion with areas of decreased T2 signal. These findings favor high-grade malignancy such as atypical teratoid rhabdoid tumor, medulloblastoma, and glioblastoma.

2. Atypical teratoid rhabdoid tumor will usually be located off-midline in the posterior fossa, which may help distinguish it from medulloblastoma. The mass is usually heterogeneous on T1, T2, and postcontrast with areas of low T2 signal reflecting highly cellular areas, which also show decreased ADC. On MR spectroscopy, significant elevation of choline is typical for a high-grade neoplasm.

3. Atypical teratoid rhabdoid tumor carries a dismal prognosis (>80% mortality) for patients younger than 3, partly due to the lack of radiation as an option, which would devastate immature, developing brains. Children older than 3 can have up to 70% survival.

4. A particular histological feature of ATRT is the rhabdoid cells, which are similar to malignant rhabdoid tumor of the kidney.

5. 50% of atypical teratoid rhabdoid tumors present in the posterior fossa, which is the most common presentation for this tumor, with 40% supratentorial and the remainder presenting both supra- and infratentorial. 15%-20% can present with dissemination.

Pearls

- Consider atypical teratoid rhabdoid tumor in large, heterogeneous CNS masses in children under 3 years of age.
- Tends to be off midline in the posterior fossa compared to medulloblastoma.
- Heterogeneous on T1, T2, and postcontrast.
- Areas of decreased attenuated diffusion coefficient likely due to hypercellularity.
- May have increased relative cerebral blood volume with dynamic susceptibility contrast perfusion imaging.

Suggested Readings

Han L, Qiu Y, Xie C, et al. Atypical teratoid/rhabdoid tumors in adult patients: CT and MR imaging features. *AJNR Am J Neuroradiol*. 2011 Jan;32(1):103-108.

Koral K, Zhang S, Gargan L, et al. Diffusion MRI improves the accuracy of preoperative diagnosis of common pediatric cerebellar tumors among reviewers with different experience levels. *AJNR Am J Neuroradiol*. 2013 Dec;34(12):2360-2365.

Warmuth-Metz M, Bison B, Dannemann-Stern E, Kortmann R, Rutkowski S, Pietsch T. CT and MR imaging in atypical teratoid/rhabdoid tumors of the central nervous system. *Neuroradiology*. 2008 May;50(5):447-452.

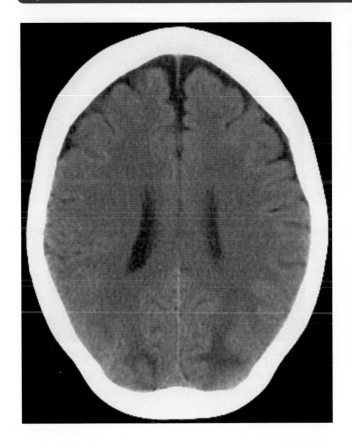 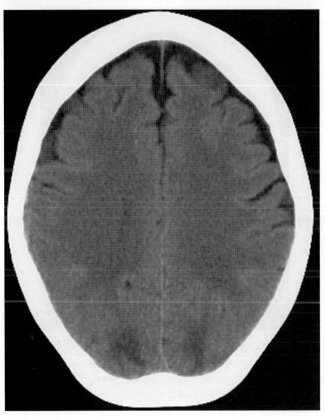

1. Which part of the brain does this entity most commonly involve?

2. What are the classic imaging findings?

3. What diseases are associated with this entity?

4. What is the presumed pathophysiology of this disorder?

5. What typically happens to the imaging finding after treatment?

Case ranking/difficulty:

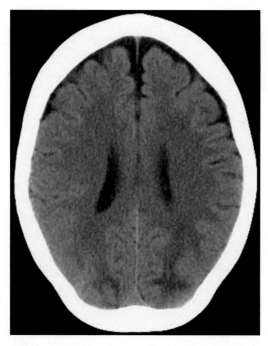

Axial CT image at the level of superior aspect of the lateral ventricular bodies demonstrates low attenuation within the white matter of the parietal lobes (*arrows*). Notice that the low attenuation relatively spares the gray matter and has a vasogenic edema pattern.

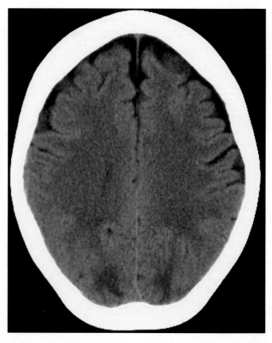

Axial CT image above the level of the lateral ventricles shows continued low attenuation within the cortex and subcortical white matter of the parietal lobes (*arrows*).

Answers

1. PRES (posterior reversible encephalopathy syndrome) is usually symmetric and may involve any part of the brain. It most commonly involves the parietal and occipital lobes.

2. PRES (posterior reversible encephalopathy syndrome) classically demonstrates bilateral symmetric vasogenic edema.

3. PRES is associated with these conditions: hypertension, toxemia of pregnancy (preeclampsia, eclampsia), posttransplant (allo-bone marrow transplant, solid organ transplant), immune suppression (cyclosporine, tacrolimus), thrombotic microangiopathy (HUS, DIC, TTP), sepsis/shock (multiorgan dysfunction syndrome, systemic inflammatory response syndrome), autoimmune disease (lupus, scleroderma, Wegener), high-dose chemotherapy, and other miscellaneous conditions.

4. PRES most likely is secondary to a failure in cerebral autoregulation.

5. PRES manifests as vasogenic edema, which usually resolves, especially in the setting of hypertension.

Pearls

- PRES (posterior reversible encephalopathy syndrome) is a transient neurotoxic state most likely secondary to dysfunctional autoregulation.
- Bilateral and symmetric distribution.
- Vasogenic edema pattern.
- Parietal and occipital lobes most commonly affected.
- Restricted diffusion is less common but has been reported.
- 25% of patients do not have hypertension.
- The vasogenic edema usually completely reverses after removal of etiology.

Suggested Readings

Bartynski WS. Posterior reversible encephalopathy syndrome, part 1: fundamental imaging and clinical features. *AJNR Am J Neuroradiol.* 2008 Jun;29(6):1036-1042.

Bartynski WS. Posterior reversible encephalopathy syndrome, part 2: controversies surrounding pathophysiology of vasogenic edema. *AJNR Am J Neuroradiol.* 2008 Jun;29(6):1043-1049.

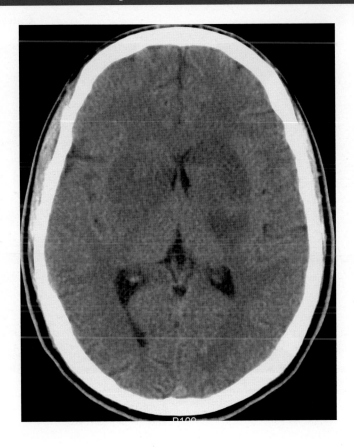

1. Where is the abnormality located?

2. What other electrolyte or hormonal imbalance can cause these findings?

3. What is the differential diagnosis for bilateral basal ganglia cytotoxic edema?

4. What are some toxic causes of this injury?

5. What diseases can cause unilateral basal ganglia findings?

Case ranking/difficulty:

Category: Intra-axial supratentorial

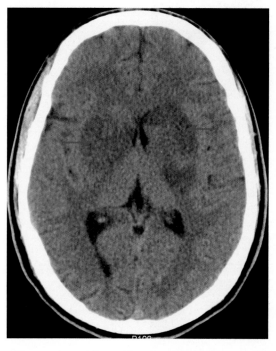

Axial CT image shows bilateral basal ganglia low attenuation (*arrows*).

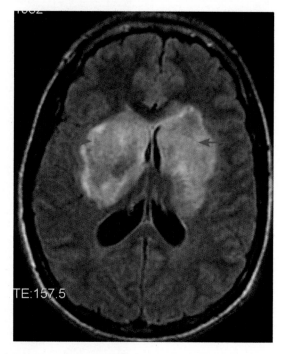

Axial FLAIR image shows bilateral basal ganglia high signal involving the caudate nuclei, internal capsules, lentiform nuclei, and thalami (*arrows*).

Answers

1. The abnormality is located within both basal ganglia.

2. The basal ganglia are susceptible to metabolic changes resulting in electrolyte imbalance. These include hyperammonemia, hypoglycemia, hyperglycemia, hyponatremia, and others.

3. The differential for bilateral basal ganglia cytotoxic edema includes toxic etiology (from CO poisoning or illicit drug use), osmotic myelinolysis (extrapontine myelinolysis), and hypoxic ischemic encephalopathy (HIE). Creutzfeldt-Jakob disease is an uncommon infectious cause of bilateral basal ganglia decreased diffusion.

4. Toxicity of the basal ganglia can occur with exposure to carbon monoxide, methanol, ethylene glycol, cyanide, heroin, opiates, and methylenedioxymethamphetamine (MDMA or ecstasy).

5. Unilateral basal ganglia findings may be seen with neoplasia, infection, and MCA infarction.

Pearls

- Toxic or metabolic etiologies should be considered with bilateral basal ganglia cytotoxic edema.
- The basal ganglia are susceptible to subtle changes in blood flow (autoregulation) and hypoxemia because of their high metabolic rate and blood supply.
- In young patients consider illicit drug abuse (heroin, opiates, ecstasy MDMA).
- Consider hypoxic ischemic injury with cortical involvement.
- Consider osmotic myelinolysis with pontine involvement.

Suggested Readings

Beltz EE, Mullins ME. Radiological reasoning: hyperintensity of the basal ganglia and cortex on FLAIR and diffusion-weighted imaging. *AJR Am J Roentgenol.* 2010 Sep;195(3 suppl):S1-S8 (Quiz S9-S11).

Hegde AN, Mohan S, Lath N, Lim CC. Differential diagnosis for bilateral abnormalities of the basal ganglia and thalamus. *Radiographics.* 2011;31(1):5-30.

Saenz RC. The disappearing basal ganglia sign. *Radiology.* 2005 Jan;234(1):242-243.

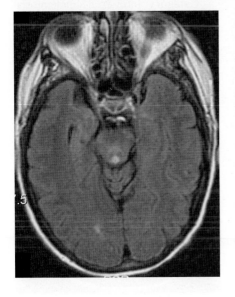 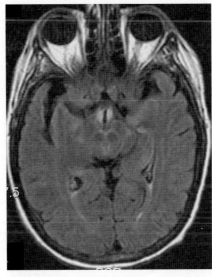 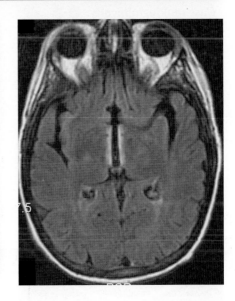

1. Where is the abnormality located?

2. What are the classic imaging findings for this entity?

3. What is the differential diagnosis?

4. What are typical presenting symptoms in this entity?

5. What is the treatment for this entity?

Case ranking/difficulty:

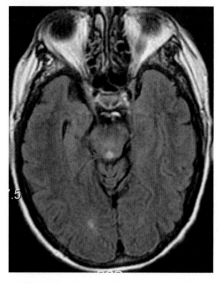

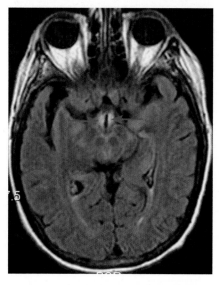

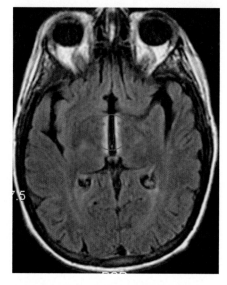

Axial FLAIR image demonstrates high signal surrounding the periaqueductal gray (*arrow*).

Axial FLAIR image demonstrates high signal involving the hypothalami (*arrows*).

Axial FLAIR image demonstrates high signal involving the border of the third ventricle and medial thalami (*circle*).

Answers

1. The abnormality is located within the periaqueductal gray, hypothalamus, and medial thalami.

2. The classic MRI findings of Wernicke encephalopathy (WE) include symmetric high T2 signal along the borders of the third ventricle and the periaqueductal gray. Also commonly involved are the medial thalamus, tectal plate, and mamillary bodies.

3. The differential diagnosis includes Wernicke encephalopathy, artery of Percheron infarct, and osmotic myelinolysis.

4. WE patients present with altered consciousness, ocular dysfunction, and ataxia.

5. This is considered a medical emergency as thiamine replacement must be given.

Pearls

- Wernicke encephalopathy (WE) is a neurologic disorder related to thiamine deficiency.
- Patients present with altered consciousness, ocular dysfunction, and ataxia.
- Key to diagnosis is high T2 signal involving the borders of the third ventricle and the periaqueductal gray.
- Contrast enhancement of the mamillary bodies is highly suggestive of WE.
- With pons involvement, consider osmotic myelinolysis.
- Artery of Percheron infarct involves the medial thalami and/or midbrain.

Suggested Readings

Hegde AN, Mohan S, Lath N, Lim CC. Differential diagnosis for bilateral abnormalities of the basal ganglia and thalamus. *Radiographics*. 2011;31(1):5-30.

Zuccoli G, Siddiqui N, Cravo I, Bailey A, Gallucci M, Harper CG. Neuroimaging findings in alcohol-related encephalopathies. *AJR Am J Roentgenol*. 2010 Dec;195(6):1378-1384.

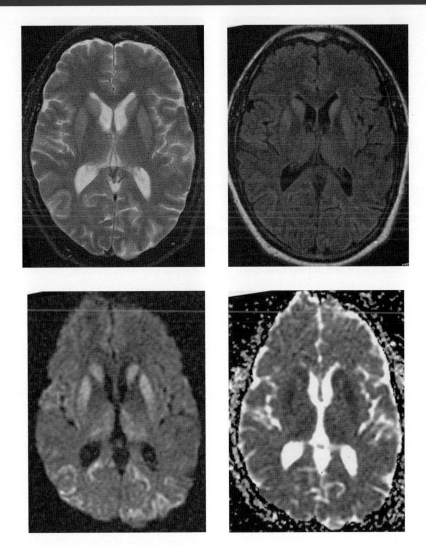

1. What are the typical MRI findings of this disease?

2. Which sequence is the most sensitive for the disease?

3. Which of these findings can be seen late in the disease?

4. What is the transmitted form of the disease?

5. What are typical clinical symptoms of the disease?

Case ranking/difficulty:

Category: Intra-axial supratentorial

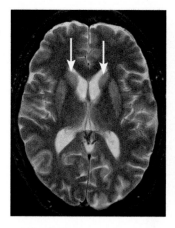

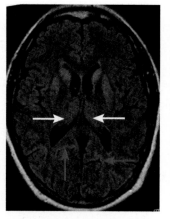

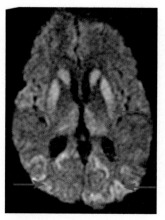

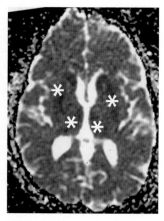

Axial T2 at the ganglionic level shows increased T2 signal of the bilateral caudate (*white arrows*) and putamina (*red arrows*).

Axial FLAIR through the ganglionic level shows T2 hyperintensity through the caudate and putamina as well as more subtle increased signal of the medial thalami (*white arrows*) and occipital parietal cortices (*red arrows*).

Axial DWI b = 1000 shows bright signal of the bilateral caudate, putamina, thalami, and occipital parietal cortices (*red arrows*).

Axial ADC shows corresponding decreased signal of the bilateral caudate, putamina, thalami (*asterisks*), and occipital cortex.

Answers

1. T2 hyperintensity associated with diffusion restriction of the basal ganglia, thalami, and cortex are typical MRI findings in Creutzfeldt-Jakob disease. As the disease progresses, cerebral atrophy is invariable.

2. Diffusion-weighted imaging is the most sensitive for early and intermediate changes of Creutzfeldt-Jakob disease. Restricted diffusion may persist beyond the usual 10-14 days seen in cytoxic edema from acute infarction.

3. As Creutzfeldt-Jakob progresses, there can be disappearance of DWI hyperintensity and development of white matter T2 hyperintensity. Cerebral atrophy always occurs as the disease progresses.

4. Creutzfeldt-Jakob disease (CJD) can be transmitted through infected beef (variant CJD) and iatrogenically from soiled instruments.

5. Rapid progression of dementia, myoclonic jerks, and akinetic mutism are clinical hallmarks of Creutzfeldt-Jakob disease.

Pearls

- Creutzfeldt-Jakob disease is a spongiform encephalopathy characterized by rapidly progressive dementia and movement abnormalities
- MRI imaging shows bilateral or unilateral T2 hyperintensity of the basal ganglia, thalami, and cerebral cortex not following a specific vascular distribution
- DWI show restricted diffusion of involved structures early in the disease and may persist greater than the expected 10-14 days for acute infarct.

Suggested Readings

Degnan AJ, Levy LM. Inherited forms of Creutzfeldt-Jakob disease. *AJNR Am J Neuroradiol*. 2013 Sep;34(9): 1690-1691.

Letourneau-Guillon L, Wada R, Kucharczyk W. Imaging of prion diseases. *J Magn Reson Imaging*. 2012 May;35(5):998-1012.

Ukisu R, Kushihashi T, Kitanosono T, et al. Serial diffusion-weighted MRI of Creutzfeldt-Jakob disease. *AJR Am J Roentgenol*. 2005 Feb;184(2):560-566.

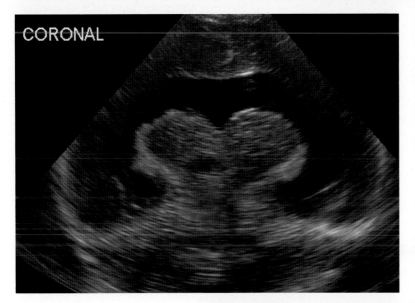

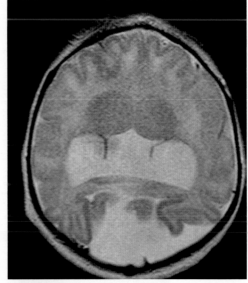

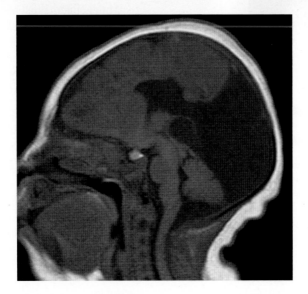

1. What is the diagnosis?

2. What are the classic imaging findings for this entity?

3. What are the different forms of this entity?

4. What are associated midline anomalies?

5. What is the vascular supply to the brain in this entity?

Case ranking/difficulty:

Category: Intra-axial supratentorial

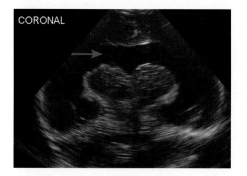

Coronal ultrasound image shows monoventricle (*green arrow*) and fusion of thalami (*blue arrow*) across the midline. Septum pellucidum is absent.

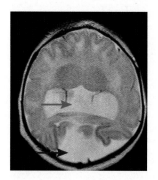

Axial T2 image shows a monoventricle (*green arrow*) and dorsal cyst (*blue arrow*) in alobar holoprosencephaly. Septum pellucidum is absent.

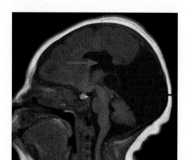

Sagittal T1 image shows monoventricle (*green arrow*) and dorsal cyst (*blue arrow*) in alobar holoprosencephaly. Corpus callosum is absent.

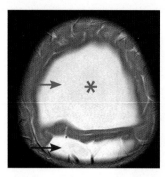

Axial T2 image shows an increase in size of the monoventricle (*green arrow*) and dorsal cyst (*blue arrow*) seen 10 months later. Septum pellucidum is absent (*red asterisk*).

Answers

1. This alobar holoprosencephaly shows crossing of gyrus across the midline. Failure of midline cleavage of the prosencephalon leads to holoprosencephaly.

2. Crossing of gyrus across the midline is the most important feature in alobar holoprosencephaly. Monoventricle, dorsal cyst, fusion of hypothalami and basal ganglia, absent interhemispheric fissure, absent falx cerebri, absent septum pellucidum, absent corpus callosum, and midline facial anomalies are typical findings. Sylvian fissure is absent or located more anteriorly and near the midline.

3. Lobar form of holoprosencephaly shows relatively well-developed frontal horns, frontal lobes, temporal horns, third ventricle, and hippocampi compared to semilobar form. Lobar form also shows nearly normal sylvian fissure; basal ganglia and interhemispheric falx may be present but hypoplastic. However, septum pellucidum is absent even in lobar form. Clinically, lobar form

is milder compared to the most severe alobar form. Middle interhemispheric variant or syntelencephaly shows absence of body of corpus callosum with fusion of posterior frontal or anterior parietal lobes across the midline. Genu and splenium of corpus callosum are present. Septum pellucidum is absent. Falx and interhemispheric fissure are hypoplastic and focally absent at the site of the fusion.

4. Midline facial anomalies are seen in holoprosencephaly: hypoplasia of premaxillary segment, single central maxillary incisor, hypotelorism, and cyclopia.

5. Anterior and middle cerebral arteries are usually absent or there is azygos anterior cerebral artery. The cerebrum is supplied by multiple small vessels arising directly from internal carotid and basilar arteries.

Pearls

- Holoprosencephaly is a congenital malformation that involves a spectrum of anomalies of midline fusion.
- The best clue for alobar holoprosencephaly is a monoventricle with fused frontal lobes.
- Severe hydrocephalus will show thinned cortical mantle.
- Midline facial anomalies are associated.

Suggested Reading

Vaz SS, Chodirker B, Prasad C, Seabrook JA, Chudley AE, Prasad AN. Risk factors for nonsyndromic holoprosencephaly: a Manitoba case-control study. *Am J Med Genet A*. 2012 Apr;158A(4):751-758.

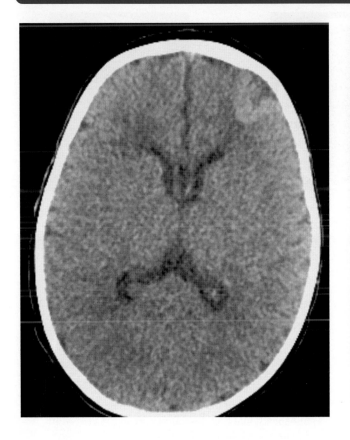 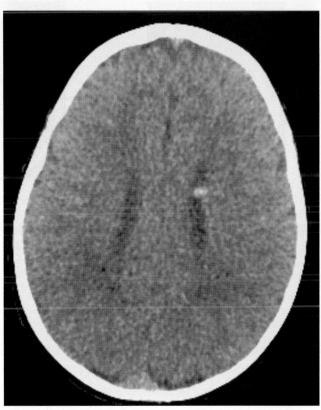

1. Where is the abnormality located?

2. What is the classic clinical triad in this entity?

3. What are other findings seen outside the CNS in this entity?

4. What are classic CNS imaging findings?

5. What are the major features in this disease?

Case ranking/difficulty:

Category: Intra-axial supratentorial

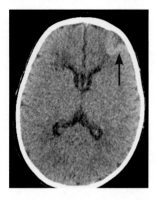

Axial CT image shows a hyperdense cortical/subcortical tuber (*blue arrow*) without vasogenic edema.

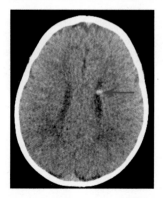

Axial CT image shows a calcified subependymal nodule (*green arrow*).

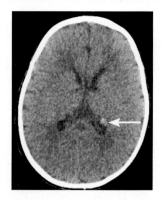

Axial CT image shows calcified subependymal nodule (*arrow*) seen in tuberous sclerosis.

Answers

1. The abnormality is located within the left frontal lobe and the left periventricular white matter.

2. Typical clinical triad in tuberous sclerosis is facial angiofibroma, mental retardation, and infantile spasm. Most patients are diagnosed by the age of 2 years.

3. Renal angiomyolipomas require monitoring by ultrasound as they can rapidly grow in size. When they reach more than 4 cm in size, there is a higher incidence of rupture and life-threatening hemorrhage. Angiomyolipoma appear echogenic on ultrasound and hypodense on CT due to fat content in the lesion. MRI also demonstrates presence of fat within the lesion using fat-saturated sequences.

   Lymphangioleiomyomatosis appear as multiple cystic lesions in the lungs with very thin walls. They are uniformly distributed within the lung parenchyma.

   Ash leaf spots are depigmented nevi in the skin.

4. The classic imaging findings include cortical tubers and calcified subependymal nodules. The cortical tubers have variable signal on T2-weighted images, depending on calcification. The subependymal nodules commonly calcify, and can be easily detected on CT secondary to calcification.

5. Definitive diagnosis of tuberous sclerosis requires at least two major features or one major + two minor features. Major features include facial angiofibromas or forehead plaque, ungual or periungual fibromas, more than three hypomelanotic macules, shagreen patch, retinal nodular hamartomas, cortical tuber, subependymal nodule, subependymal giant cell astrocytoma, cardiac rhabdomyoma, lymphangioleiomyomatosis, and renal angiomyolipoma.

Pearls

- Tuberous sclerosis (TS) is a neurocutaneous syndrome that has autosomal dominant inheritance (via either gene 9q34 or 16p13).
- Lymphangioleiomyomatosis and renal angiomyolipoma are major features of TS but either one alone do not make a definitive diagnosis.
- Subependymal nodules calcify after first year of life and are easily seen on CT scan.
- Subependymal nodules in neonatal ultrasound appear as an echogenic area and mimic subependymal hemorrhage or subependymal heterotopia.
- Subependymal nodules in unmyelinated brain appear hyperintense on T1 and hypointense on T2 whereas in myelinated brain they appear isointense.
- FLAIR is sensitive for visualization of cortical tubers.
- Retinal hamartomas, if present, appear after the first few months of life and are usually multiple and bilateral.

Suggested Reading

Roach ES, Gomez MR, Northrup H. Tuberous sclerosis complex consensus conference: revised clinical diagnostic criteria. *J Child Neurol.* 1998 Dec;13(12):624-628.

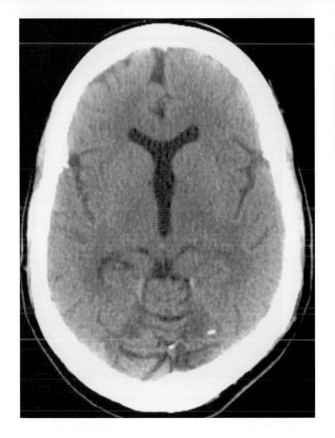 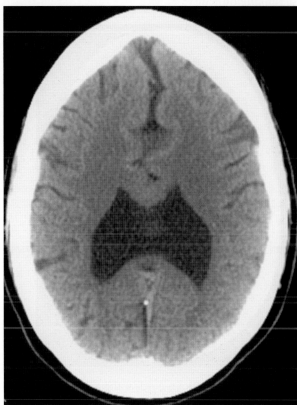

1. Where is the abnormality located?

2. What are the classic imaging findings?

3. What are possible genetic causes?

4. What is the etiology of this entity?

5. What are possible clinical findings in patients with this malformation?

Case ranking/difficulty:

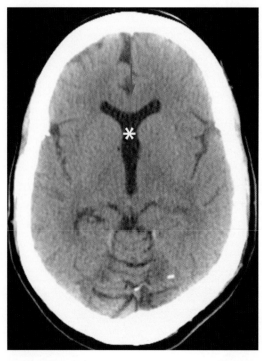

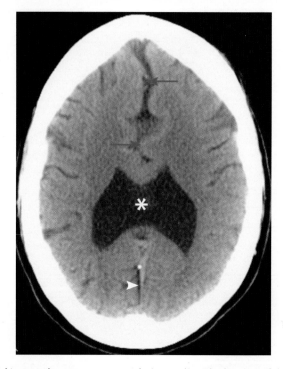

Axial CT image shows a monoventricle without septum pellucidum (*asterisk*). Note the genu of the corpus callosum is present (*arrow*).

Axial image shows monoventricle (*asterisk*) with absence of the falx cerebri anteriorly and interdigitation of the interhemispheric fissure (*arrows*). A posterior falx is present (*arrowhead*).

Answers

1. Holoprosencephalies involve lack of separation or development of midline structures. Absence of the septum pellucidum and monoventricle are typically seen within the whole spectrum.

2. Absence of the septum pellucidum, monoventricle, partial agenesis of the corpus callosum, and underdevelopment of the frontal lobes are at least typically seen with lobar holoprosencephaly, the mildest form.

3. 25%-50% of holoprosencephalies involve cytogenetic abnormalities, including trisomies 13 or 9, or deletions involving chromosomes 1, 2, 3, 7, 11, or 18.

4. This congenital malformation results from lack of separation of the embryonic forebrain or prosencephalon.

5. Patients with holoprosencephaly spectrum may be normal, or have seizures, hypothalamic/pituitary dysfunction, developmental delay, mental retardation, and dystonia and hypotonia from central nuclei fusion. Phenotypical presentation is variable depending on the amount of brain malformation. The treatment for this entity is typically supportive.

Pearls

- In semilobar holoprosencephaly, there is partial separation of the prosencephalon and therefore partial formation of midline structures.
- Mildest spectrum of holoprosencephalies.
- Absence of the septum pellucidum with monoventricle.
- Partial agenesis of the corpus callosum, splenium typically present.
- At least posterior presence of the falx cerebri and interhemispheric fissure.
- +/− partial fusion of midline structures and presence of dorsal cyst.
- Facial anomalies typically are not as severe as alobar holoprosencephaly.

Suggested Reading

Cayea PD, Balcar I, Alberti O, Jones TB. Prenatal diagnosis of semilobar holoprosencephaly. *AJR Am J Roentgenol.* 1984 Feb;142(2):401-402.

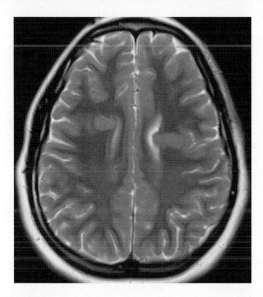
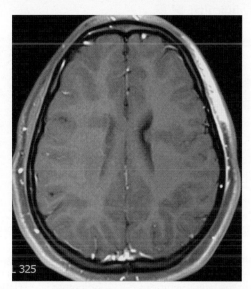
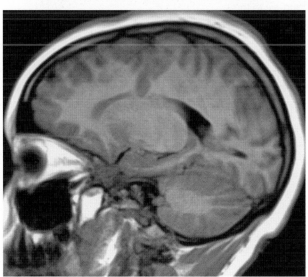
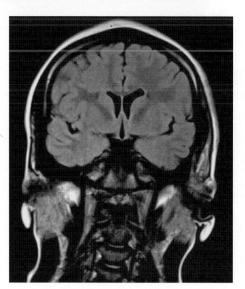

1. Which part of the brain does this entity most commonly involve?

2. What are the classic imaging findings for this entity?

3. What malformations are associated with this entity?

4. What is the etiology of this entity?

5. How is this entity treated?

Case ranking/difficulty: **Category:** Intra-axial supratentorial

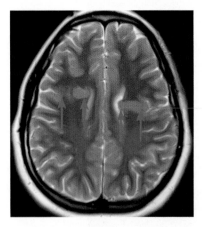

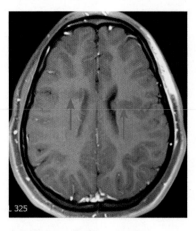

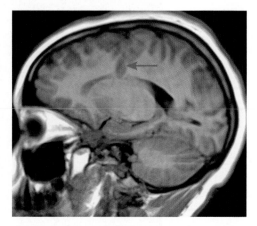

Axial T2 image shows linear clefts lined by gray matter isointense tissue extending from the cortex to the lateral ventricles with nipple-like outpouching (*arrows*). There is no CSF within the cleft, consistent with a "closed-lip" type schizencephaly.

Axial T1 image with contrast shows nonenhancing, gray matter isointense lined clefts extending from the cortical surface to the lateral ventricles bilaterally (*arrows*).

Sagittal T1 noncontrast shows the gray matter lined cleft extending through the right frontal lobe (*arrow*).

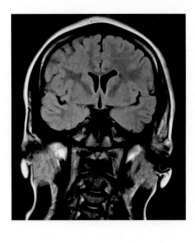

Coronal FLAIR image shows the right frontal cleft enface (*arrow*) and isointense to gray matter.

Pearls

- Schizencephaly is an abnormal cleft lined by gray matter extending from the pia matter of the cerebral cortex to the ventricular ependyma.
- In open-lip schizencephaly there is a readily apparent cerebral spinal fluid (CSF) tract that is lined by gray matter.
- Closed-lip schizencephaly demonstrates no visible CSF cleft between the approximated gray matter, and there is often a dimple or defect where the tract enters the lateral ventricle.
- Secondary to in utero insult, commonly infection, or vascular vs genetic abnormality.
- Up to 50% may be bilateral and most commonly parasylvian in location.
- Patients can present with seizures, developmental delay, and motor defects.
- Best imaged with multiplanar MRI.

Answers

1. Schizencephaly can occur anywhere, but is more common involving the parasylvian frontal or parietal lobes.

2. Classic imaging findings are an abnormal cleft lined by gray matter extending from the pial surface of the cortex to the ependymal surface of the ventricle.

3. Associated malformations include septo-optic dysplasia with absence of the septum pellucidum and hypoplasia of the optic nerves, gray matter heterotopia, pachygyria, polymicrogyria, and lissencephaly.

4. This entity is thought to be secondary to an in utero insult, commonly infection, or vascular vs genetic abnormality.

5. Supportive care is given with control of seizures and hydrocephalus if present.

Suggested Readings

Oh KY, Kennedy AM, Frias AE, Byrne JL. Fetal schizencephaly: pre- and postnatal imaging with a review of the clinical manifestations. *Radiographics*. 2010 Oct;25(3):647-657.

Patel AC, Cohen HL, Hotson GC. US case of the day. Open-lip schizencephaly with an area of heterotopic gray matter and associated absence of the septa pellucida. *Radiographics*. 2002 Oct;17(1):236-239.

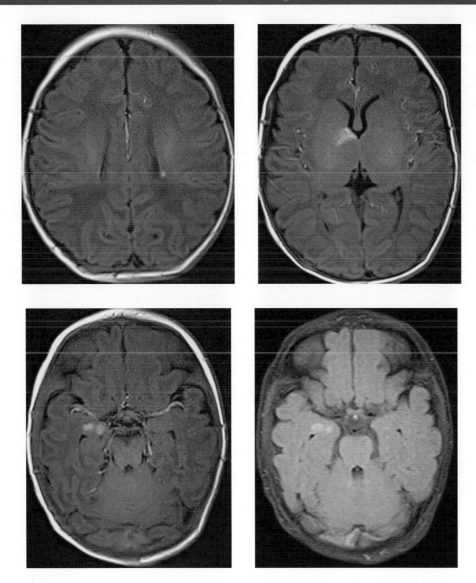

1. What are the diagnostic criteria for this disease?

2. What are typical clinical presentation(s)?

3. What is the differential diagnosis?

4. What are the characteristic radiographic features?

5. Is follow-up imaging recommended for this disease?

Case ranking/difficulty:

Category: Intra-axial supratentorial

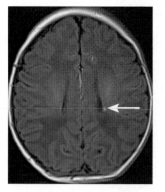

Axial T1 noncontrast image demonstrates a focus of T1 hyperintensity in the left periventricular white matter (*white arrow*).

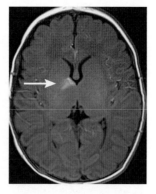

Axial T1 noncontrast image demonstrates a wedge-shaped T1 hyperintensity in the right caudal thalamic groove (*white arrow*).

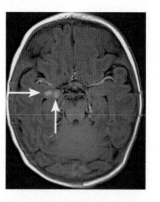

Axial T1 noncontrast image demonstrates two foci of T1 hyperintensity in the right medial temporal lobe/amygdala (*white arrows*).

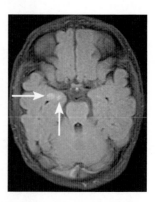

Axial T2 FLAIR image demonstrates two foci of T2 FLAIR hyperintensity in the right medial temporal lobe/amygdala (*white arrows*)

Answers

1. Neurocutaneous melanosis is a rare noninherited condition, characterized by cutaneous congenital melanocytic nevi (giant or multiple small lesions) and melanocyte deposition in the central nervous system.

2. Most patients are asymptomatic. Symptomatic patients present at an early age and are related to melanocyte deposition in the CNS causing increased intracranial pressure secondary to poor CSF circulation. Symptomatic patients typically have extremely poor prognosis.

3. Differential diagnosis of T1 hyperintense lesions includes lipoma, dermoid, and hemorrhage.

4. Characteristic imaging is T1 hyperintensity with susceptibility artifacts in SWI/GRE sequences secondary to melanocyte deposition. Parenchymal lesions are stable over time; a few case reports show regression. Leptomeningeal melanosis can show enhancement with progression to melanoma.

5. Patients with neurocutaneous melanosis need to be followed to assess for malignant transformation to melanoma. In one study this occurred in over half of the patients.

Pearls

- Rare genetic disorder, 100+ case reports.
- Giant or multiple melanocytic nevi in the skin with parenchymal and/or leptomeningeal melanosis of the central nervous system.
- Most patients are asymptomatic.

- Symptoms are related to increased intracranial pressure secondary to impaired CSF flow from leptomeningeal melanosis.
- Extremely poor prognosis in symptomatic patients.
- 5%-15% lifetime risk of malignant transformation of giant cutaneous nevi.
- More than half of patients with neurocutaneous melanosis will have leptomeningeal malignant melanoma.
- No definite treatment.
- Characteristic radiographic findings include T1 hyperintense lesions with no contrast enhancement of parenchymal lesions.
- Parenchymal lesions are usually located in the amygdala, cerebellum, brain stem, inferior frontal lobes, and thalami.
- Leptomeningeal melanosis is typically diffuse and can have enhancement.
- GRE/SWI shows blooming artifacts.
- 10% associated with Dandy-Walker malformation.
- Recommend screening MRI of the central nervous system (brain and spine) and skin examination for malignant degeneration.

Suggested Readings

Demirci A, Kawamura Y, Sze G, Duncan C. MR of parenchymal neurocutaneous melanosis. *AJNR Am J Neuroradiol.* 1995 Mar;16(3):603-606.

Ginat DT, Meyers SP. Intracranial lesions with high signal intensity on T1-weighted MR images: differential diagnosis. *Radiographics.* 2012;32(2):499-516.

Smith AB, Rushing EJ, Smirniotopoulos JG. Pigmented lesions of the central nervous system: radiologic-pathologic correlation. *Radiographics.* 2009;29(5):1503-1524.

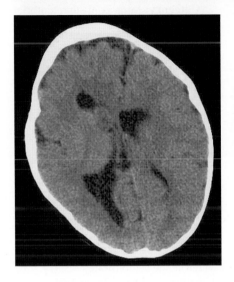 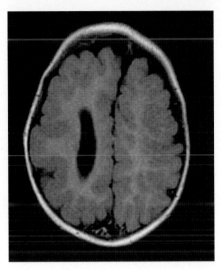 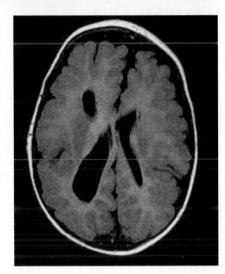

1. What is the differential diagnosis?

2. What are the typical radiographic findings of
   the affected hemisphere?

3. What is the typical clinical presentation?

4. What are common syndromic associations with
   this finding?

5. What is the treatment for this disease?

Case ranking/difficulty:

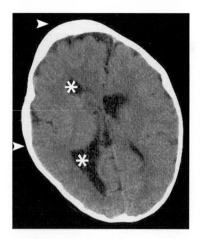 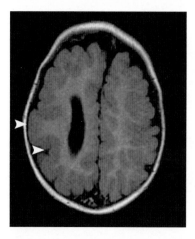 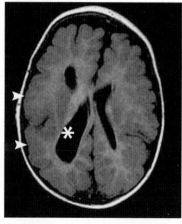

Axial noncontrast CT image demonstrates diffuse enlargement of the right cerebral hemisphere with enlarged right lateral ventricle (*white asterisks*) and right-sided calvarium thickening (*white arrowheads*).

Axial FLAIR image demonstrates hemihypertrophy of the right cerebral hemisphere associated with pachygyria (*white arrowheads*).

Axial FLAIR image demonstrates hemihypertrophy of the right cerebral hemisphere associated with pachygyria (*white arrowheads*). Also noted is enlargement of the right lateral ventricle (*white asterisk*).

Answers

1. Differential diagnosis of hemimegalencephaly include disorders that enlarge the hemisphere (gliomatosis cerebri), or hemiatrophy diseases making the normal hemisphere appear large (Rasmussen encephalitis, Dyke-Davidoff-Masson syndrome, Sturge-Weber syndrome).

2. The affected hemisphere usually demonstrates increased size of the lateral ventricle, shallow sulci with enlarged gyri, thickened calvarium, white matter gliosis, association with developmental venous anomalies, cortical malformation, and gray matter heterotopia, as well as contralateral displacement of the posterior falx.

3. The majority (90%) of patients present with focal or generalized seizures. Developmental delay, hemiparesis, and hemianopia are usually also evident.

4. Syndromic associations (47%) with hemimegalencephaly include Klippel-Trenaunay syndrome, proteus syndrome, epidermal nevus syndrome, and hypomelanosis of Ito.

5. Hemispherectomy may help control intractable seizures; anticonvulsive therapy is usually ineffective in hemimegalencephaly.

Pearls

- Rare congenital cortical malformation with hamartomatous overgrowth of cerebral hemisphere of unknown etiology.
- The affected hemisphere may have focal or diffuse cortical malformation and migrational anomalies.
- Typical clinical presentations are infantile spasm, developmental delay, hemiparesis, and hemianopia.
- May be isolated or have syndromic association (47%).
- Diagnostic clues are increased parenchymal brain volume and ipsilateral ventricle volume, with associated migrational anomalies.
- Treatment is targeted to control epilepsy.

Suggested Readings

Abdel Razek AA, Kandell AY, Elsorogy LG, Elmongy A, Basett AA. Disorders of cortical formation: MR imaging features. *AJNR Am J Neuroradiol.* 2009 Jan;30(1):4-11.

Broumandi DD, Hayward UM, Benzian JM, Gonzalez I, Nelson MD. Best cases from the AFIP: hemimegalencephaly. *Radiographics.* 2004 Aug;24(3):843-848.

Sato N, Yagishita A, Oba H, et al. Hemimegalencephaly: a study of abnormalities occurring outside the involved hemisphere. *AJNR Am J Neuroradiol.* 2007 Apr;28(4):678-682.

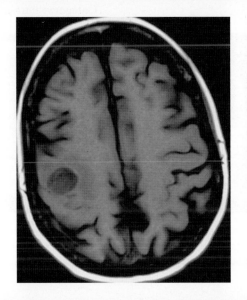
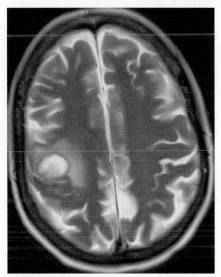
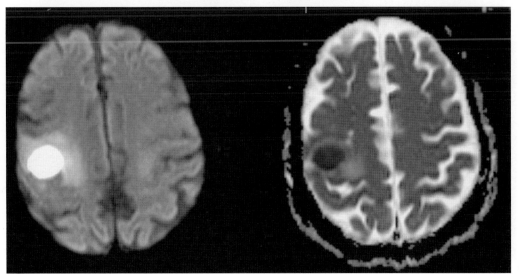

1. Where is the abnormality located?

2. What is the most common presenting symptom?

3. What is the differential diagnosis?

4. What etiologies can cause this entity?

5. What is the treatment for this entity?

Case ranking/difficulty: Category: Intra-axial supratentorial

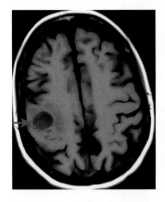

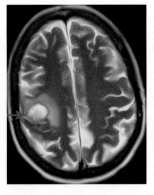

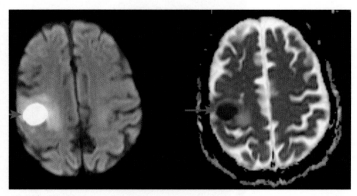

Axial T1 image shows a round lesion with low to intermediate signal lesion centrally within the right frontal lobe (*arrow*).

Axial T2 image shows a round, T2 hyperintense lesion with T2 dark rim and surrounding T2 hyperintensity representing edema (*arrow*).

Axial DWI and ADC shows the lesion with central high signal on DWI (*green arrow*) and corresponding low ADC signal (*red arrow*). This is indicative of "restricted diffusion."

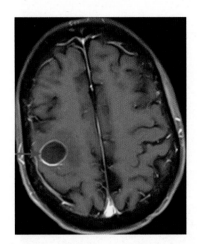

Axial postcontrast T1 shows ring enhancement (*arrow*).

Pearls

- The most common pathogens are *Staphylococcus* and *Streptococcus*.
- Abscess rim has low T2 signal.
- Most abscesses are solitary.
- Rim enhancement may be thicker along the gray matter interface and thinner along the side that abuts the white matter.
- Multiple rim enhancing lesions, think metastasis.
- GBM typically do not have smooth rim enhancement.
- Toxoplasma abscess does not typically restrict diffusion.

Suggested Readings

Chong-Han CH, Cortez SC, Tung GA. Diffusion-weighted MRI of cerebral toxoplasma abscess. *AJR Am J Roentgenol.* 2003 Dec;181(6):1711-1714.

Smirniotopoulos JG, Murphy FM, Rushing EJ, Rees JH, Schroeder JW. Patterns of contrast enhancement in the brain and meninges. *Radiographics.* 2007;27(2):525-551.

Answers

1. The abnormality is located within the posterior frontal lobe and involves the precentral gyrus.

2. The most common symptoms include headache (>90%) and fever (50%).

3. The differential diagnosis includes metastasis, abscess, and GBM.

4. This entity may be secondary to trauma, immunocompromised status, sinus/ear infection, postop, and septicemia.

5. The treatment is antibiotic therapy. When lesions are large (>3 cm), surgical drainage may be needed.

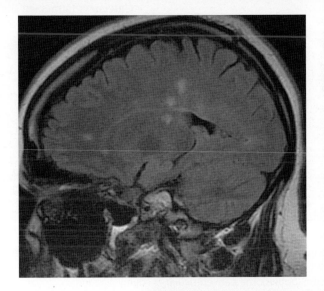
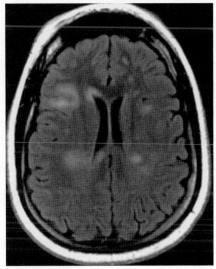

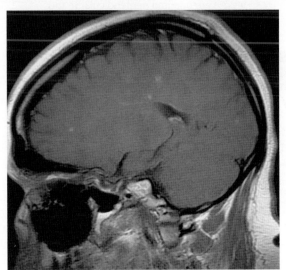

1. Where is the abnormality located?

2. What are the classic imaging findings for this entity?

3. What is the most sensitive MR sequence for detecting lesions of all ages in this entity?

4. What anatomical structures are affected by lesions in this entity?

5. What is the treatment for this entity?

Case ranking/difficulty:

Category: Intra-axial supratentorial

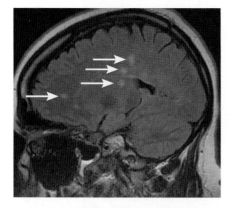

Sagittal FLAIR image shows multiple high signal periventricular lesions (*arrows*), some of which approach the callosal-septal margin.

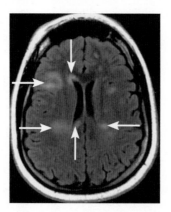

Axial FLAIR image shows multiple high signal periventricular lesions are present and a couple within the anterior and posterior corpus callosum (*arrows*). The periventricular lesions are oriented perpendicular to the ventricles, termed "Dawson fingers."

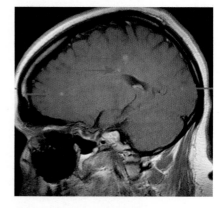

Sagittal T1 postcontrast shows enhancement of the periventricular lesions (*arrows*), indicating active demyelination.

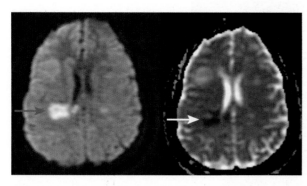

Axial DWI and ADC show one of the periventricular lesions on the right demonstrates restricted diffusion (*green arrow*). Note the low signal on the ADC image (*white arrow*). This indicates early acute demyelination.

Answers

1. The abnormality is located within the white matter.

2. On MRI, there is variable signal, usually hypointense on T1 and hyperintense on T2 within the white matter. Characteristic lesions at the level of the lateral ventricles orientated perpendicular to the long axis are termed "Dawson fingers" and are a classic finding for multiple sclerosis.

3. FLAIR is the most sensitive standard MR sequence for detecting demyelinating lesions of all ages.

4. Multiple sclerosis is a demyelinating disease that may involve the brain (predominantly white matter), spinal cord, and cranial nerves.

5. The treatment for MS includes corticosteroids and other immunosuppressants.

Pearls

- High-field (3T) MRI is more sensitive for detecting demyelinating plaques.
- Large MS lesions may mimic tumor; key is "incomplete" ring enhancement (horseshoe appearance).
- Utilize fat saturation sequences for optic neuritis.
- Approximately half of optic neuritis patients develop MS.
- 80%-90% of MS patients have CSF oligoclonal bands.
- In young patients with febrile prodrome consider Marburg variant, which presents with an acute, fulminant demyelinating mass.
- With only optic nerve and spinal cord involvement consider neuromyelitis optica (Devic disease).
- Corpus callosum and deep gray nuclei involvement consider Susac syndrome.

Suggested Readings

Eisele P, Szabo K, Griebe M, et al. Reduced diffusion in a subset of acute MS lesions: a serial multiparametric MRI study. *AJNR Am J Neuroradiol*. 2012 Aug;33(7):1369-1373.

Filippi M, Rocca MA. MR imaging of multiple sclerosis. *Radiology*. 2011 Jun;259(3):659-681.

Given CA, Stevens BS, Lee C. The MRI appearance of tumefactive demyelinating lesions. *AJR Am J Roentgenol*. 2004 Jan;182(1):195-199.

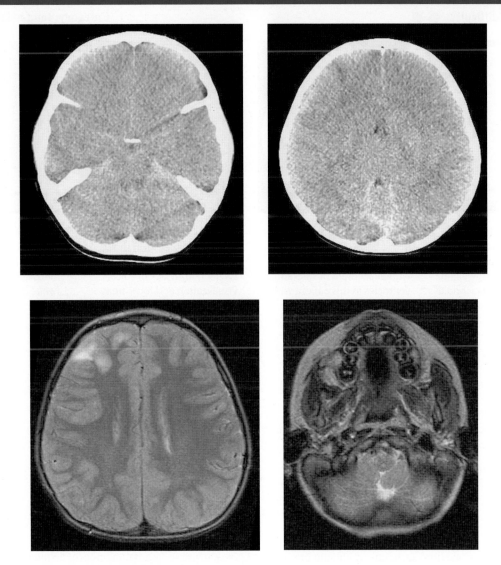

1. What is the prognosis for this disease?

2. What can be seen in specific MRI sequences of this disease?

3. What is the differential diagnosis of this finding?

4. What MRI findings can be seen with viral encephalitides?

5. What is the most common pathogen of sporadic viral encephalitis?

Case ranking/difficulty: **Category:** Intra-axial supratentorial

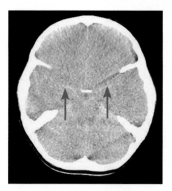

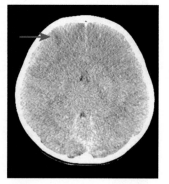

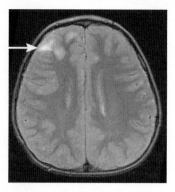

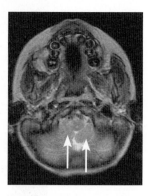

Axial CT image at the level of the midbrain shows diffuse effacement of the basilar cisterns and cerebral swelling. There is "pseudosubarachnoid" sign (*red arrows*).

Axial CT image at the level of the basal ganglia shows diffuse cerebral swelling with effacement of sulci and ventricles in this patient with La Crosse viral encephalitis. Focal hypodensity from more severe edema is seen in the right frontal lobe (*red arrow*).

Axial T2 image at the supraganglionic level shows diffuse cerebral gray matter swelling from lack of sulcal visualization and focal areas of right frontal cortical edema (*white arrow*) in this patient with La Crosse viral encephalitis.

Axial T2 image at the skull base shows cerebellar tonsillar herniation from diffuse cerebral edema (*white arrows*).

Answers

1. Although dependent on the specific pathogen, as a whole, viral encephalitides can have high morbidity and mortality, especially without treatment.

2. Viral encephalitides will typically show T2 hyperintensity from inflammatory swelling with some diffusion restriction. Contrast enhancement can be seen but is not obligatory for the diagnosis. Hemorrhage is uncommon in the majority of viral encephalitides.

3. With diffuse brain swelling, ischemia, traumatic brain injury, and viral encephalitides should be considered. Status epilepticus can also show diffuse swelling. The clinical history is helpful to distinguish these entities.

4. Although with a predilection for gray matter (including basal ganglia) diffuse inflammation, white matter lesions and brainstem involvement can be characteristic of some specific pathogens. Ring-enhancing lesions are not usual for viral encephalitis.

5. The herpes virus, specifically the herpes simplex 1 virus, is the most common sporadic cause of viral encephalitis with 70% mortality if not treated.

Pearls

- Viral encephalitides have high morbidity and mortality especially in certain age groups, depending on the specific pathogen.
- Herpes is the most common cause of sporadic viral encephalitis.
- MRI usually shows a preference for gray matter involvement, although white matter can be commonly involved with specific pathogens.
- Diffuse inflammation, poorly delineated T2 hyperintensity, and areas of diffusion restriction +/− enhancement are typical.
- The cerebellum can be affected in isolation or conjunction.
- Rapid diagnosis with treatment using available antivirals can significantly improve outcome.

Suggested Readings

Gupta RK, Soni N, Kumar S, Khandelwal N. Imaging of central nervous system viral diseases. *J Magn Reson Imaging*. 2012 Mar;35(3):477-491.

Kirolğu Y, Calli C, Yunten N, et al. Diffusion-weighted MR imaging of viral encephalitis. *Neuroradiology*. 2006 Dec;48(12):875-880.

Parmar H, Ibrahim M. Pediatric intracranial infections. *Neuroimaging Clin N Am*. 2012 Nov;22(4):707-725.

65-year-old female with progressive memory decline, confusion, and agitation over several weeks

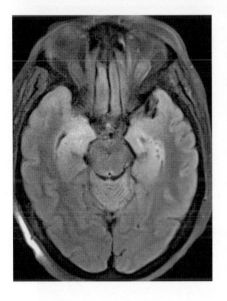 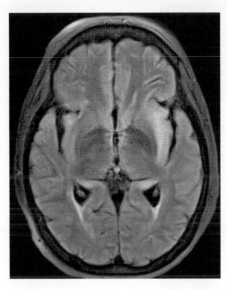 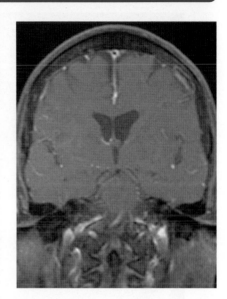

1. What is the differential for these MRI findings?

2. What is the usual anatomy affected in this disease?

3. What is the pathophysiology of the disease?

4. What is the treatment for this disease?

5. What are other related syndromes with similar pathophysiology as this disease?

Case ranking/difficulty:

Category: Intra-axial supratentorial

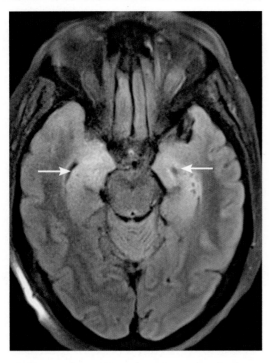

Axial FLAIR image shows bilateral swelling and T2 hyperintensity of the medial temporal lobes (*white arrow*).

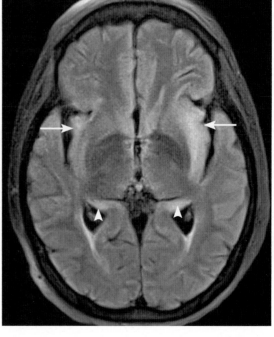

Axial FLAIR image shows involvement of the bilateral insular cortex (*white arrows*) and tails of the hippocampi (*arrowheads*). This patient was eventually diagnosed with small cell lung cancer.

Answers

1. The differential for bilateral swelling of the medial temporal lobes includes limbic encephalitis, herpes encephalitis, and status epilepticus. Clinical history should be helpful to distinguish between these entities. If herpes encephalitis cannot be excluded, rapid treatment with acyclovir must be considered.

2. Limbic encephalitis affects the medial temporal lobes, insular cortex, and inferior frontal lobes.

3. Paraneoplastic syndromes are thought to be immune mediated with autoantibodies or cytotoxic T-cell activity. Anti-Hu autoantibodies are found in the majority of cases of limbic encephalitis, which is associated with small cell lung cancer.

4. Limbic encephalitis is a paraneoplastic syndrome caused by autoimmune factors. Treatment with immunomodulators and suppressive agents such as corticosteroids, as well as plasmapheresis has shown some benefits; however, no clinical trial has been performed. Symptoms of paraneoplastic syndromes generally improve as the primary neoplasm is treated.

5. Both Lambert-Eaton and opsoclonus-myoclonus are paraneoplastic syndromes.

Pearls

- Limbic encephalitis is the most common paraneoplastic syndrome involving the CNS.
- Small cell lung cancer is classically implicated in limbic encephalitis, although other neoplasms can cause it as well.
- Clinical presentation usually involves subacute presentation with progressive cognitive decline over weeks to months.
- MRI findings of bilateral medial temporal lobe, insular cortex, and inferior frontal lobe involvement are typical with T2 hyperintensity and swelling.
- Patchy enhancement and restricted diffusion have been described but are variable.

Suggested Readings

Demaerel P, Van Dessel W, Van Paesschen W, Vandenberghe R, Van Laere K, Linn J. Autoimmune-mediated encephalitis. *Neuroradiology*. 2011 Nov;53(11):837-851.

Urbach H, Soeder BM, Jeub M, Klockgether T, Meyer B, Bien CG. Serial MRI of limbic encephalitis. *Neuroradiology*. 2006 Jun;48(6):380-386.

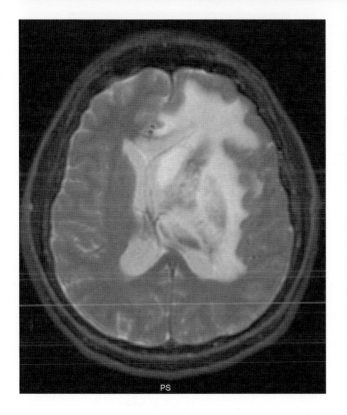
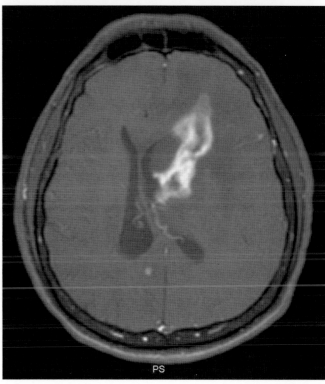

1. Where is the abnormality located?

2. What are the classic imaging findings for this entity?

3. What is the differential diagnosis?

4. What is the typical clinical presentation?

5. What is the treatment for this entity?

Case ranking/difficulty: 🌑🌑

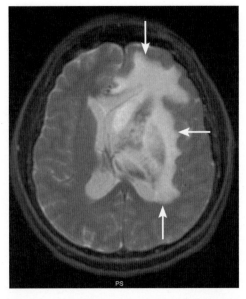

Axial T2 image shows extensive vasogenic edema centered in the left basal ganglia, and extending to the hemispheric white matter (*arrows*). The vasogenic edema results in subfalcine herniation from left to right. Notice the compression of the left lateral ventricle.

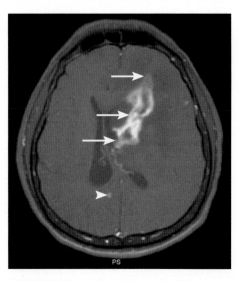

Axial T1 postcontrast demonstrates an irregular peripherally enhancing lesion within the left periventricular basal ganglia and white matter extending to the subependymal surface and into the subcortical white matter of the left frontal lobe (*arrows*). A focus of leptomeningeal enhancement is seen posteriorly involving the right occipital lobe (*arrowhead*).

Answers

1. The abnormality is located in the left periventricular region involving the superior aspect of the left basal ganglia. Toxoplasmosis most commonly involves the basal ganglia.

2. On CT imaging, the lesions are usually low density. On MRI, lesions are low T1 signal with corresponding high or mixed T2 signal. After administration of contrast, the lesions will show rim or ring enhancement.

3. The differential diagnosis includes toxoplasma encephalitis (cerebral toxoplasmosis), lymphoma, and glioma.

4. Toxoplasmosis is secondary to *Toxoplasmosis gondii*, which is an intracellular protozoan. The most common symptom is headache. Other common symptoms include fever, altered mental status, seizures, sensory disturbances, motor weakness, and speech disturbance.

5. The treatment for this entity is medical treatment with pyrimethamine and sulfadiazine. The duration of therapy is 6 weeks and pyrimethamine requires folinic acid to prevent toxicity.

Pearls

- Toxoplasmosis is secondary to *Toxoplasmosis gondii*, which is an intracellular protozoan.
- It may be transmitted to humans via undercooked pork, contaminated vegetables, or cat feces.
- Toxoplasmosis is the most likely infection with ring-enhancing lesions involving the basal ganglia in AIDS patients.
- "Target" sign with central nodular enhancement within the ring enhancement is suggestive of toxo.
- A solitary mass is more likely to be lymphoma in HIV/AIDS.
- Consider PML or HIV encephalopathy in nonenhancing lesions of the subcortical white matter in AIDS patients.
- Immunocompromised patients with basilar meningeal enhancement consider tuberculosis.
- With thallium, lymphoma is "hot," but toxo is not.

Suggested Readings

Hegde AN, Mohan S, Lath N, Lim CC. Differential diagnosis for bilateral abnormalities of the basal ganglia and thalamus. *Radiographics*. 2011;31(1):5-30.

Lee GT, Antelo F, Mlikotic AA. Best cases from the AFIP: cerebral toxoplasmosis. *Radiographics*. 2009;29(4):1200-1205.

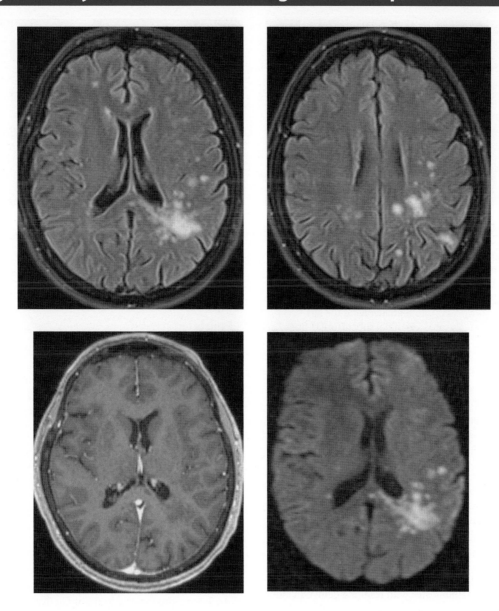

1. What is the differential diagnosis?

2. What are typical imaging findings for this entity?

3. What is the etiology of this disease?

4. What are associated risk factors for this entity?

5. What is the treatment for this disease?

Case ranking/difficulty:

Category: Intra-axial supratentorial

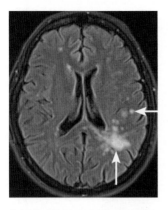

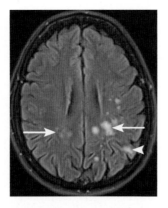

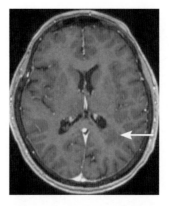

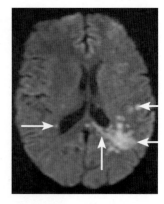

Axial FLAIR image shows patchy white matter lesions primarily in the left parietal lobe extending toward the splenium of the corpus callosum, which is confluent and appears mass like (*arrows*).

Axial FLAIR image at the corona radiata shows the patchy white matter lesions to be bilateral (*arrows*) but asymmetric, predominantly on the left. A lesion is seen involving the left parietal subcortical U-fiber (*arrowhead*).

Axial T1 postcontrast image shows no enhancement of the white matter lesions (*arrow*).

Axial DWI b = 1000 image shows diffusion restriction of the white matter lesions (*arrows*).

Answers

1. In an immunosuppressed patient, the differential includes progressive multifocal leukoencephalopathy (PML), HIV encephalitis, and immune reconstitution inflammatory syndrome (IRIS). In immunocompetent patients, ADEM or MS should be considered.

2. Typical MRI imaging findings for PML include patchy, bilateral asymmetric white matter lesions, which involve the subcortical U-fibers. Lesions may become confluent and mass like. Enhancement is atypical. DWI shows diffusion restriction in acute lesions.

3. PML is an opportunistic infection of the JC papovavirus involving the oligodendrocytes with resulting demyelination.

4. Immunosuppression is the greatest risk factor for PML, primarily including AIDS, transplantation, and chemotherapy. PML was initially described associated with hematologic and lymphoid malignancies. Rheumatologic diseases are also associated.

5. No specific treatment for PML currently exists. HAART in AIDS patients prolongs survival but increases the risk for IRIS.

Pearls

- Opportunistic infection by the JC papovavirus of oligodendrocytes with widespread demyelination.
- Greatest risk factor is immunosuppression.
- Variable-size T2 hyperintense and T1 hypointense white matter lesions, which may become confluent and mass like.
- Subcortical U-fibers are typically involved.
- Lesions may be bilateral but asymmetric.
- Acute lesions can demonstrate diffusion restriction.
- Enhancement is not typical.

Suggested Readings

Buckle C, Castillo M. Use of diffusion-weighted imaging to evaluate the initial response of progressive multifocal leukoencephalopathy to highly active antiretroviral therapy: early experience. *AJNR Am J Neuroradiol*. 2010 Jun;31(6):1031-1035.

Post MJ, Thurnher MM, Clifford DB, Nath A, Gonzalez RG, Gupta RK, Post KK. CNS-immune reconstitution inflammatory syndrome in the setting of HIV infection, part 1: overview and discussion of progressive multifocal leukoencephalopathy-immune reconstitution inflammatory syndrome and cryptococcal-immune reconstitution inflammatory syndrome. *AJNR Am J Neuroradiol*. 2013 Jul;34(7):1297-1307.

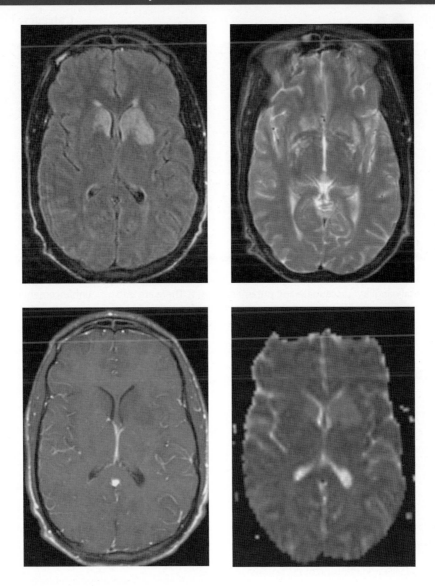

1. What is the differential diagnosis?

2. What CNS structures are most commonly involved?

3. What anatomic structure is the primary method of spread?

4. Prior to HAART therapy, what percentage of AIDS patients had this disease?

5. What is the treatment for this disease?

Case ranking/difficulty:

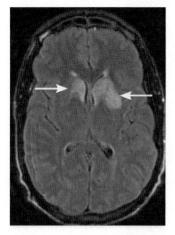

Axial FLAIR image shows increased asymmetric signal of the basal ganglia (*arrows*).

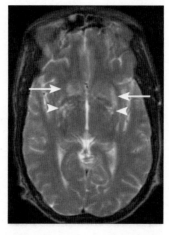

Axial T2 image shows abnormal signal of the caudate and putamen (*arrows*). There are also enlarged perivascular spaces (*arrowheads*) not completely suppressed on FLAIR (*not shown*).

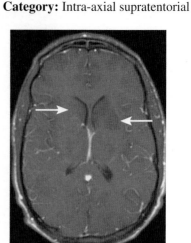

Axial T1 postcontrast shows no enhancement of the basal ganglia lesions (*arrows*).

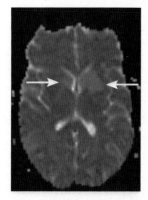

Axial DWI ADC image shows facilitated diffusion of the lesions (*arrows*).

Answers

1. Differential for bilateral asymmetric basal ganglia lesions without diffusion restriction includes cryptococcosis, viral encephalitis, and CNS lymphoma.

2. CNS cryptococcosis typically involves deep structures such as the deep gray nuclei, white matter, and brainstem.

3. CNS cryptococcosis typically spreads through the perivascular spaces, reaching deep brain structures in addition to causing meningitis.

4. 10% of patients with AIDS had cryptococcosis prior to the onset of HAART therapy. *Cryptococcus* is the third most common CNS infection in AIDS patients after HIV and toxoplasmosis.

5. Antifungals such as amphotericin B are used as the mainline of treatment. Maintenance therapy with fluconazole is indicated in AIDS patients.

Pearls

- *Cryptococcus* infection is the third most common CNS infection in AIDS patients.
- Cryptococci typically involves the lungs, which spread hematogenously to the CNS with deposition in the leptomeningeal and perivascular spaces.
- Perivascular spaces are filled with fungi and mucinous material forming gelatinous pseudocysts and cryptococcomas.
- Deep gray nuclei, brainstem, cerebellum, and white matter can be involved.
- MRI imaging shows dilated perivascular spaces with T2 hyperintense lesions with variable FLAIR suppression, and typically nonenhancement with weakened immune status.

Suggested Readings

Khandelwal N, Gupta V, Singh P. Central nervous system fungal infections in tropics. *Neuroimaging Clin N Am.* 2011 Nov;21(4):859-866, viii.

Sanossian N, Shatzmiller RA, Djabiras C, Liebeskind DS. FLAIR vascular hyperintensity preceding stroke in cryptococcal meningitis. *J Neuroimaging.* 2013 Jan;23(1):126-128.

9-year-old male with disorientation, developmental regression, and altered mental status

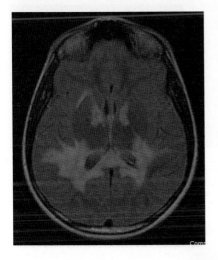
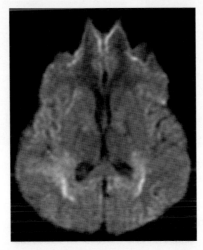
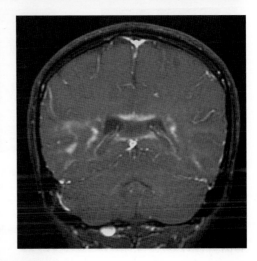
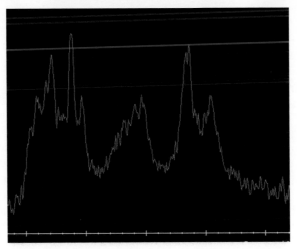

1. What are the typical imaging characteristics of this entity?

2. What is the symptomatic pathophysiological process of this disease?

3. What is typically seen on MRI spectroscopy within the affected white matter?

4. What is the genetic inheritance and age- and gender-based phenotypes for this disease?

5. What is the MR scoring system of this disease?

Case ranking/difficulty:

Category: Intra-axial supratentorial

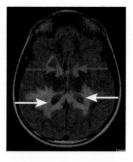 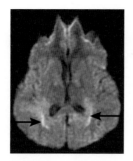 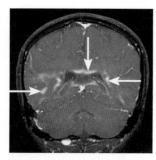 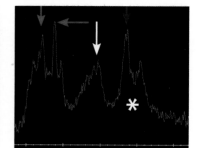

Symmetric T2 prolongation involving the splenium (*blue arrow*), periatrial (*white arrows*), and capsular white matter (*red arrows*) is seen in this classic pattern of x-linked adrenoleukodystrophy.

Peripheral areas of diffusion restriction (*black arrows*) are indicative of acute demyelination.

Postcontrast enhancement (*white arrows*) of the intermediate zone of demyelination is typical of progressive X-ALD.

MRI spectroscopy of the involved white matter demonstrates decrease in NAA (*white arrow*), elevation of choline (*red arrow*) and myo-inositol (*green arrow*) with significant presence of lactate (*blue arrow*) and lipid breakdown products and very long chain fatty acid molecules in the 0.9 to 2.4 ppm range (*asterisk*).

Answers

1. Posterior symmetric, confluent involvement of the parietal, occipital, and temporal white matter is classic with subcortical U fibers usually spared early. The splenium is typically involved. The "leading-edge" enhancement, which correlates with the intermediate zone of inflammation, is an imaging sign correlating with disease progression.

2. X-ALD is an inherited peroxisomal metabolism disorder where there is failure of oxidation of very long chain fatty acids. While metabolites are deposited in all tissues, including the liver, only the CNS myelin, adrenal cortex, and Leydig cell of the testes lead to symptomatology.

3. While the MRI spectroscopic profile is nonspecific, elevation of lactate, choline, and myo-inositol is a typical finding. NAA is decreased within the abnormal appearing white matter. Decrease in NAA in normal-appearing white matter may reflect progression. Lipids are typically elevated, which reflects the deposition of very long chain fatty acids.

4. Classic adrenoleukodystrophy is x-linked, with the expected male predominance. Up to 50% of carrier females will have adult-onset symptoms, usually adrenomyeloneuropathy-like symptoms with predominantly spinal and peripheral nerve involvement, as well as adrenal failure. Variant adult-onset forms are less common, although with increasing recognition, the percentage will likely increase. Adult-onset forms typically present with adrenomyeloneuropathy.

5. The Loes MRI scoring system correlates with disease progression:
   - Pattern 1 is the typical posterior white matter involvement associated with late childhood onset.
   - Pattern 2 has a frontal white matter predominance with similar progression as pattern 1.
   - Pattern 3 involves the corticospinal tracts usually seen in adults with slower progression.
   - Pattern 4 includes the cerebellar white matter in addition to the corticospinal tract and is seen in the adolescent-onset form.
   - Pattern 5 has fulminant frontal and posterior involvement with rapid progression.

Pearls

- Posterior, symmetric, and central involvement of the splenium, periatrial, and capsular white matter is typical.
- Intermediate zone of enhancement and peripheral zone of diffusion restriction is typical as the demyelination progresses.

Suggested Readings

Kim JH, Kim HJ. Childhood X-linked adrenoleukodystrophy: clinical-pathologic overview and MR imaging manifestations at initial evaluation and follow-up. *Radiographics*. 2005 Jul;25(3):619-631.

Vijay K, Ouyang T. Anterior pattern disease in adrenoleukodystrophy. *Pediatr Radiol*. 2010 Dec;40(suppl 1):S157.

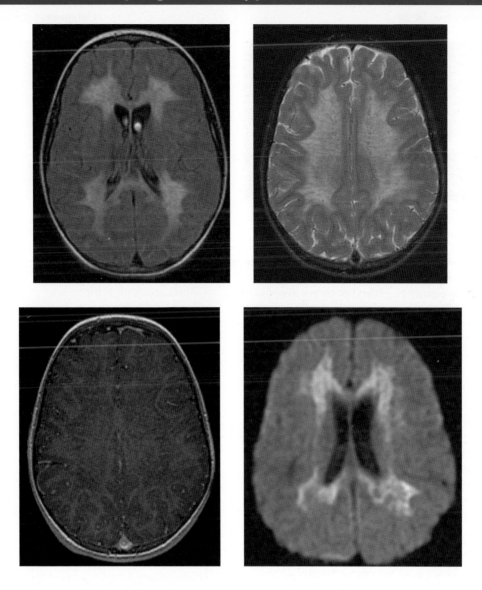

1. What are the typical MRI findings of this disease?

2. What is the pattern of white matter involvement as the disease progresses?

3. What is the pathophysiology of this disease?

4. What are the risk factors for this disease?

5. What is the usual clinical presentation of the common form of this disease?

Case ranking/difficulty:

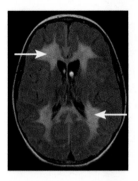

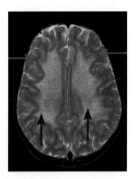

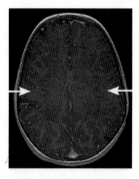

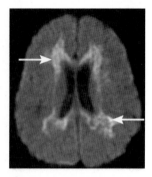

Axial T2 FLAIR shows diffuse white matter demyelination with T2 hyperintensity in a symmetric, confluent distribution in a "butterfly" pattern with both anterior and posterior involvement (*white arrows*). Demyelination of the corpus callosum is seen later in the disease (*red arrows*).

T2 axial image above the ventricles demonstrates confluent symmetric involvement of the centrum semiovale. There is sparing of the subcortical U fibers (*red arrows*) as well as the perivenular myelin (*blue arrows*), giving the appearance of a "tigroid" pattern.

Postcontrast imaging shows no enhancement, due to the lack of inflammation seen with this disease. Note the sparing of the subcortical U-fibers, seen early in the disease (*white arrows*).

There is decreased diffusion seen in the areas of active demyelination (*white arrows*).

Answers

1. Metachromatic leukodystrophy (MLD) classically is confluent, symmetric, and involves both anterior and posterior portions of the cerebral hemispheres in a "butterfly" pattern. Decreased diffusion can be seen in active demyelination but a lack of histological inflammation corresponds with a lack of contrast enhancement. Sparing of the perivenular myelin can lead to "leopard" spots and "tigroid" stripes within the affected white matter.

2. Metachromatic leukodystrophy typically spares the subcortical U-fibers, internal capsule, and deep callosal fibers early in the disease. As the disease progresses, these white matter structures are usually involved. Corticospinal tract involvement in the brainstem can be seen in the late phase of the disease. Histological demyelination of the Schwann cells of the peripheral nervous system is a typical finding of all subtypes of metachromatic leukodystrophy.

3. MLD is a lysosomal storage disorder with defect of arylsulfatase-A, located at 22q13, leading to the accumulation of sulfatides. These deposit symptomatically in the CNS, PNS, and gallbladder, but can also be seen asymptomatically in other abdominal organs. There are three main clinical forms of MLD: late infantile, juvenile, and adult onset, with the late infantile being the most common of the three.

4. Risk factors for MLD include Navajo Indian ancestry, Habbanite Jewish ancestry, or a relative with the disease.

5. The late infantile form is the most common presentation of MLD. Insidious onset of symptoms begins around 2 years of age with gait disturbance, weakness, hypotonia, and ataxia as common presenting signs. Abdominal pain can be seen with sulfatide deposition in the gallbladder.

Pearls

- Bilateral symmetric and confluent "butterfly" pattern of demyelination of the hemispheric cerebral white matter.
- Lack of white matter enhancement due to lack of inflammation. Cranial nerves have been described to demonstrate enhancement.
- Subcortical and capsular white matter typically spared early in the disease.
- "Tigroid" appearance of the spared perivenular myelin.

Suggested Readings

Martin A, Sevin C, Lazarus C, Bellesme C, Aubourg P, Adamsbaum C. Toward a better understanding of brain lesions during metachromatic leukodystrophy evolution. *AJNR Am J Neuroradiol.* 2012 Oct;33(9):1731-1739.

Sener RN. Metachromatic leukodystrophy: diffusion MR imaging findings. *AJNR Am J Neuroradiol.* 2002 Sep;23(8):1424-1426.

van der Voorn JP, Pouwels PJ, Kamphorst W, et al. Histopathologic correlates of radial stripes on MR images in lysosomal storage disorders. *AJNR Am J Neuroradiol.* 2005 Mar;26(3):442-446.

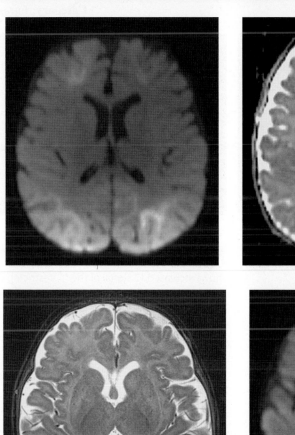

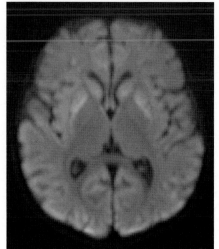

1. What are the typical MRI findings of this disease?

2. What is the method of inheritance of this disease?

3. What is the pathophysiology of this disease?

4. What are clinical symptoms and prognosis of this disease?

5. What diseases can show elevation of NAA on MR spectroscopy?

Case ranking/difficulty:

Category: Intra-axial supratentorial

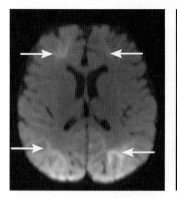

Axial DWI b = 1000 images show bright diffusion signal in the subcortical U-fibers of the frontal and occipital lobes (*white arrows*).

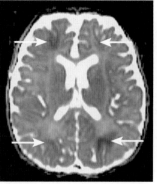

Axial ADC map confirms restricted diffusion of the subcortical white matter (*white arrows*).

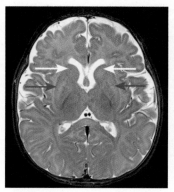

Axial T2 through the ganglionic level on follow-up imaging in 3 months of the same patient shows increased T2 signal of the bilateral caudate (*white arrows*) and putamen (*red arrows*).

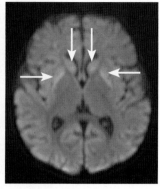

Corresponding axial DWI b = 1000 through the ganglionic level shows restricted diffusion of the corpus striatum (*white arrows*).

Answers

1. Canavan disease MRI findings have typically been described to involve the subcortical U-fibers early with progression centrally, but sparing the central white matter tracts of the corpus callosum and internal capsules early. Central gray structures such as the thalami and globi pallidi can be involved. Elevation of NAA is a hallmark of this disease.

2. Canavan disease is autosomal recessive with defect of the enzyme aspartoacylase, and predominantly seen in Ashkenazi Jewish populations.

3. Canavan disease is associated with mutations of the ASPA gene on chromosome 17. The ASPA gene encodes aspartylaminase enzyme, which breaks down N-acetyl aspartic acid. In Canavan disease, NAA deposition leads to toxicity of the CNS and can be detected in the urine.

4. Patients with Canavan disease typically present within the first year of life with macrocephaly, hypotonia, seizures, spasticity, and other signs of neurologic deterioration, leading to death in the first decade. A clinical subtype with a different mutation of the ASPA gene may have delayed onset, slower progression, and longer survival. No effective treatment currently exists, although ongoing trials with gene therapy and acetate supplementation may hold promise.

5. In addition to Canavan disease, Pelizaeus Merzbacher, a primary hypomyelination syndrome, can show mild increase in NAA with absolute measurements. Salla disease leads to a buildup of N-acetylneuraminic acid (free sialic acid), which has similar resonance with NAA. In addition, Salla disease may show increased creatine, which has not been reported in Canavan disease.

Pearls

- Typical descriptions of Canavan disease include early involvement of the subcortical U-fibers with progression, sparing the central white matter tracts such as the internal capsule and corpus callosum.
- Central gray matter involvement usually involves the thalami and globi pallidi, although caudate and putamen have been reported.
- MR spectroscopy shows the typical relative elevation of N-acetylaspartate (NAA), which is relatively specific.

Suggested Readings

Brismar J, Brismar G, Gascon G, Ozand P. Canavan disease: CT and MR imaging of the brain. *AJNR Am J Neuroradiol.* 1997 Jan;11(4):805-810.

Engelbrecht V, Scherer A, Rassek M, Witsack HJ, Mödder U. Diffusion-weighted MR imaging in the brain in children: findings in the normal brain and in the brain with white matter diseases. *Radiology.* 2002 Feb;222(2):410-418.

Hanefeld FA, Brockmann K, Pouwels PJ, Wilken B, Frahm J, Dechent P. Quantitative proton MRS of Pelizaeus-Merzbacher disease: evidence of dys- and hypomyelination. *Neurology.* 2005 Sep;65(5):701-706.

6-month old with history of prematurity, necrotizing enterocolitis, developmental delay, and spasticity. Had minor head trauma with abnormal imaging findings

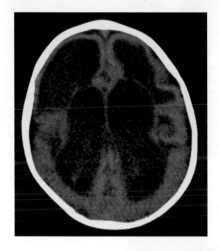
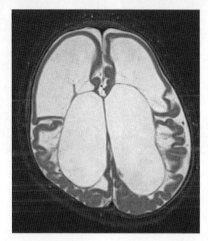
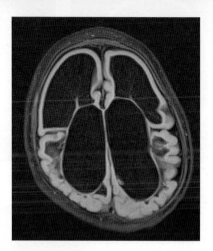

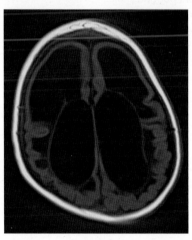
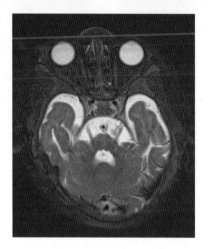

1. What are MRI findings that have been proposed as obligatory criteria for this diagnosis?

2. What is the genetic basis of the disease?

3. What other organ systems have been described to present with pathology with this disease?

4. What clinical factors cause episodes of deterioration?

5. Which group has a higher risk of this disease?

Case ranking/difficulty:

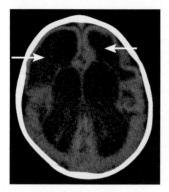

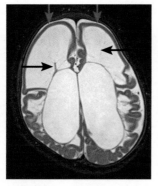

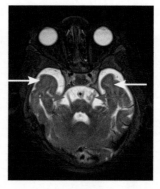

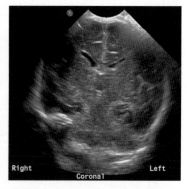

Axial CT for head trauma shows severe hypodensity of the frontal white matter (*white arrows*), which has the same density as CSF in the dilated lateral ventricles.

Axial T2 image shows diffuse abnormal white matter involving both central and peripheral subcortical fibers with high T2 signal intensity following CSF. There are hypointense radial bands of tissue traveling through the affected white matter (*black arrows*). The frontal gyri are lissencephalic (*red arrows*) but with normal thickness and intensity.

Axial T2 image of the pons shows relative sparing of the temporal lobes (*white arrows*). There is prominence of the fourth ventricles from pontine and cerebellar atrophy. The bilateral fifth cranial nerves appear prominent (*red arrows*).

Coronal ultrasound at birth shows a normal volume of white matter.

Answers

1. Diffuse involvement of the cerebral white matter with progression to CSF signal is a hallmark of this disease. FLAIR suppression is key to imaging diagnosis. White matter fluid-filled space without complete collapse and without contrast enhancement is typical, with the temporal lobes relatively spared. Cerebellar white matter can be involved, demonstrating atrophy and T2 hyperintensity without rarefaction to CSF signal.

2. Vanishing white matter disease is autosomal recessive with mutations involving the EIF2B protein complex. This complex is involved in regulating RNA translation to prevent protein misfolding in times of cellular stress.

3. In adult-onset forms of vanishing white matter, premature ovarian failure has been described in a few cases.

4. Episodes of deterioration in vanishing white matter disease are precipitated by a recent history of stressors.

5. Cree leukoencephalopathy is a subgroup of vanishing white matter disease, which presents in the infant with rapid decline. This group of people lives predominantly in the northern Quebec and Manitoba regions. Carrier rates in this population are higher than general at 1 in 10 in a study of 50 unaffected Cree adults.

Pearls

- Rarefaction of white matter following CSF signal with suppression on FLAIR is characteristic.
- Disease progresses from central to peripheral without sparing of subcortical U-fibers.
- Relative sparing of the temporal lobes.
- No rarefaction of cerebellum or brainstem; however, these structures may show atrophy and T2 prolongation.

Suggested Readings

Senol U, Haspolat S, Karaali K, Lüleci E. MR imaging of vanishing white matter. *AJR Am J Roentgenol.* 2000 Sep;175(3):826-828.

van der Knaap MS, Pronk JC, Scheper GC. Vanishing white matter disease. *Lancet Neurol.* 2006;5:413.

Vermeulen G, Seidl R, Mercimek-Mahmutoglu S, et al. Fright is a provoking factor in vanishing white matter disease. *Ann Neurol.* 2005;57:560.

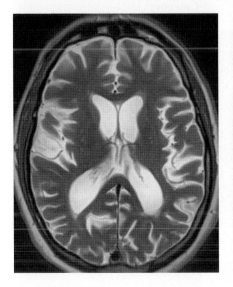
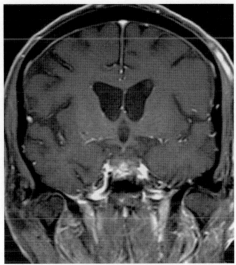
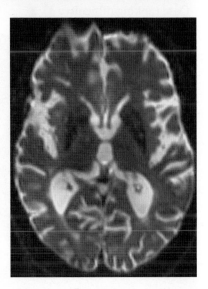

1. What are the described MRI findings for this disease?

2. What is the cause of decreased T2 signal of the striatum in this disease?

3. What are the classic clinical symptoms of this disease?

4. What is the genetic inheritance of this disease?

5. What are the organ systems affected in this disease?

Case ranking/difficulty: **Category:** Intra-axial supratentorial

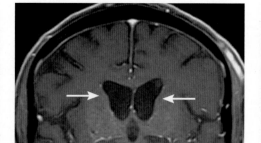

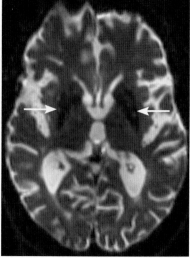

Axial T2 image through the ganglionic level shows caudate atrophy with increased T2 signal (*white arrows*), as well as diffuse cerebral atrophy.

Coronal T1 with contrast demonstrates dilatation of the frontal horns from caudate atrophy (*white arrows*).

Axial DWI b = 0 images demonstrate T2 hypointensity (T2*) from iron deposition in the bilateral putamen and globi pallidi (*white arrows*).

Answers

1. Caudate atrophy, with increased T2 signal from gliosis, is the hallmark of Huntington disease. Diffuse cerebral atrophy and decreased T2 signal of the striatum are typical associated findings.

2. Decreased T2 signal in Huntington disease within the corpus striatum is due to iron deposition. Iron deposition in the globus pallidus is a normal function of aging, so care should be made not to overcall iron deposition in this structure.

3. Huntington disease typically presents with variable severity of the triad of chorea, dementia, and psychosis (personality changes).

4. Huntington disease is inherited in an autosomal dominant fashion with trinucleotide repeat mutations of the huntingtin protein gene on chromosome 4p16.3. The greater the number of trinucleotide repeats, the worse the disease. There is complete penetrance of the mutation.

5. In addition to the brain, abnormal Huntingtin protein causes pathology in the gonads, heart, lungs, and liver.

Pearls

- Huntington disease is an autosomal dominant inherited disease characterized by choreiform movements.
- MRI demonstrates caudate atrophy with increased T2 signal from gliosis.
- Diffuse cerebral atrophy is also seen with decreased T2 signal of the striatum from iron deposition.
- No treatment exists with most patients dying within two decades from disease onset.

Suggested Readings

Hobbs NZ, Barnes J, Frost C, et al. Onset and progression of pathologic atrophy in Huntington disease: a longitudinal MR imaging study. *AJNR Am J Neuroradiol.* 2010 Jun;31(6):1036-1041.

Mahalingam S, Levy LM. Genetics of Huntington disease. *AJNR Am J Neuroradiol.* 2014;35(6):1070-1072.

54-year-old male with progressive balance problems, falls, and speech difficulty

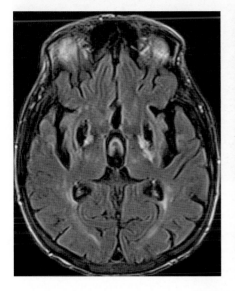
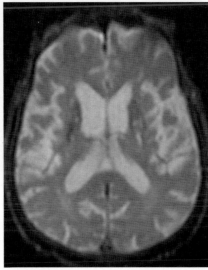
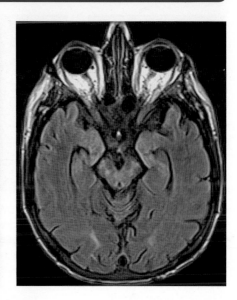
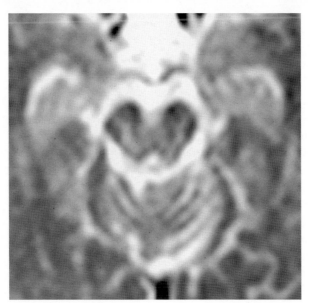

1. What are the MRI findings in this disease?

2. What causes the "face of the giant panda" sign?

3. What is the genetic basis of this disease?

4. What is the pathophysiology of this disease?

5. What are treatment options for this disease?

Wilson disease

Case ranking/difficulty:

Category: Intra-axial supratentorial

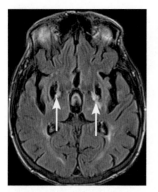

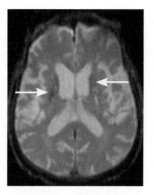

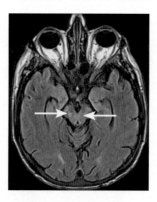

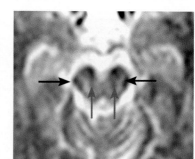

Axial FLAIR shows suppression of the central putamen lesions with surrounding hyperintensity. This is consistent with late cystic degeneration. There is bilateral hyperintensity of the globi pallidi and left internal capsule (*white arrows*).

Axial b = 0 DWI image shows the decreased signal from copper deposition in the bilateral caudate and putamen (*white arrows*).

Axial FLAIR through the midbrain demonstrates focal T2 hyperintensity of the midbrain (*white arrows*).

Axial b = 0 DWI zoomed in image of the midbrain demonstrates the face of the giant panda sign with tegmental T2 hyperintensity, T2 hypointensity of the red nuclei (*red arrows*), and cerebral peduncles (*black arrows*). This is characteristic in Wilson disease.

Answers

1. Bilateral symmetric T2 hyper- and hypointensities of the basal ganglia and thalami are hallmarks of Wilson disease from copper deposition. T2 hyperintensity of the midbrain causing a "face of the giant panda" sign is also characteristic. T2 hyperintense lesions in the cerebral and cerebellar white have also been described. No enhancement is typically seen.

2. The "face of the giant panda" sign is characteristic of Wilson disease when the midbrain tegmentum becomes edematous with increased T2 signal. The normal T2 hypointense signal of the red nuclei from iron deposition makes the eyes of the panda while the cerebral peduncles make the ears.

3. Wilson disease is an autosomal recessive disease with mutations of the ATP7B gene on chromosome 13q14-q21, which encodes an ATPase copper transporting peptide.

4. Wilson disease is a disorder of copper transportation, with the inability to excrete excess copper leading to deposition in the liver and other organ systems causing free radicals and cellular damage.

5. Wilson disease can be treated by restricting dietary intake of copper, impairing the absorption of copper with zinc, and chelating excess copper with penicillamine. Orthotopic liver transplant can cure Wilson disease.

Pearls

- Wilson disease is an autosomal recessive disease with impairment of copper transport, leading to copper deposition in the liver and other organs.
- MRI findings of the brain primarily involve the basal ganglia and thalami with mixed T2 hyperintensity from swelling and atrophy, as well as hypointensity from copper deposition.
- The "face of the giant panda" sign from T2 hyperintensity of the midbrain with normal hypointensity of the red nuclei is characteristic.
- Patchy white matter T2 hyperintensity of the cerebrum and cerebellum can also be seen.
- Treatment with chelating agents can reverse MRI findings.

Suggested Readings

Aggarwal A, Bhatt M. Update on Wilson disease. *Int Rev Neurobiol*. 2013 Nov;110(110):313-348.

Trocello JM, Woimant F, El Balkhi S, et al. Extensive striatal, cortical, and white matter brain MRI abnormalities in Wilson disease. *Neurology*. 2013 Oct;81(17):1557.

11-year-old female with delayed onset of walking and progressive loss of function

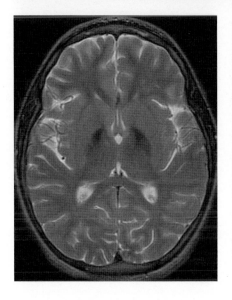 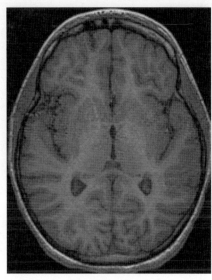 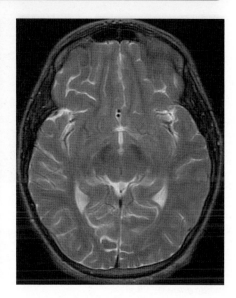

1. What disease is the eye of the tiger sign associated with?

2. What causes decreased signal of the globi pallidi in this disease?

3. What areas other than the globi pallidi can show decreased T2 signal?

4. What is the treatment of this disease?

5. What are typical clinical symptoms of the disease?

Case ranking/difficulty: 🦋🦋   **Category:** Intra-axial supratentorial

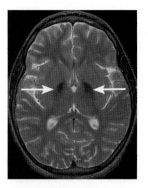 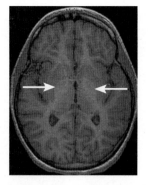 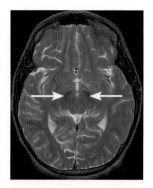 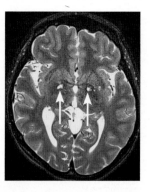

Axial T2 image of the ganglionic level shows significant T2 hypointensity of the bilateral globi pallidi from pathologic iron deposition (*white arrows*).

Axial T1 image of the ganglionic level shows T1 shortening of the globi pallidi (*white arrows*) blending in with myelinated white matter.

Axial T2 of the midbrain shows greater than expected decreased signal of the cerebral peduncles from iron deposition in the substantia nigra (*white arrows*).

Axial T2 image of a patient with "eye of the tiger" sign seen with PANK2 mutations shows central globi pallidi T2 hyperintensity (*white arrows*), thought to represent cystic degeneration within the iron deposition.

Answers

1. The "eye of the tiger" sign is specific for pantothenate kinase-associated neurodegeneration with PANK2 mutation.

2. Neurodegeneration with brain iron accumulation all demonstrate abnormal deposition of iron in the globi pallidi.

3. Typical locations for normal or pathologic iron deposition other than the globi pallidi are the dentate nuclei, substantia nigra, red nucleus, and putamen.

4. Aceruloplasminemia is the only subtype of neurodegeneration with brain iron accumulation that can be treated with iron chelation. Palliative care of extrapyramidal symptoms, which develop in these diseases, are indicated.

5. Extrapyramidal signs such as dysarthria and dystonia are common symptoms. Ataxia and vision loss from retinal degeneration are also common symptoms.

Pearls

- Neurodegeneration with brain iron accumulation (NBIA) is an umbrella term that includes pantothenate kinase–associated degeneration (PKAN), previously known as Hallervorden-Spatz.
- Decreased T2 signal and susceptibility on T2* imaging from iron deposition are seen symmetrically within the globi pallidi, substantia nigra, and variably in the dentate nuclei, corpus striatum, and cortex.
- The "eye of the tiger" sign with central T2 hyperintensity within the T2 dark globi pallidi is specific for PANK2 mutation of PKAN.
- Care must be made to distinguish pathology from normal iron deposition of the globi pallidi with aging, especially on 3T.

Suggested Readings

Guillerman RP. The eye-of-the-tiger sign. *Radiology*. 2000 Dec;217(3):895-896.

Hayflick SJ, Hartman M, Coryell J, Gitschier J, Rowley H. Brain MRI in neurodegeneration with brain iron accumulation with and without PANK2 mutations. *AJNR Am J Neuroradiol*. 2010 Mar;27(6):1230-1233.

Kruer MC, Boddaert N, Schneider SA, et al. Neuroimaging features of neurodegeneration with brain iron accumulation. *AJNR Am J Neuroradiol*. 2012 Mar;33(3):407-414.

23-month-old male with loss of milestones, developmental regression, and macrocephaly

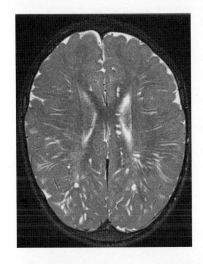
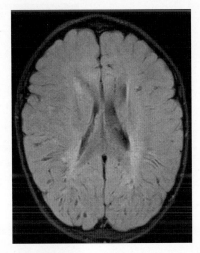
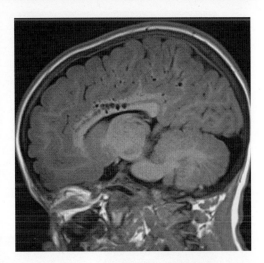
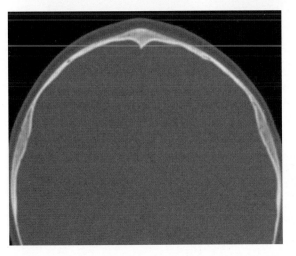
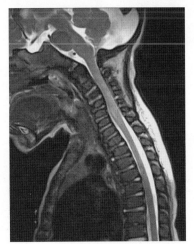
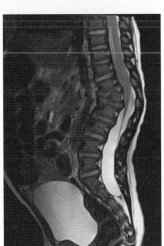

1. What are the brain findings of this disease?

2. What can be seen within the spine of this disease?

3. What is the metabolite deposited in the organs?

4. What is the treatment for this disease?

5. What are common initial presenting symptoms?

Case ranking/difficulty:

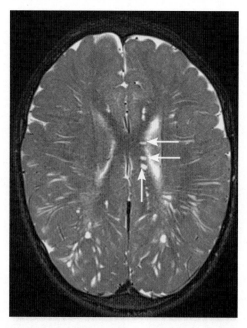

Axial T2 image of the supraganglionic brain shows numerous dilated perivascular spaces, including extension into the corpus callosum (*white arrows*).

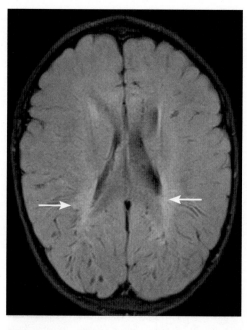

Axial FLAIR of the supraganglionic brain demonstrates suppression of the numerous dilated perivascular spaces with adjacent periventricular white matter T2 hyperintensity (*white arrows*).

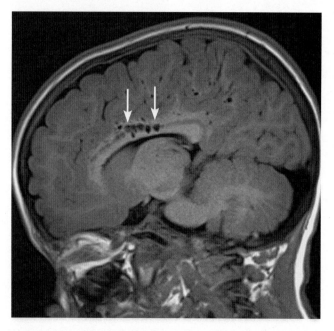

Sagittal T1 just left of midline shows involvement of the corpus callosum (*white arrows*), which is not usually involved in normal variant dilated perivascular spaces.

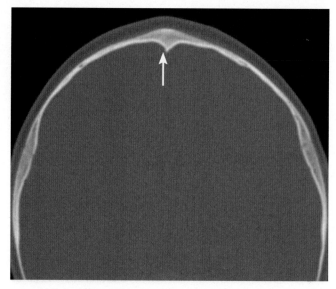

CT of the frontal skull shows ridging from metopic suture synostosis (*white arrow*).

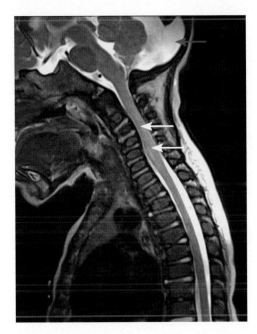

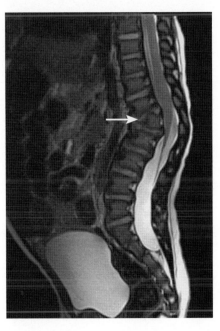

Sagittal T2 image of the upper spine shows cervical stenosis with increased T2 signal in the cord (*white arrows*). Note large cystic space of the posterior fossa (*red arrow*). Mega cisterna magna is associated with mucopolysaccharidoses.

Sagittal T2 image of the lower spine shows a gibbus deformity and focal kyphosis at L1 (*white arrow*).

Answers

1. Mucopolysaccharidoses demonstrate dilated perivascular spaces from glycosaminoglycan (GAG) deposition with T2 hyperintensities of the surrounding white matter. All mucopolysaccharidoses can demonstrate this finding with the exception of Morquio syndrome (MPS4).

2. Within the spine, cranial cervical junction stenosis causing cervical myelopathy can be caused by deposition of GAG around the dens, atlantoaxial instability, and a short arch of C1. Lumbar gibbus deformity with kyphosis can be seen in the most severe forms. Anterior wedging of the vertebral bodies is a skeletal dysplasia in mucopolysaccharidoses.

3. Heparan, dermatan, and chondroitin sulfate are all glycosaminoglycans and are deposited in different types of mucopolysaccharidoses.

4. Bone marrow transplant and recombinant enzyme therapy can be used to treat mucopolysaccharidoses. With the most severe form MPS1H (hurler) the disease is fatal within a decade.

5. A wide range of symptoms can be seen with mucopolysaccharidoses including macrocephaly, developmental delay, corneal clouding, gargoylism, and sensorineural hearing loss.

Pearls

- Mucopolysaccharidoses are a group of inherited metabolic disease that fail to break down glycosaminoglycans (GAG).
- Type 1H (Hurler) is the prototype and most severe form.
- All organ systems can be involved.
- In the CNS, GAG is deposited in the perivascular spaces leading to dilatation and adjacent white matter T2 hyperintensity.
- Skeletal changes include metopic suture beaking, lumbar gibbus deformity, and cranial cervical stenosis.

Suggested Readings

Kwee RM, Kwee TC. Virchow-Robin spaces at MR imaging. *Radiographics*. 2010 Aug;27(4):1071-1086.

Zafeiriou DI, Batzios SP. Brain and spinal MR imaging findings in mucopolysaccharidoses: a review. *AJNR Am J Neuroradiol*. 2013 Jan;34(1):5-13.

20-year-old female with new-onset left facial droop and sudden vision loss, history of headaches and seizures, prior strokes

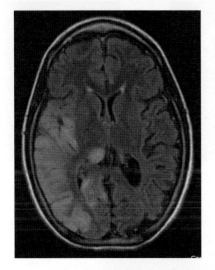
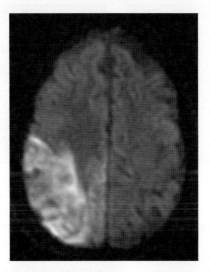
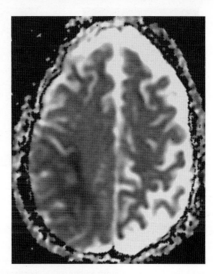
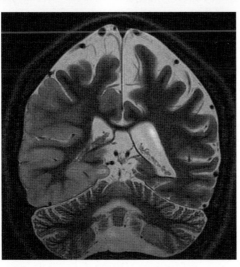
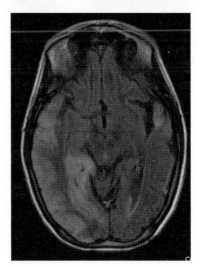

1. What are the typical MRI findings of this disease?

2. What is the differential diagnosis for this appearance?

3. What is the clinical presentation of this disease?

4. What is the pathogenesis of the disease?

5. What is the inheritance of this disease?

Case ranking/difficulty:

Category: Intra-axial supratentorial

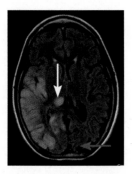

Axial FLAIR image through the ganglionic level shows T2 hyperintensity and swelling of the right temporal lobe, insula, and occipital lobe. In addition, the pulvinar region of the thalamus is also involved (*white arrow*) in these stroke-like lesions. This involves both the PCA and MCA arterial distributions. Note the atrophy of the left occipital lobe from prior stroke-like involvement (*red arrow*).

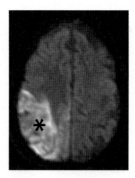

Axial DWI b = 1000 image above the ganglionic level shows right posterior parietal bright signal from an acute stroke-like lesion (*asterisk*).

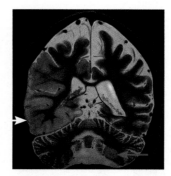

Coronal T2 image shows right temporal and occipital hyperintensity and swelling from acute stroke-like lesion (*white arrow*). Note the focal hyperintensity and swelling in the inferior left cerebellar hemisphere (*red arrow*), which showed no diffusion restriction consistent with a subacute lesion.

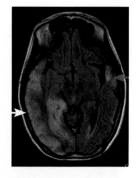

Axial FLAIR image shows the right temporal and occipital acute stroke-like lesion (*white arrow*) as well as a chronic lesion of the left temporal lobe tip with gliosis (*red arrow*).

Answers

1. MELAS typically will have multiple stroke-like lesions primarily involving the posterior cerebrum and basal ganglia with different stages of evolution. Angiography is typically normal.

2. Leigh disease, MERRF, and vasculitis can give multiple areas of parenchymal cytotoxic edema at different times. Embolic stroke, especially with multiple emboli, can give multiple vascular distribution infarcts and can give strokes of different ages if the embolic source is not treated.

3. The clinical presentation is varied with myopathy inducing exercise intolerance, migraines, diabetes, hearing loss, failure to thrive for infantile presentation, neuropsychiatric illness (such as depression), and blindness (either from cortical blindness or from optic atrophy).

4. Pathogenesis of MELAS is not exactly known but is thought to involve oxidative phosphorylation deficiency of the brain and vessel wall cells.

5. MELAS, as a mitochondrial DNA disorder, is inherited through maternal mitochondria. Familial inheritance is more common than sporadic mutations. 80% of MELAS patients will have mutation of MT-TL1.

Pearls

- MELAS (mitochondrial myopathy, encephalopathy, lactic acidosis, and stroke-like episodes) has variable phenotype and different clinical presentations.
- MRI of MELAS shows stroke-like lesions indistinguishable from vascular infarction but typically does not follow a vascular distribution.
- Stroke-like lesions usually involve the posterior cerebrum and basal ganglia.
- There may be multiple stroke-like lesions demonstrating differing ages of evolution.
- Consider MELAS for unexplained strokes in a young patient.

Suggested Readings

Abe K, Yoshimura H, Tanaka H, Fujita N, Hikita T, Sakoda S. Comparison of conventional and diffusion-weighted MRI and proton MR spectroscopy in patients with mitochondrial encephalomyopathy, lactic acidosis, and stroke-like events. *Neuroradiology*. 2004 Feb;46(2):113-117.

Kim IO, Kim JH, Kim WS, Hwang YS, Yeon KM, Han MC. Mitochondrial myopathy-encephalopathy-lactic acidosis-and strokelike episodes (MELAS) syndrome: CT and MR findings in seven children. *AJR Am J Roentgenol*. 1996 Mar;166(3):641-645.

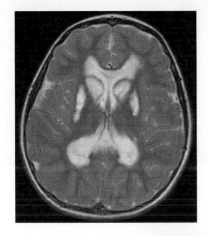
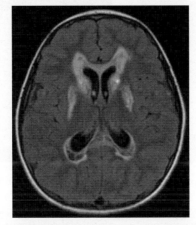
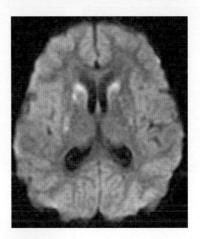

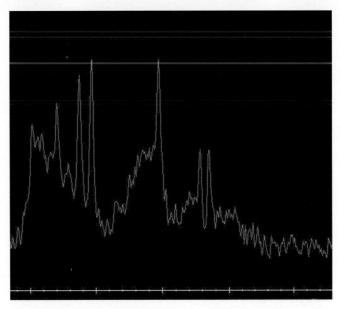

1. What is the differential diagnosis?

2. What is the significance of the diffusion restriction in this case?

3. What is the most common genetic defect for this group of diseases?

4. What is the prognosis of this disease?

5. What is the mode of genetic inheritance?

Case ranking/difficulty: **Category:** Intra-axial supratentorial

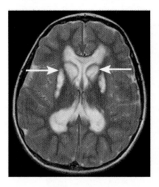 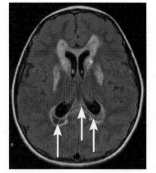 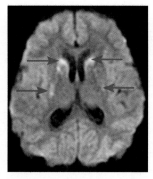 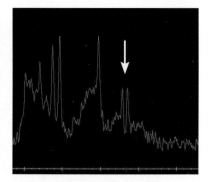

Axial T2 image through the ganglionic level of a patient with non-SURF1 Leigh syndrome shows T2 hyperintensity of the bilateral caudate and putamen (*white arrows*) as well as the corpus callosum and periventricular white matter (*red arrows*). The bilateral caudate heads appear swollen, while the putamina appear atrophic.

Axial FLAIR image through the ganglionic level shows bilateral symmetric caudate and putamen hyperintensity as well as callosal and periventricular white matter involvement. Note the cavitation of the splenium and periatrial white matter (*white arrows*).

Axial b = 1000 DWI image shows decreased diffusion corresponding to bright signal of the bilateral caudate heads and some spots in the putamina (*red arrows*). This correlates with more acute injury.

MR spectroscopy of the basal ganglia shows a prominent lactate doublet peak at 1.4 ppm (*white arrow*).

5. Leigh syndrome genetic mutations can be both mitochondrial and nuclear with inheritance including mitochondrial, autosomal recessive, and x-linked.

Answers

1. The differential for bilateral, relatively symmetric basal ganglia swelling, and diffusion restriction includes anoxic injury and metabolic disease, which includes non-SURF1 Leigh syndrome, Krabbe, and Glutaric aciduria. The white matter involvement is commonly seen with Krabbe, and is uncommon for Leigh syndrome. This patient has a non-SURF1 Leigh syndrome. SURF1 mutation Leigh syndrome characteristically does not involve the basal ganglia.

2. In this case of Leigh syndrome, metabolic stressors cause increased mitochondrial demand, which cannot be met by dysfunctional mitochondrial respiration, leading to deterioration.

3. Leigh syndrome is a genetically heterogeneous group of diseases that causes defects in mitochondrial respiration. The most common genetic defect are SURF1 mutations, which contribute to cytochrome C oxidase (COX).

4. Leigh syndrome typically presents within the first year of life with progressive deterioration to death in childhood for most patients. The SURF1 mutation Leigh syndrome has an earlier onset with rapid progression and dismal prognosis. Episodes of deterioration seem to coincide with metabolic stressors, such as infection.

Pearls

- Leigh syndrome is a genetically heterogeneous group of metabolic neurodegenerative disorders with abnormality of mitochondrial respiration.
- SURF1 mutations are the most common of the Leigh syndromes that show characteristic symmetric involvement of the subthalamic nuclei, cerebellum, and lower brainstem. There is worse prognosis and rapid deterioration to death.
- Non-SURF1 Leigh disease usually involves the bilateral basal ganglia, thalami, cerebral peduncles, and midbrain tegmentum.
- Acute areas of involvement typically show T2 hyperintensity from swelling and diffusion restriction without significant enhancement.
- No treatment is available with most cases progressing to death in childhood.

Suggested Readings

Arii J, Tanabe Y. Leigh syndrome: serial MR imaging and clinical follow-up. *AJNR Am J Neuroradiol.* 2000 Sep;21(8):1502-1509.

Rossi A, Biancheri R, Bruno C, et al. Leigh syndrome with COX deficiency and SURF1 gene mutations: MR imaging findings. *AJNR Am J Neuroradiol.* 2003 Sep;24(6):1188-1191.

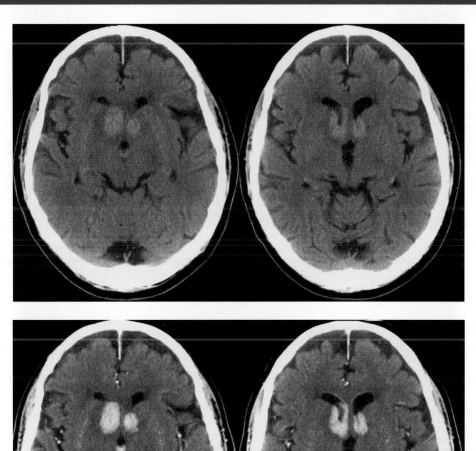

1. Where is the abnormality located?

2. What are the classic imaging findings of this entity on MRI?

3. What is the differential diagnosis?

4. What is the significance of high attenuation on noncontrast CT with this entity?

5. What is the treatment for this entity?

Case ranking/difficulty:

Category: Intra-axial supratentorial

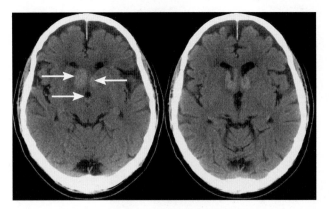

Axial CT images without contrast shows high-density masses along both ependymal surfaces of the basal ganglia. Similar attenuation is seen in the interpeduncular cistern (*arrows*). Surrounding mass effect is seen within the basal ganglia

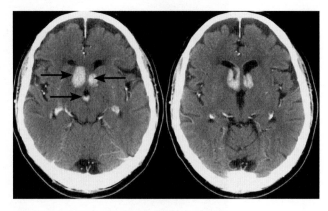

Axial CT postcontrast shows the high-density areas now demonstrate enhancement along both ependymal surfaces of the basal ganglia and in the interpeduncular cistern (*arrows*).

3. The differential diagnosis includes lymphoma, glioma, and metastasis.

4. Non-Hodgkin lymphoma CNS metastasis classically demonstrates high density on CT. This is likely secondary to the high cellularity.

5. The treatment typically is intrathecal chemotherapy.

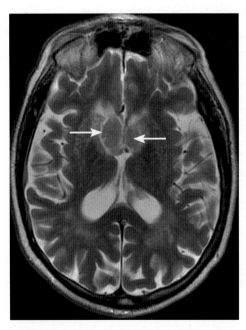

Axial T2 image shows the high-density areas on CT with corresponding low T2 signal (*arrows*).

Pearls

- Non-Hodgkin lymphoma with CNS metastasis occurs in 5% to 9% of patients.
- Metastatic CNS lymphoma commonly involves dura and leptomeninges; parenchymal lesions can also occur.
- When parenchymal lesions are seen, it is usually secondary to infiltration of perivascular spaces.
- Lymphoma typically has low T2 signal and high density on CT.
- Lymphoma may restrict diffusion on DWI.
- After administration of contrast, homogeneous enhancement is seen.

Answers

1. The abnormality is located along the ependymal surfaces of the anterior horns of the lateral ventricle, basal ganglia, and third ventricle.

2. CNS metastasis of non-Hodgkin lymphoma typically shows isointense to hypointense T1 signal and hypointense T2 signal on MRI. After administration of contrast, homogeneous enhancement is seen. Diffusion-weighted imaging may demonstrate restriction.

Suggested Readings

Comert M, Bassullu N, Kaya E, Kocak A. Intracranial involvement in a patient with Hodgkin's lymphoma. *Singapore Med J*. 2011 Sep;52(9):e180-e183.

Slone HW, Blake JJ, Shah R, Guttikonda S, Bourekas EC. CT and MRI findings of intracranial lymphoma. *AJR Am J Roentgenol*. 2005 May;184(5):1679-1685.

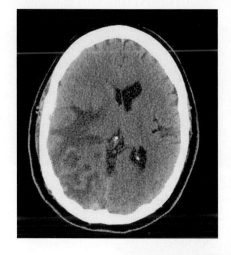
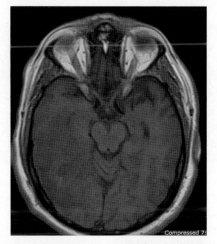
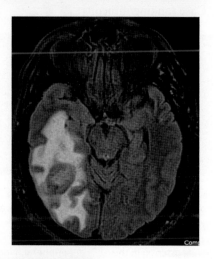

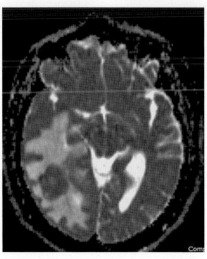
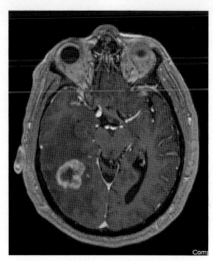

1. What is the differential diagnosis?

2. What is the most common age group in this tumor?

3. What is an imaging diagnostic clue in this disease?

4. Where is the common location of this tumor?

5. What is the prognosis of this disease?

Case ranking/difficulty: **Category:** Intra-axial supratentorial

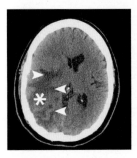

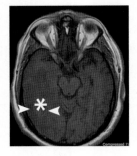

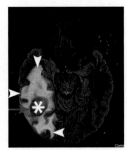

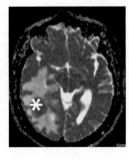

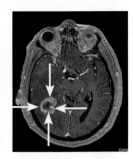

Noncontrast CT image demonstrates a hyperdense mass with a hypodense center (*white asterisk*) in the right temporo-occipital lobe with surrounding vasogenic edema (*white arrowheads*).

Axial T1 image demonstrates a T1 hypointense lesion (*white asterisk*) with faint peripheral hyperintensity (*white arrowheads*) in the right temporo-occipital lobe. This may represent blood products.

Axial T2 FLAIR image demonstrates mass (*white asterisk*) with surrounding vasogenic edema or tumor infiltration (*white arrowheads*) in the right temporo-occipital lobe. The rim of the mass is dark while the center is T2 hyperintense likely representing necrosis (*red arrow*).

Axial DWI ADC image shows the mass has restricted diffusion, likely representing hypercellularity in a high-grade neoplasm (*asterisk*).

Axial T1 postcontrast image demonstrates an irregular thick rim enhancing lesion (*white arrows*) in the right temporo-occipital lobe.

Answers

1. Gliosarcoma and glioblastoma multiforme are indistinguishable on imaging. Peripheral location with dural and skull invasion is a clue to suggest gliosarcoma. Metastasis, abscess, and lymphoma can also be included in the differential.

2. Gliosarcoma occurs most commonly in males (1.6:1, male:female), typically fifth to sixth decade.

3. A diagnostic clue for gliosarcoma is intra-axial peripheral location with dural and skull invasion. Glioblastoma will rarely have dural and skull invasion. Hemangiopericytoma can appear similarly as an extraaxial mass with dural and skull invasion.

4. In decreasing order of frequency, gliosarcoma most commonly occurs in temporal > parietal > frontal > occipital lobes. Cerebellar hemisphere occurrence has been reported in the literature.

5. The prognosis of gliosarcoma is poor, with median survival 6-12 months. Extracranial metastasis to lungs, liver, and lymph nodes is seen in 15%-30%, atypical for primary CNS neoplasms.

Pearls

- Rare, primary intra-axial brain tumor (WHO grade IV).
- Considered as a histological variant of glioblastoma multiforme (GBM).
- Two histological components: glial and mesenchymal (sarcomatous) components.
- Predilection toward the temporal lobes.
- Unlike other primary CNS neoplasms, 15%-30% metastasis to lungs, liver, and lymph nodes via the blood stream.
- Radiographic features are indistinguishable from GBM, a heterogenous rim enhancing mass with central necrosis or hemorrhage associated with more propensity for dural and/or skull invasion.
- Poor prognosis with median survival of 6-12 months.
- Treatment options include surgical resection, chemotherapy, and radiation.

Suggested Reading

Lee YY, Castillo M, Nauert C, Moser RP. Computed tomography of gliosarcoma. *AJNR Am J Neuroradiol.* 2000 Feb;6(4):527-531.

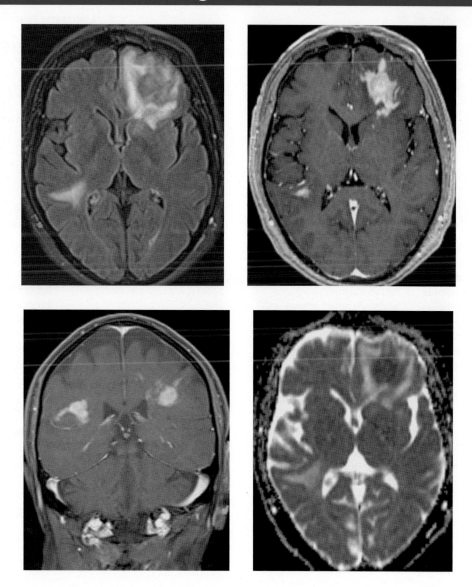

1. What are the differential diagnoses?

2. What is the greatest risk factor for this disease?

3. What are differences in imaging between the immunodeficient and immunocompetent individuals with this disease?

4. What imaging studies can be helpful in distinguishing this disease from glioblastoma?

5. What is the prognosis for this disease?

Case ranking/difficulty:

Category: Intra-axial supratentorial

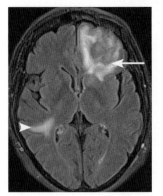

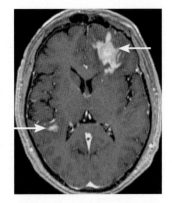

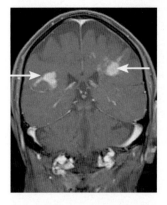

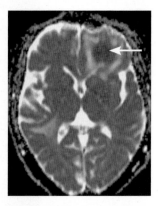

Axial FLAIR image shows a left frontal mass with central hypointensity and surrounding T2 hyperintensity (*arrow*). This extends to the ventricular margin with focal mass effect. A second T2 hyperintense lesion is seen in the right temporal parietal lobe subcortical white matter (*arrowhead*).

Axial T1 postcontrast image shows intense enhancement of the central portions of the multifocal noncontiguous masses is noted (*arrows*).

Coronal T1 postcontrast image shows flame-shaped irregular enhancement of the bilateral parietal lobe lesions (*arrows*).

Axial DWI ADC map shows central decreased diffusion (*arrow*) corresponding to hypercellularity or high nuclear to cytoplasmic ratio in this case of multifocal lymphoma.

Answers

1. In this case of primary multifocal CNS lymphoma, the differential includes progressive multifocal leukoencephalopathy, metastatic disease, tumefactive demyelination, and multifocal GBM.

2. The greatest risk factor for primary CNS lymphoma is immunodeficiency of which 95% is associated with the presence of the Epstein-Barr virus genome.

3. Primary CNS lymphoma typically demonstrates intense enhancement in immunocompetent individuals and ring enhancement in immunocompromised individuals.

4. The vast majority of glioblastoma will show central necrosis, while central necrosis is a less common feature for CNS lymphoma in immunocompetent individuals. Primary CNS lymphoma shows lower CBV, ADC, and FA values compared to GBM; however, this is based on relatively few studies. Overshoot of the baseline from first pass bolus on time to signal intensity curves of MRI DSC perfusion seem to be characteristic of lymphomas compared to GBM or metastatic disease.

5. Treatment with chemotherapy and radiation helps prolong survival, although most patients succumb to disease recurrence. Age greater than 60 years and involvement of the deep brain regions are some of the poor prognostic factors. Corticosteroid administration can show dramatic imaging improvement, although all patients demonstrate recurrence of disease once corticosteroids are stopped.

Pearls

- Primary CNS Lymphoma (PCNSL) is predominantly a B-cell non-Hodgkin lymphoma that presents in the CNS without systemic involvement at diagnosis.
- Immunodeficiency is the greatest risk for developing PCNSL.
- Incidence increases with age in immunocompetent individuals.
- PCNSL has a predilection for central periventricular structures such as basal ganglia, thalami, white matter including the corpus callosum.
- Multifocal disease can be seen in 25%.
- Intense enhancement is seen with immunocompetent individuals with ring enhancement in immunocompromised patients.
- Decreased ADC is typically seen either from high nuclear to cytoplasmic ratio or from hypercellularity.

Suggested Readings

Berger JR. Mass lesions of the brain in AIDS: the dilemmas of distinguishing toxoplasmosis from primary CNS lymphoma. *AJNR Am J Neuroradiol.* 2003 Apr;24(4):554-555.

Johnson BA, Fram EK, Johnson PC, Jacobowitz R. The variable MR appearance of primary lymphoma of the central nervous system: comparison with histopathologic features. *AJNR Am J Neuroradiol.* 1997 Mar;18(3):563-572.

Yamashita K, Yoshiura T, Hiwatashi A, et al. Differentiating primary CNS lymphoma from glioblastoma multiforme: assessment using arterial spin labeling, diffusion-weighted imaging, and 18F-fluorodeoxyglucose positron emission tomography. *Neuroradiology.* 2013 Feb;55(2):135-143.

13-year-old male with seizures

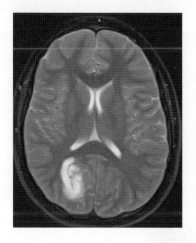
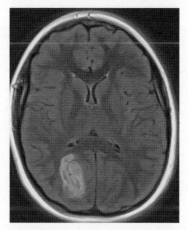
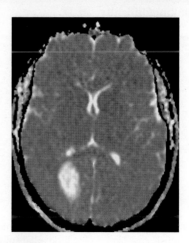

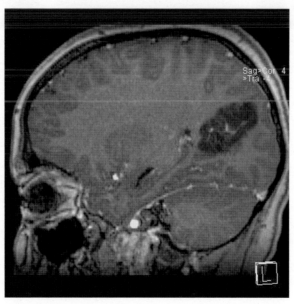

1. What is the differential diagnosis?

2. What is the embryological structure of origin for this tumor?

3. What are typical MRI findings of this tumor?

4. What is the typical clinical presentation?

5. What is the prognosis for this disease?

Case ranking/difficulty:

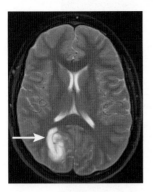

Axial T2 image shows a T2 hyperintense, cyst-like cortically based lesion (*arrow*) in the right parietal occipital lobe, which is well circumscribed.

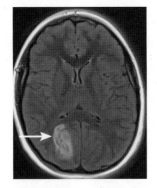

Axial FLAIR image shows little adjacent edema with increased to isointense signal of the tumor (*arrow*). The tumor is mildly wedge shaped and points toward the lateral ventricle.

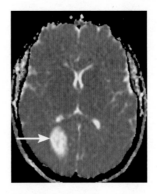

Axial DWI ADC map shows increased diffusion of the tumor (*arrow*).

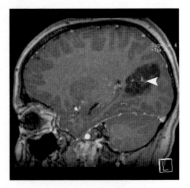

Sagittal T1 postcontrast image shows the lesion involving the cortex spanning the parietal occipital fissure without significant enhancement. The central linear enhancing structures represent cortical vessels (*arrowhead*).

Answers

1. The differential for a cortically based T2 hyperintense, cystic appearing lesion includes dysembryoplastic neuroepithelial tumor, cortical dysplasia of Taylor, and neuroepithelial cyst.

2. The origin of dysembryoplastic neuroepithelial tumors is thought to be dysplastic cells that originate in the germinal matrix and migrate out to the cortex.

3. Dysembryoplastic neuroepithelial tumors typically appear as bubbly, cyst-like, well-circumscribed, cortically based lesions without adjacent edema. There is a characteristic bright FLAIR rim sign of the cyst-like lesions, which usually are wedge shaped and point toward the lateral ventricles.

4. Patients with dysembryoplastic neuroepithelial tumors typically present with complex partial seizures.

5. Dysembryoplastic neuroepithelial tumors are indolent, with cure from complete surgical resection. Recurrence and malignant transformation are rare.

Pearls

- Dysembryoplastic neuroepithelial tumors (DNET) are benign WHO grade I cortically based tumors that typically present with complex partial seizures in the second to third decade of life.
- The typical appearance is a bubbly, cyst-like cortically based lesion that is wedge shaped and points toward the lateral ventricles.
- The cyst-like lesions are typically T2 bright with isointense to hypointense FLAIR signal, and FLAIR bright rim to the cyst-like lesions.
- There is usually no adjacent edema.
- Enhancement occurs in only 30% of lesions with nodular and ring enhancement.
- Recurrence is rare and may show atypical enhancement, but remains benign.
- Complete surgical resection is curative.
- Malignant degeneration is rare.

Suggested Readings

Campos AR, Clusmann H, von Lehe M, et al. Simple and complex dysembryoplastic neuroepithelial tumors (DNT) variants: clinical profile, MRI, and histopathology. *Neuroradiology.* 2009 Jul;51(7):433-443.

Fernandez C, Girard N, Paz Paredes A, Bouvier-Labit C, Lena G, Figarella-Branger D. The usefulness of MR imaging in the diagnosis of dysembryoplastic neuroepithelial tumor in children: a study of 14 cases. *AJNR Am J Neuroradiol.* 2003 May;24(5):829-834.

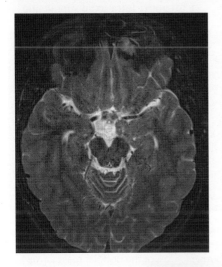
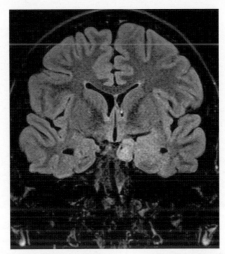
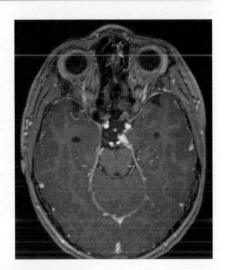

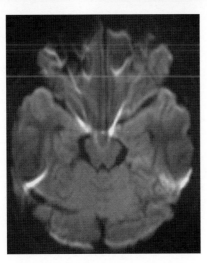
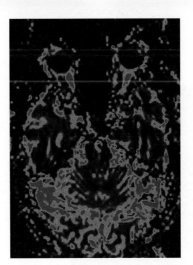

1. What is the differential diagnosis?

2. What are typical findings for this tumor?

3. What part of the brain is most commonly
   involved for this tumor?

4. What is the typical clinical presentation?

5. What is the prognosis for this disease?

Case ranking/difficulty:  **Category:** Intra-axial supratentorial

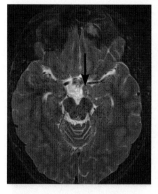

Axial T2 image shows an isointense mass projecting from the left uncus into the suprasellar cistern (*arrow*).

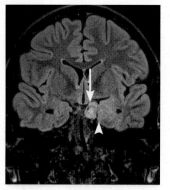

Coronal FLAIR image shows mild hyperintensity of the nodule (*arrow*) projecting from the uncus with associated thickening of the parahippocampal cortex (*arrowhead*).

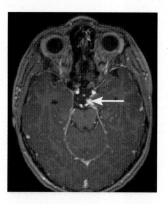

Axial T1 postcontrast shows homogeneous enhancement of the nodular mass (*arrow*).

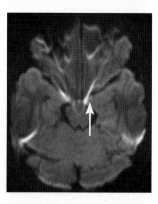

Axial DWI b = 1000 image shows no diffusion restriction of the nodular mass (*arrow*).

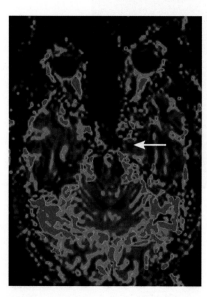

Color CBV map from dynamic susceptibility contrast perfusion imaging shows no increased perfusion of the tumor (*arrow*).

4. Temporal lobe seizures are the most common (90%) presentation of gangliogliomas. Gangliogliomas are the most common neoplastic cause of temporal lobe seizures.

5. Gangliogliomas are typically WHO grade I-II tumors with complete surgical resection being curative. 94% recurrence-free survival at 7.5 years has been reported.

Pearls

- Gangliogliomas are the most common neoplastic cause of temporal lobe epilepsy.
- Gangliogliomas are the most common mixed glial-neuronal tumors.
- Gangliogliomas are primarily a tumor of children and young adults with 80% of patients less than 30 years of age.
- Most common location is the temporal lobe (>75%).
- Morphology of the tumor can be solid with gyral thickening or cyst with mural nodule.
- Enhancement is variable, with calcification common.
- Prognosis is excellent with complete surgical resection.
- Malignant degeneration is rare of the glial component.

Answers

1. The differential for a well-circumscribed tumor in the temporal lobe includes ganglioglioma, pilocytic astrocytoma, pleomorphic xanthoastrocytoma, and oligodendroglioma.

2. Gangliogliomas can have a solid nodular appearance that can cause gyral thickening or a circumscribed cyst with mural nodule.

3. Greater than 75% of gangliogliomas occur in the temporal lobe followed by the frontal and parietal lobes.

Suggested Readings

Adachi Y, Yagishita A. Gangliogliomas: characteristic imaging findings and role in the temporal lobe epilepsy. *Neuroradiology*. 2008 Oct;50(10):829-834.

Shin JH, Lee HK, Khang SK, et al. Neuronal tumors of the central nervous system: radiologic findings and pathologic correlation. *Radiographics*. 2003 Jan;22(5):1177-1189.

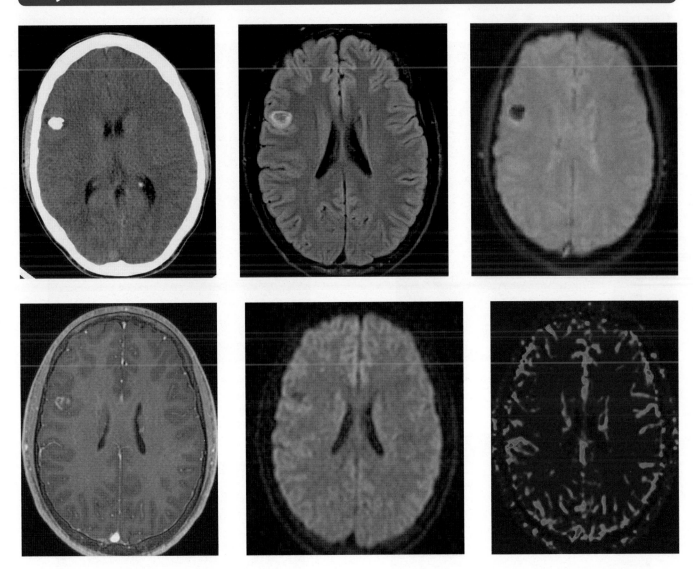

1. What is the differential diagnosis?

2. What is the most common location for this tumor?

3. Where does the tumor usually originate?

4. What are the typical imaging characteristics of this tumor?

5. What is the prognosis for the disease?

Case ranking/difficulty:

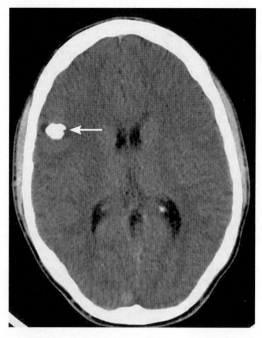

Axial T1 image shows a well-circumscribed densely calcified lesion in the right frontal lobe (*arrow*).

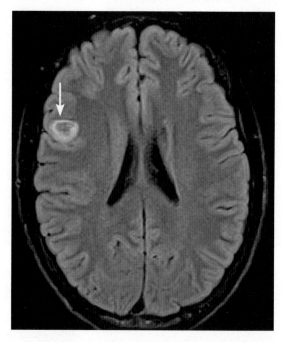

Axial FLAIR image shows a well-circumscribed T2 hyperintense lesion in the cortical subcortical region of the right frontal lobe without surrounding T2 hyperintensity. The central aspect of the lesion shows decreased T2 signal likely due to calcification (*arrow*).

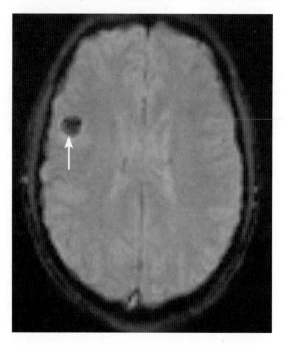

Axial GRE image shows significant hypointensity without blooming artifact of the lesion from calcification (*arrow*).

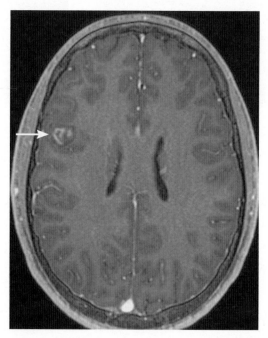

Axial T1 postcontrast image shows heterogeneous internal enhancement (*arrow*).

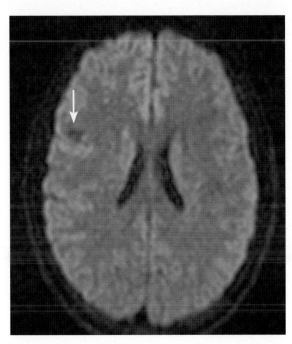

Axial DWI b = 1000 image shows no restricted diffusion of the tumor (*arrow*).

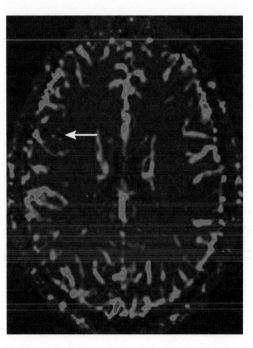

Axial color CBV map from dynamic susceptibility contrast perfusion technique shows relative low perfusion in the tumor (*arrow*). Oligodendrogliomas can show high CBV and is a confounding tumor on perfusion imaging, which can be mistaken for a high-grade neoplasm.

Answers

1. The differential of a well-circumscribed cortically based mass should include oligodendroglioma, ganglioglioma, and pleomorphic xanthoastrocytoma. Given the calcification, late-stage neurocysticercosis could be considered.

2. 50%-65% of oligodendrogliomas are located in the frontal lobe.

3. Oligodendrogliomas are usually cortical with subcortical extension.

4. Oligodendrogliomas are usually well demarcated with minimal adjacent edema. They are commonly T2 hyperintense with variable heterogeneous enhancement. 70%-90% will show some calcification. Oligodendrogliomas can be confounding tumors on perfusion imaging as low-grade tumors can show increased cerebral blood volume.

5. Although the median survival is longer in grade II oligodendrogliomas compared to grade II astrocytomas, most patients succumb to the tumor due to recurrence and malignant transformation to anaplastic oligodendroglioma. Complete surgical resection and 1p, 19q deletions (80% of oligodendrogliomas) are associated with more favorable prognosis as these deletions are associated with increased sensitivity of tumor cells to treatment.

Pearls

- Oligodendrogliomas are WHO grade II tumors that have a tendency to progress to the grade III anaplastic variant.
- These are tumors of young to middle-aged adults.
- They occur most commonly in the frontal lobes involving the cortex and subcortical white matter.
- They are usually circumscribed with little adjacent edema but may also uncommonly present in an infiltrative pattern.
- Oligodendrogliomas are typically T2 hyperintense with variable heterogeneous enhancement.
- Progression to enhancement of a previously nonenhancing tumor may suggest malignant degeneration.
- 70%-90% of oligodendrogliomas will have calcification.
- Increased CBV on perfusion imaging can be seen, which may mistake this tumor for a more higher-grade neoplasm.
- MR spectroscopy may be helpful to distinguish grade II and grade III tumors with the presence of lactate in the higher-grade neoplasm.

Suggested Readings

Chawla S, Krejza J, Vossough A, et al. Differentiation between oligodendroglioma genotypes using dynamic susceptibility contrast perfusion-weighted imaging and proton MR spectroscopy. *AJNR Am J Neuroradiol*. 2013 Aug;34(8):1542-1549.

Khalid L, Carone M, Dumrongpisutikul N, et al. Imaging characteristics of oligodendrogliomas that predict grade. *AJNR Am J Neuroradiol*. 2012 May;33(5):852-857.

16-year-old male with history of slurred speech, blurred vision, and altered mental status

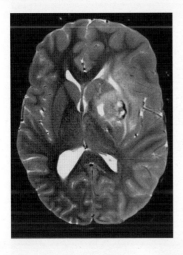
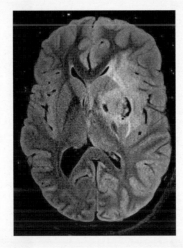
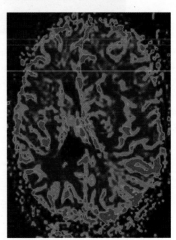

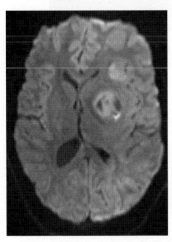
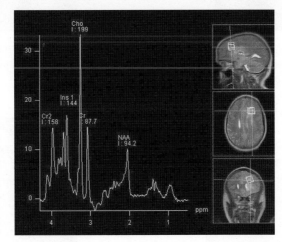
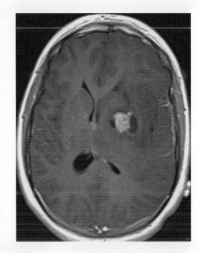

1. What is the differential for these MRI findings in a child?

2. What MRI findings correlate with malignancy?

3. Compared to medulloblastoma (cerebellar PNET) what is the prognosis for this disease?

4. What are the typical imaging characteristics of this tumor?

5. What imaging is necessary for staging prior to surgery?

Case ranking/difficulty: 　　　　　　**Category:** Intra-axial supratentorial

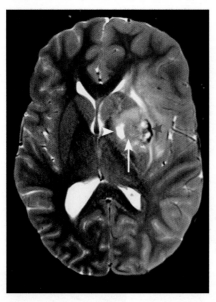

Axial T2 image shows a heterogeneous mass centered in the left basal ganglia with surrounding infiltrative T2 hyperintensity. Note the central T2 hypointensity (*white arrow*) that can be seen with highly cellular tumors. There is also a small focal area of hemorrhage (*red arrowhead*) and cystic necrosis (*white arrowhead*).

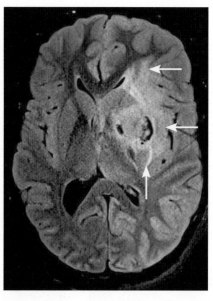

Axial FLAIR image shows the infiltrative adjacent T2 prolongation likely representing tumor infiltration with associated mass effect (*arrows*).

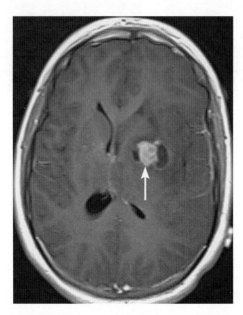

Axial T1 postcontrast shows the central heterogeneous enhancement (*arrow*).

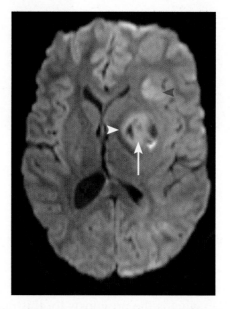

Axial DWI b = 1000 image shows focal areas of diffusion restriction in the central enhancing component (*white arrow*), the medial rim (*white arrowhead*), and an anterior region that is nonenhancing (*red arrowhead*). These correlate with areas of high cellularity and tumor infiltration.

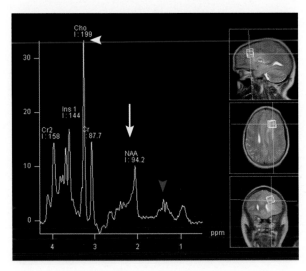

MRI spectroscopy at 30 TE of the nonenhancing region shows significant elevation of choline (*white arrowhead*), decreased NAA (*white arrow*), and the presence of a lactate doublet (*red arrowhead*), consistent with a malignant tumor profile.

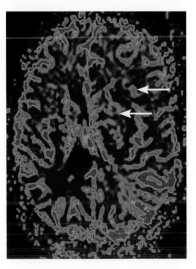

Axial color CBV image from dynamic susceptibility contrast perfusion imaging shows areas of increased perfusion, which correspond to the areas of diffusion restriction (*arrows*).

Answers

1. The differential for a heterogeneous hemispheric mass with malignant features in a child includes glioblastoma multiforme, primitive neuroectodermal tumor, atypical teratoid rhabdoid tumor, and choroid plexus carcinoma with significant parenchymal invasion.

2. T2 hypointensity and decreased diffusion correlate with hypercellular areas of neoplasms, which correspond to higher-grade malignancy. This can be seen in this case of primitive neuroectodermal tumor.

3. Medulloblastomas with similar histology to supratentorial PNET are also considered infratentorial or cerebellar PNET. However, prognosis is significantly worse for supratentorial PNET than medulloblastoma. Furthermore, younger children with supratentorial PNET tend to do worse than older children, which may be a reflection of underutilization of radiotherapy in very young children.

4. Supratentorial PNETs are typically large at presentation, with heterogeneous enhancement and areas of hemorrhage and cystic necrosis.

5. Spine imaging with contrast is necessary prior to surgery to evaluate for drop metastases. Supratentorial PNET, similar to medulloblastoma, has a propensity for CSF dissemination.

Pearls

- Supratentorial primitive neuroectodermal tumors (S-PNET) are uncommon malignant, poorly differentiated WHO grade IV embryonal tumors that share significant pathology with medulloblastoma.
- Compared to medulloblastoma (Cerebellar PNET), S-PNET patients generally have worse outcome, suggesting different oncogene expression.
- Hemispheric S-PNET is typically large and heterogeneous at presentation and may show significant infiltration, or surprisingly little adjacent T2 prolongation for size.
- Cystic necrosis, hemorrhage, and calcification are common.
- Heterogeneous enhancement is typical.
- Solid components will show decreased T2 and decreased diffusion corresponding with high cellularity.
- CSF seeding is common, which necessitates spine imaging prior to surgery.

Suggested Readings

Erdem E, Zimmerman RA, Haselgrove JC, Bilaniuk LT, Hunter JV. Diffusion-weighted imaging and fluid attenuated inversion recovery imaging in the evaluation of primitive neuroectodermal tumors. *Neuroradiology*. 2001 Nov;43(11):927-933.

Klisch J, Husstedt H, Hennings S, von Velthoven V, Pagenstecher A, Schumacher M. Supratentorial primitive neuroectodermal tumours: diffusion-weighted MRI. *Neuroradiology*. 2000 Jun;42(6):393-398.

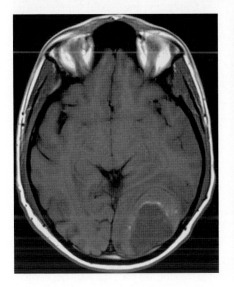 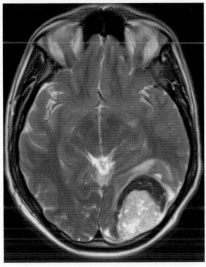 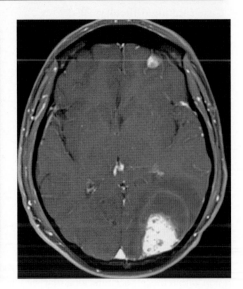

1. Where is the abnormality located?

2. What are the classic imaging findings for this entity?

3. What is the differential diagnosis?

4. What is the significance of low T1 signal in this entity?

5. What is the significance of the high T1 signal with this lesion?

Case ranking/difficulty:

Category: Intra-axial supratentorial

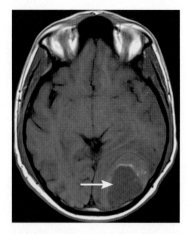

Axial T1 image shows a parenchymal lesion within the left occipital lobe that is of mixed T1 signal with peripheral T1 predominantly isointense signal (*arrow*).

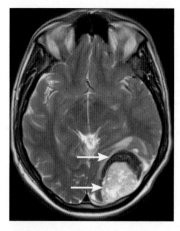

Axial T2 image shows the lesion is of mixed T2 signal but mostly hyperintense to brain with a rim of low signal (*arrows*): The peripheral blood product is primarily acute in nature.

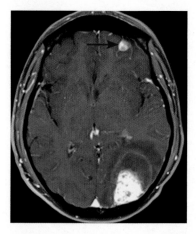

Axial T1 postcontrast shows the intra-axial lesion within the left occipital lobe has central enhancement (*red arrow*). A second focus of enhancement is seen within the left frontal lobe, which is much smaller (*blue arrow*).

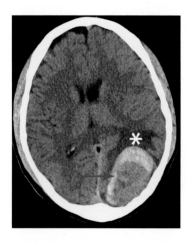

Axial CT image shows the peripheral hemorrhage of the left occipital mass (*red arrow*) with adjacent edema (*asterisk*).

Pearls

- Hematomas on MRI have variable signal depending on the age of the blood.
- T2* imaging blooming confirms blood products.
- Intermediate T1, Dark T2 = acute, deoxyhemoglobin.
- Bright T1, Dark T2 = early subacute, intracellular methemoglobin.
- Bright T1, Bright T2 = late subacute, extracellular methemoglobin.
- Dark T1, Dark T2 = chronic, hemosiderin.
- Follow-up MRI should be considered in patients without a diagnosis of cancer in order to exclude an underlying tumor.
- Melanoma, renal cell, choriocarcinoma, and thyroid metastases are prone to hemorrhage ("Mr. CT").
- A hemorrhagic metastasis is likely to be lung or breast carcinoma due to higher incidence of these cancers.

Answers

1. The abnormality is located within the left occipital lobe.

2. The classic imaging findings for hemorrhagic metastases are multiple intra-axial lesions with associated hemorrhage. On CT, high density is seen, and on MRI, the findings are variable and depend on the age of the blood products.

3. The differential diagnosis includes metastasis, abscess, and hematoma.

4. Chronic blood is identified by low signal on both T1 and T2 secondary to magnetic susceptibility from hemosiderin and ferritin, which coincides with a bleed that is weeks to years in age.

5. On MRI, the appearance of hyperintense T1 signal indicates methemoglobin, which signifies subacute hemorrhage.

Suggested Readings

Chan JH, Peh WC. Methemoglobin suppression in T2-weighted pulse sequences: an adjunctive technique in MR imaging of hemorrhagic tumors. AJR *Am J Roentgenol.* 1999 Jul;173(1):13-14.

Janick PA, Hackney DB, Grossman RI, Asakura T. MR imaging of various oxidation states of intracellular and extracellular hemoglobin. *AJNR Am J Neuroradiol.* 1993 May;12(5):891-897.

Toh CH, Wei KC, Ng SH, Wan YL, Lin CP, Castillo M. Differentiation of brain abscesses from necrotic glioblastomas and cystic metastatic brain tumors with diffusion tensor imaging. *AJNR Am J Neuroradiol.* 2011 Oct;32(9):1646-1651.

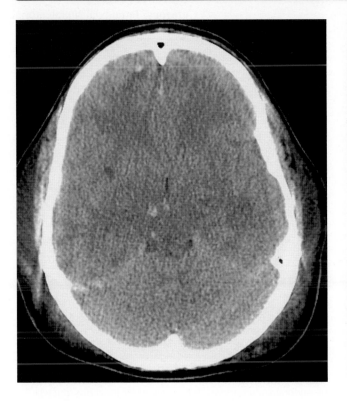
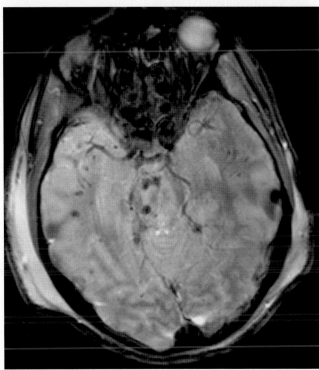

1. Where is the CT abnormality located?

2. Where are lesions most commonly located in this entity?

3. What is the most sensitive MR sequence for this entity?

4. What is the etiology for these lesions?

5. What causes the high CT attenuation?

Case ranking/difficulty:

Category: Intra-axial supratentorial

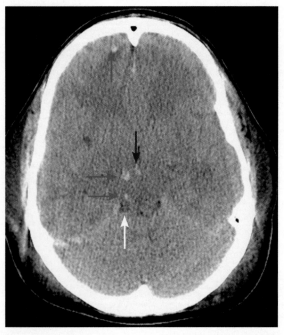

Axial CT shows small foci of hyperattenuation. Two within the midbrain (*red arrows*) and one within the right frontal lobe (*green arrow*). A small amount of subarachnoid blood is present in the interpeduncular cistern (*blue arrow*). Note the paucity of sulci and poor definition of the ambient cistern indicating elevated ICP (*white arrow*).

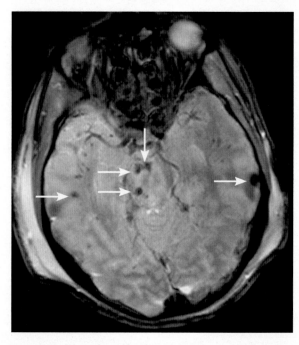

Axial T2 GRE shows multiple, small foci of low signal are seen within the midbrain and temporal lobes gray-white junctions (*arrows*).

Answers

1. Hyperattenuation is seen within the midbrain and right frontal lobe.

2. The classic lesion locations in diffuse axonal injury include the gray-white junctions, dorsolateral midbrain, and corpus callosum (splenium the most common).

3. The most sensitive MR sequences for this entity are GRE (gradient recalled echo) and SWI (susceptibility-weighted imaging), which are T2* weighted sequences.

4. This entity is secondary to traumatic brain injury.

5. The cause of high CT attenuation is blood products.

Pearls

- Diffuse axonal injury (DAI) is caused by a high-velocity traumatic event resulting in a tensile strain injury.
- DAI occurs secondary to the different densities of white and gray matter, which accelerate and decelerate at different rates.
- The resultant hemorrhages manifest most commonly at the gray-white junctions, midbrain, corpus callosum (splenium most common), ependymal lining, and superior cerebellar peduncles.
- These hemorrhages are usually less than 1 cm in size.
- Use GRE and SWI images for easier detection.
- A negative CT with a low GCS, consider follow-up MRI to exclude DAI.
- DAI location triad: gray-white junction, corpus callosum, and dorsolateral midbrain.

Suggested Readings

Aiken AH, Gean AD. Imaging of head trauma. *Semin Roentgenol.* 2010 Apr;45(2):63-79.

Blitstein MK, Tung GA. MRI of cerebral microhemorrhages. *AJR Am J Roentgenol.* 2007 Sep;189(3):720-725.

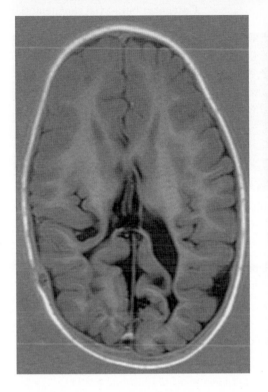

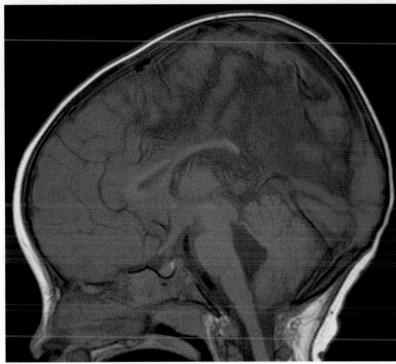

1. Where is the abnormality located?

2. What are the findings in this entity?

3. What is the best modality to diagnose this entity?

4. What are the causes of this finding?

5. What is in the differential for periatrial hyperintense FLAIR signal in infants and young children?

Case ranking/difficulty:

Category: Intra-axial supratentorial

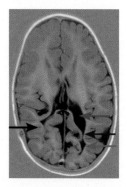

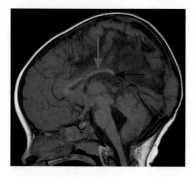

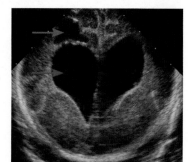

Axial T1 image shows undulating, irregular walls (*green arrow*) of lateral ventricles (*red arrow*) due to thinning of periventricular white matter (*blue arrows*). White matter is so thinned that the sulci and gyri (*black arrow*) almost reach the ventricles. Ventricles have collapsed after shunt placement.

Sagittal T1 image shows thinning of the splenium (*blue arrow*) and posterior part of the body (*green arrow*) of the corpus callosum due to decreased number of crossing fibers from loss of white matter.

Coronal ultrasound at 10 weeks of age shows cystic change (*green arrow*) in the periventricular white matter. Ventricles are dilated (*red arrow*).

Answers

1. The abnormality is located within the white matter.

2. White matter injury of prematurity (W-MIP) is a better terminology for periventricular leukomalacia as any white matter may be affected: deep, subcortical, or periventricular. In addition to white matter, neuronal and axonal injury may also involve the thalami, basal ganglia, brain stem, cerebellum, and cerebral cortex. Volume loss of the periventricular white matter and corpus callosum with ex-vacuo dilatation of ventricles and irregular margins of the ventricles is typically seen in the chronic stage.

3. MRI is the best modality to detect white matter injury. Ultrasound diagnoses cavitary white matter injury but underdiagnoses noncavitary white matter injury.

4. Most of the time, the periventricular white matter injury is due to hypoxic ischemic injury in premature neonates. Premature neonates are also at risk for intraventricular hemorrhage. Hence, many of the infants with W-MIP may have past history of intraventricular hemorrhage that may be seen as old hemorrhagic products on gradient/susceptibility MR sequence. However, periventricular white matter injury can also occur in other situations like infection, metabolic disease, hydrocephalus, and congenital heart disease.

5. Other than white matter injury from hypoxic ischemic injury, terminal myelination zones in the periatrial white matter can also be a normal cause of T2 hyperintensity in the periventricular white matter. Transependymal seepage of CSF in hydrocephalus can also cause hyperintense T2 signal in periventricular regions.

Pearls

- Periventricular leukomalacia is a white matter injury of prematurity and the sequela of a watershed infarction.
- Three types of white matter injury of prematurity in order of increasing severity of clinical manifestations: diffuse noncavitary, focal/multifocal noncavitary, and focal/multifocal cavitary.
- MRI shows hyperintense punctate T1 foci in early stages followed by some hypointensities within these hyperintense foci due to liquefactive necrosis.
- Necrosis may lead to small cavitations that may coalesce and form larger cavities.
- Imaging in the chronic stage shows diffuse white matter loss, angular and wavy ventricular margins, and periventricular gliosis.

Suggested Readings

Izbudak I, Grant PE. MR imaging of the term and preterm neonate with diffuse brain injury. *Magn Reson Imaging Clin N Am*. 2011 Nov;19(4):709-31; vii.

Sie LT, van der Knaap MS, van Wezel-Meijler G, Taets van Amerongen AH, Lafeber HN, Valk J. Early MR features of hypoxic-ischemic brain injury in neonates with periventricular densities on sonograms. *AJNR Am J Neuroradiol*. 2000 May;21(5):852-861.

Volpe JJ. Hypoxic-ischemic encephalopathy: neuropathology and pathogenesis. In: Volpe JJ, ed. *Neurology of the Newborn*. Philadelphia, PA: Saunders-Elsevier; 2008.

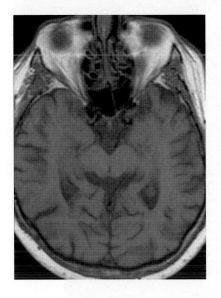
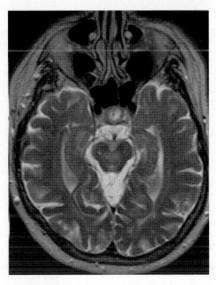
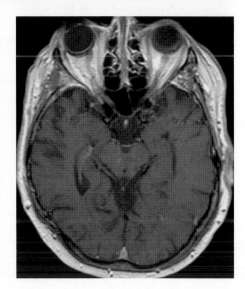

1. Where is the abnormality located?

2. What are the classic imaging findings for this entity?

3. What is the differential diagnosis?

4. What is the significance of low signal on MRI GRE images with this entity?

5. What is the treatment for this entity?

Case ranking/difficulty:

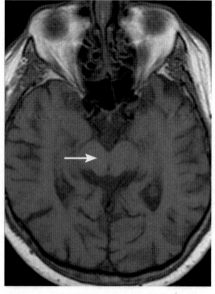

Axial T1 image does not show any findings. The (*arrow*) denotes where the lesion will be seen on the other sequences.

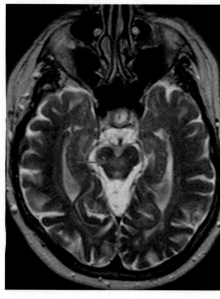

Axial T2 image shows increased signal in the right midbrain near the red nucleus (*arrow*).

3. The differential diagnosis includes glioma, capillary telangiectasia, and metastasis.

4. Hemorrhage is only seen when associated with cavernous malformations. Decreased T2* is thought to be deoxyhemoglobin within dilated capillaries.

5. No treatment is needed. These are considered "no touch" vascular malformations.

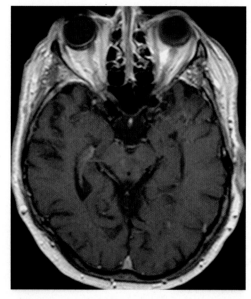

Axial T1 postcontrast image shows correlating faint enhancement (*arrow*).

Pearls

- Capillary telangiectasia is a benign vascular malformation that is usually asymptomatic and does not require treatment.
- The most common location is in the brain stem (most often the pons).
- Faint brain stem "brush-like or stipple" enhancement.
- Usually subcentimeter in size.
- When mass effect is present consider tumor (metastasis or glioma).

Answers

1. The abnormality is located within the midbrain.

2. The classic appearance on MRI is almost nonperceptable on T1 and T2. T2 may demonstrate high signal, but the hallmark finding is "brush-like" enhancement.

Suggested Reading

Castillo M, Morrison T, Shaw JA, Bouldin TW. MR imaging and histologic features of capillary telangiectasia of the basal ganglia. *AJNR Am J Neuroradiol.* 2001 Sep;22(8):1553-1555.

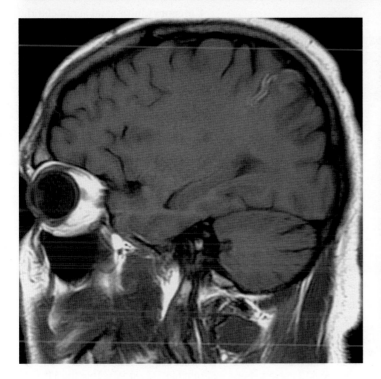

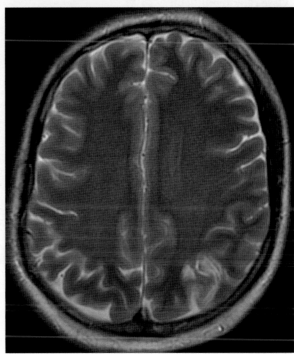

1. Where is the abnormality located?

2. What are the classic imaging findings for this entity?

3. What are possible causes for this entity?

4. What time course after an ischemic event does this entity appear?

5. What is the treatment for this entity?

Case ranking/difficulty:

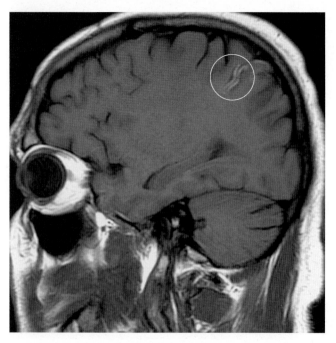

Sagittal T1 image shows gyriform high signal within the left parietal cortex with volume loss (*circle*).

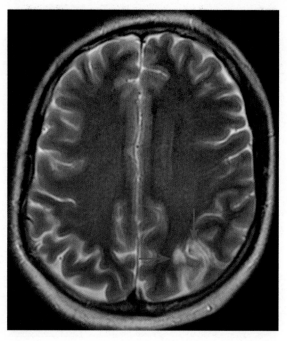

Axial T2 images shows gyriform high T2 signal within the left parietal cortex (*green arrow*). There is associated volume loss and gliosis (*red arrow*).

Answers

1. The abnormality is located in the parietal lobe.

2. On CT, there is usually linear gyriform high density within the cortical gray matter. On MRI, this is recognized by gyriform high T1 signal involving the gray matter with corresponding volume loss.

3. Cortical laminar necrosis can be a subacute sequela of an ischemic event, but has also been described with chemotherapy or immunosuppressive treatment.

4. Cortical laminar necrosis can typically appear 2 weeks after an ischemic event.

5. No treatment is necessary for this entity. Workup for stroke or other causes of cortical injury may be necessary.

Pearls

- Cortical laminar necrosis (CLN) can be seen in the subacute phase of cytotoxicity of the cortex, most commonly the sequela of an ischemic event.
- CLN can also be seen with chemotherapy or immunosuppressive treatment.
- This insult occurs in the third layer of the cortex.
- If ring enhancement is seen, consider metastasis.
- If mass effect is present, consider neoplasm.

Suggested Reading

Ginat DT, Meyers SP. Intracranial lesions with high signal intensity on T1-weighted MR images: differential diagnosis. *Radiographics*. 2012;32(2):499-516.

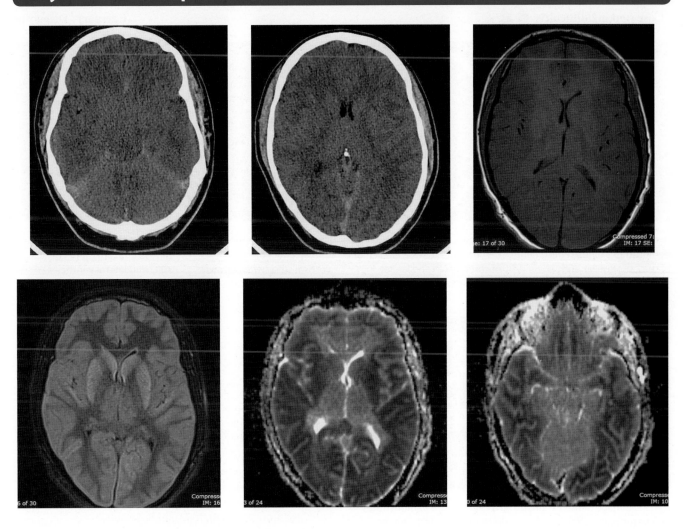

1. What are common causes of this finding?

2. What is the most sensitive imaging modality?

3. What is the differential diagnosis?

4. In mild-to-moderate ischemic injury, where are the expected location of abnormalities?

5. What structures are more susceptible to ischemic injury due to high metabolic activity?

Case ranking/difficulty: **Category:** Diagnostic

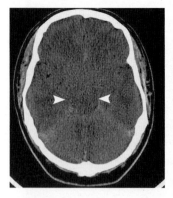

Axial noncontrast CT demonstrates diffuse effacement of sulci, suprasellar, and quadrigeminal cisterns (*white arrowheads*).

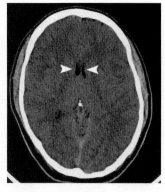

Axial noncontrast CT demonstrates diffuse effacement of cortical sulci and lateral ventricles (*white arrowheads*).

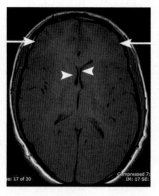

Axial T1 image demonstrates diffuse effacement of cortical sulci (*white arrows*) and lateral ventricles (*white arrowheads*).

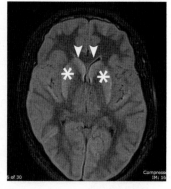

Axial FLAIR image demonstrates diffuse effacement of cortical sulci and lateral ventricles (*white arrowheads*). The basal ganglia appear increased in T2 hyperintensity (*asterisks*).

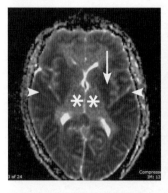

DWI ADC image demonstrates diffuse restricted diffusion of the cortices (*white arrowheads*) and basal ganglia (*white arrow*) bilaterally, relatively sparing bilateral thalami (*white asterisks*).

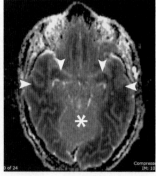

DWI ADC image demonstrates diffusion restricted cortices and hippocampi bilaterally (*white arrowheads*), sparing the cerebellum (*white asterisk*).

Pearls

- Cardiac arrest and cerebrovascular disease are the most common causes of hypoxia in the adult.
- Highly variable radiographic findings depend on severity and duration of insult, and type and timing of imaging studies.
- Mild-to-moderate global ischemia usually results in watershed zone infarcts.
- Severe ischemia primarily affects gray matter structures due to high metabolic activity.
- CT findings include diffuse cerebral edema, effacement of the cortical sulci, loss of gray-white differentiation, reverse gray-white attenuation, and white cerebellum sign.
- DWI and MRS are the most sensitive modalities with DWI becoming positive in the first hour.

Answers

1. Hypoxic ischemic injury in adults is more often a result of cardiac arrest or cerebrovascular disease. Drowning and asphyxia remain common causes in older children.

2. DWI is the most sensitive imaging modality and becomes positive in the first hour after an ischemic event.

3. Hypertensive encephalopathy, toxic/metabolic encephalopathy, and CJD are the differential diagnoses.

4. In mild-to-moderate hypoxic events, the watershed zone is the typical location due to lowest perfusion in the distal field of vascular supply.

5. Gray matter and deep gray nuclei are areas at risk from a severe hypoxic event due to high number of dendritic synapses and high metabolic activity.

Suggested Reading

Huang BY, Castillo M. Hypoxic-ischemic brain injury: imaging findings from birth to adulthood. *Radiographics.* 2008 Aug;28(2):417-439; quiz 617.

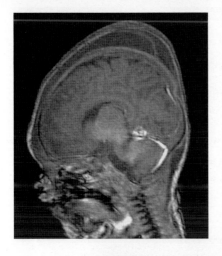
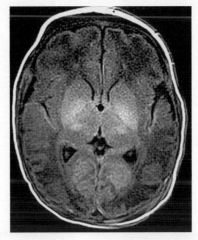
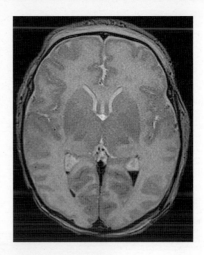

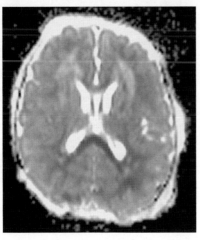
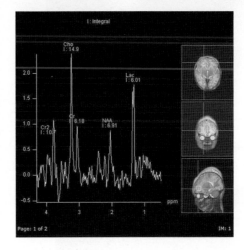

1. What structures are affected in mild-to-moderate injury?

2. What is the most common cause of this disease?

3. When is DWI most helpful in this disease and what is typically seen?

4. What can be seen in the subacute phase on T1 and T2 imaging?

5. What imaging findings correlate with worse prognostic outcome?

Case ranking/difficulty:

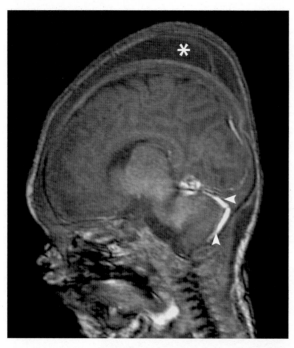

Sagittal T1 image demonstrates a large cephalhematoma (*white asterisk*) in the vertex as well as a thin layer of T1 shortening along the tentorium cerebelli and posterior fossa (*white arrowheads*), representing subdural blood from birth trauma.

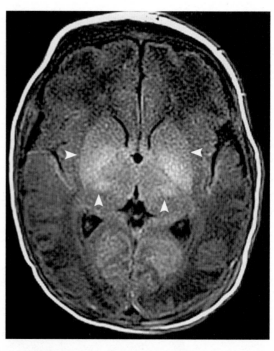

Axial T1 image at the level of the basal ganglia demonstrates greater than expected T1 hyperintensity of the putamen and ventrolateral thalami (*arrowheads*) indicating subacute ischemic injury.

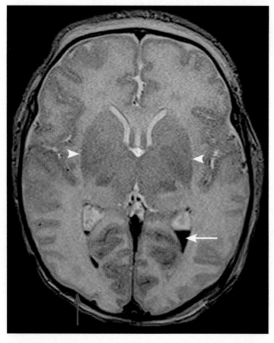

Axial T2 image shows T2 hypointensity of the putamen and ventrolateral thalami from subacute injury (*arrowheads*). Note the layering intraventricular blood (*arrow*), and areas of gyral swelling from edema (*red arrows*).

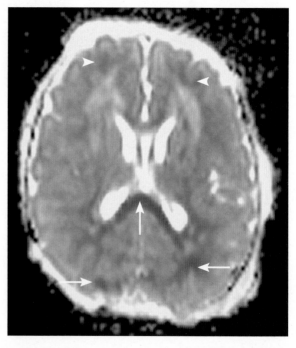

Axial ADC image demonstrates resolving restricted diffusion involving subcortical white matter diffusely of the bilateral cerebral hemispheres (*white arrowheads*) with more intense restriction in the splenium of the corpus callosum and parietal subcortical white matter (*white arrows*). This is indicative of delayed cellular death of severe diffuse ischemic injury.

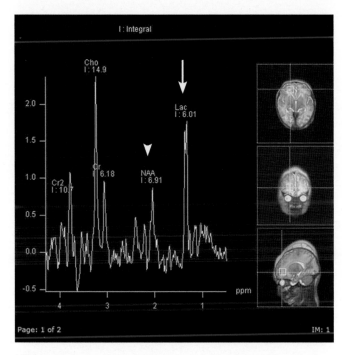

MR spectroscopy with voxel placement in the right periventricular white matter (TE 270 ms) demonstrates decreased NAA (*white arrowhead*) with increased lactate peaks (*white arrow*).

Answers

1. Mild-to-moderate hypoperfusion injury in hypoxic ischemic injury of the term neonate affects intravascular watershed zones, including the cortex and parasagittal white matter.

2. Perinatal asphyxia secondary to difficult birth is the most common cause of hypoxic ischemic injury of the term neonate.

3. ADC pseudonormalization occurs faster in neonates than in adults, within 5-7 days versus 7-10 days. DWI is more sensitive than T1/T2 images in the acute phase of hypoxic ischemic injury, especially in the background of normal unmyelinated white matter. DWI abnormality can increase after the first few days of injury from delayed cell death.

4. In the subacute phase of hypoxic ischemic injury (starting 3-6 days), affected brain structures show T1 hyperintensity and T2 hypointensity. As ADC begins to pseudonormalize in this phase, careful evaluation of T1 and T2 changes is important to understand the extent of injury.

5. Severe hypoperfusion injury involves the deep gray matter, perirolandic cortex, brainstem, and cerebellum. These findings, along with decreasing NAA and increasing lactate, correlate with poor outcome.

Pearls

- Perinatal asphyxia is the most important cause of hypoxic ischemic injury.
- Mild-to-moderate hypoperfusion usually affects intervascular watershed zones along parasagittal locations, including cortex and white matter.
- Severe hypoperfusion usually affects gray matter including ventrolateral thalami, posterior putamina, hippocampi, corticospinal tracts, and sensorimotor cortex.
- DWI performed between 24 hours and 5 days of life is more sensitive for the detection of cytotoxic edema, with faster pseudonormalization compared to adults.
- Subacute (3-6 days) changes typically show increased T1 and decreased T2 signal.
- Chronic changes will show progression to volume loss, cystic encephalomalacia, and gliosis.
- MR spectroscopy is the most sensitive in detection of metabolic derangement of brain injury with decreasing NAA and increasing lactate peaks correlating with worse prognosis.

Suggested Readings

Chao CP, Zaleski CG, Patton AC. Neonatal hypoxic-ischemic encephalopathy: multimodality imaging findings. *Radiographics*. 2006 Oct;26(suppl 1):S159-S172.

Liauw L, van der Grond J, van den Berg-Huysmans AA, Palm-Meinders IH, van Buchem MA, van Wezel-Meijler G. Hypoxic-ischemic encephalopathy: diagnostic value of conventional MR imaging pulse sequences in term-born neonates. *Radiology*. 2008 Apr;247(1):204-212.

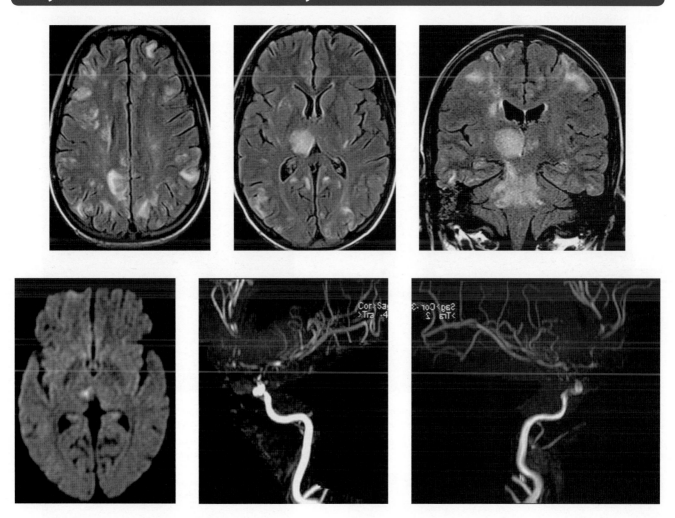

1. What is the differential diagnosis?

2. What is the typical clinical profile?

3. How often is there CNS involvement in this disease?

4. What are the patterns of radiographic features?

5. How often does angiography of any modality demonstrate vasculitic changes of this disease?

Case ranking/difficulty:

Category: Intra-axial supratentorial

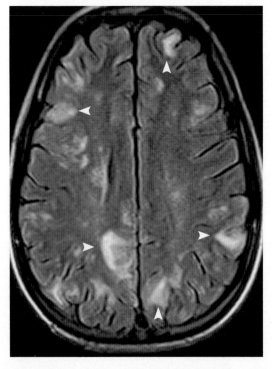

Axial FLAIR image demonstrates multifocal FLAIR hyperintensities predominantly involving the cortex and juxtacortical/subcortical white matter of the bilateral cerebral hemispheres (*white arrowheads*).

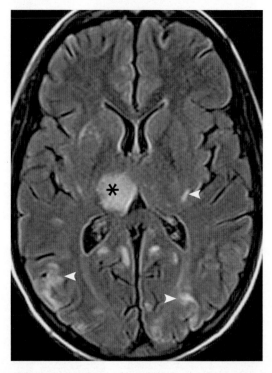

Axial FLAIR image demonstrates multifocal FLAIR hyperintensities predominantly involving the cortex and juxtacortical/subcortical white matter of the temporal occipital lobes (*white arrowheads*) as well as in the right thalamus (*black asterisk*).

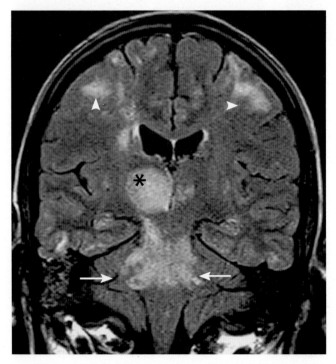

Coronal FLAIR image again demonstrates bilateral cortical and subcortical hyperintensities (*white arrowheads*) also involving the right thalamus (*black asterisk*) and pons (*white arrows*).

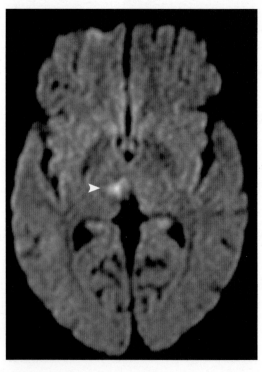

DWI image demonstrates restricted diffusion in the left thalamus (*white arrowhead*) from focal infarct.

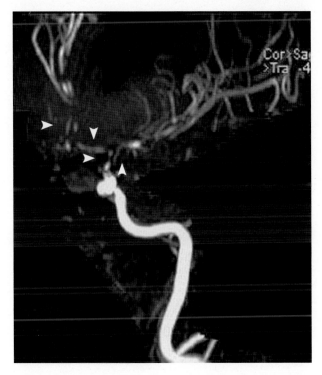

MRA MIP image of the left internal carotid artery demonstrates diffuse irregular narrowing of the precavernous, cavernous internal carotid artery as well as A1 and M1 segments (*white arrowheads*), consistent with vasculitis.

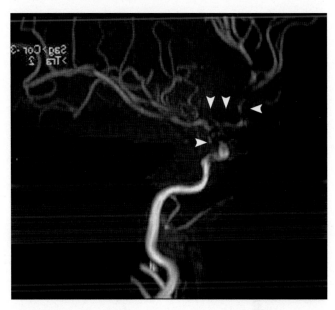

MRA MIP image of the right internal carotid artery demonstrates diffuse irregular narrowing of the precavernous, cavernous internal carotid artery as well as A1 and M1 segments (*white arrowheads*), consistent with vasculitis.

Answers

1. This is a case of systemic lupus erythematosus. Differential diagnosis of the appearance of multiple T2 hyperintense lesions affecting the gray matter and subcortical white matter is broad and includes ADEM, Susac syndrome, inherited stroke disorder such as CADASIL, and vasculitides such as Behcet disease.

2. The classic presentation of SLE is a woman of child-bearing age with fever, joint pain, and malar rash.

3. CNS involvement occurs in approximately 75% of SLE patients.

4. MRI of neuropsychiatric SLE is often normal. However, when imaging findings are positive, there are four recognized patterns: (1) focal infarcts are seen in patients with increased anticardiolipin and lupus anticoagulant antibodies; (2) multiple T2 hyperintensities of the white matter can be seen in microinfarctions; (3) focal areas of T2 hyperintensity in the gray matter— "migratory" edematous areas; and (4) diffuse steroid-responsive subcortical lesions associated with antineurofilament antibodies.

5. Vasculitis demonstrated on any angiographic modality from lupus is rare. Although catheter angiography remains the gold standard for anatomic vessel evaluation, vasculitic changes from SLE are rarely demonstrated.

Pearls

- Multisystem autoimmune connective tissue disease.
- 75% of cases have CNS involvement.
- Most common presentation is organic encephalopathy (35%-75% of case series) including acute confusion, lethargy, coma, chronic dementia, depression, or psychosis.
- Other clinical presentations include acute or subacute mental status changes secondary to diffuse cerebritis, PRES, seizure, cranial nerve involvement, stroke, peripheral neuropathy, myopathy, spinal cord involvement, and fatigue.
- Neuropsychiatric involvement of lupus often has normal imaging.
- DWI images demonstrate restricted diffusion in ischemia or infarct and increased diffusion in vasogenic edema.
- Vasculitis associated with lupus is rarely demonstrated on angiography.

Suggested Readings

Luyendijk J, Steens SC, Ouwendijk WJ, et al. Neuropsychiatric systemic lupus erythematosus: lessons learned from magnetic resonance imaging. *Arthritis Rheum*. 2011 Mar;63(3):722-732.

Steup-Beekman GM, Zirkzee EJ, Cohen D, et al. Neuropsychiatric manifestations in patients with systemic lupus erythematosus: epidemiology and radiology pointing to an immune-mediated cause. *Ann Rheum Dis*. 2013 Apr;72(suppl 2):ii76-ii79.

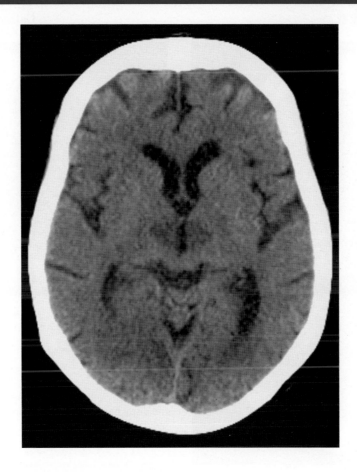

1. What is the differential diagnosis?

2. What is the typical clinical syndrome of entity?

3. What structures are usually involved?

4. Where does the artery of Percheron arise?

5. Which modality is most sensitive for acute infarction?

Case ranking/difficulty:

Category: Intra-axial supratentorial

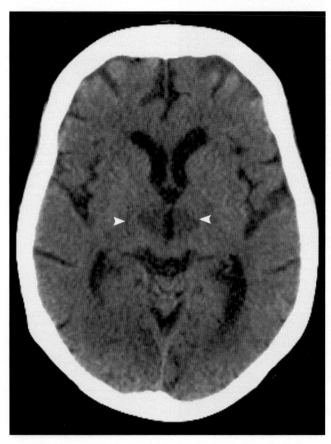

Axial noncontrast CT image demonstrates hypodensity foci in bilateral paramedian thalami (*white arrowheads*).

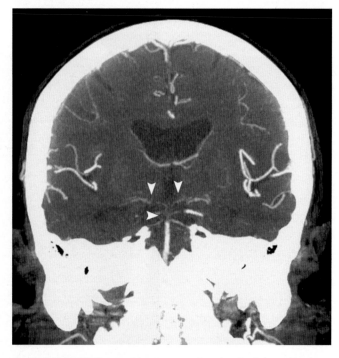

Coronal CTA MIP image demonstrates intraluminal thrombus in the distal basilar artery extending to the bilateral P1 segments (*white arrowheads*).

Answers

1. Differential diagnosis of bilateral thalamic hypodensity includes artery of Percheron infarct, deep venous thrombosis, Wernicke encephalopathy, and top of basilar infarction.

2. Top of basilar infarction is a recognized syndrome with visual and oculomotor deficits, somnolence, or behavioral changes.

3. Structures supplied by the distal basilar artery include the midbrain and thalami while the PCA distribution (occipital and paramedian parietal lobes) is typically also involved.

4. Artery of Percheron is a rare anatomical variation in the brain in which a single arterial trunk arises from the posterior cerebral artery (PCA) to supply paramedian thalami and the rostral midbrain bilaterally.

5. Diffusion-weighted imaging is the most sensitive for infarct in the acute phase, lasting up to 7-10 days.

Pearls

- Top of basilar infarct is a clinically recognizable syndrome.
- Visual, oculomotor deficits, somnolence, and behavioral changes.
- Relative absence of motor deficits.
- Involves rostral midbrain, thalamus, and posterior cerebral lobes.
- Hypodensity on CT and restricted diffusion on MRI.
- CTA or MRA is helpful to evaluate extension of intraluminal thrombus.
- Bilateral paramedian thalamic lesions can also suggest artery of Percheron infarct or Wernicke encephalopathy.

Suggested Reading

Matheus MG, Castillo M. Imaging of acute bilateral paramedian thalamic and mesencephalic infarcts. *AJNR Am J Neuroradiol.* 2007 May;24(10):2005-2008.

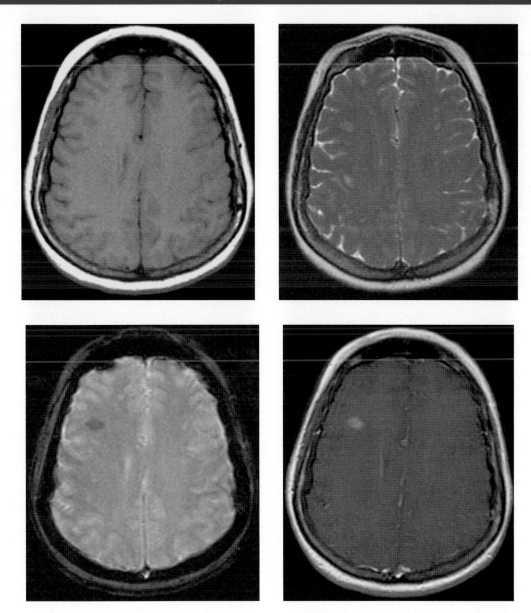

1. What is the differential diagnosis?

2. What is the typical clinical presentation?

3. What are typical radiographic features?

4. What are the most common locations for this lesion?

5. What is the treatment for this entity?

Case ranking/difficulty: **Category:** Intra-axial supratentorial

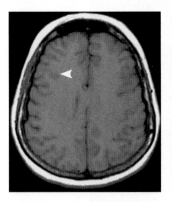 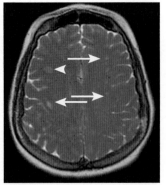 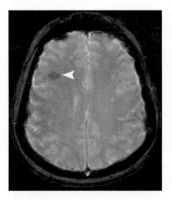 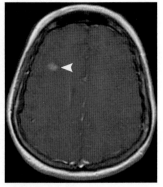

Axial T1 image demonstrates a focus of T1 isointensity in the right frontal subcortical white matter (*white arrowhead*).	Axial T2 image demonstrates a focus of T2 hyperintensity in the right frontal subcortical white matter (*white arrowhead*). Also noted are few foci of T2 hyperintensity in bilateral centrum semiovale (*white arrows*), consistent with gliosis related to small vessel disease.	Axial GRE image demonstrates a focus of susceptibility artifact in the right frontal subcortical white matter (*white arrowhead*).	Axial T1 postcontrast image demonstrates amorphous contrast enhancement without adjacent edema in the right frontal subcortical white matter (*white arrowhead*).

Answers

1. In this case of capillary telangiectasia, the differential diagnosis includes AVM, cavernoma, and metastasis.

2. Most patients with capillary telangiectasia are asymptomatic and incidentally found on neuroimaging.

3. Capillary telangiectasias are best seen on postcontrast images with intense brush-like enhancement and T2* images with susceptibility artifact from blood pooling. T1 may be normal or slightly hypointense to white matter with slight increased T2 signal. There is no surrounding edema.

4. Most common locations are pons, midbrain, cerebellum, dentate nuclei, and spinal cord.

5. No treatment or follow-up is required. Hemorrhage occurs only when associated with other vascular malformations.

Pearls

- Area of abnormal capillaries interspersed within brain parenchyma.
- Second most common vascular malformation after DVA (developmental venous anomaly).
- Can be single or multiple lesions and may demonstrate areas of microhemorrhage if associated with DVA and/or cavernous malformation.

- Most common locations are in the pons, middle cerebellar peduncles, dentate nuclei, and spinal cord.
- Usually asymptomatic.
- MRI with GRE/SWI and contrast is the most sensitive.
- Typical radiographic features include T1 normal to subtle hypointensity, T2 slight hyperintensity with blooming/susceptibility artifact from blood pooling, and brush-like contrast enhancement.
- No mass effect to adjacent brain parenchyma.
- No treatment required.

Suggested Readings

El-Koussy M, Schroth G, Gralla J, et al. Susceptibility-weighted MR imaging for diagnosis of capillary telangiectasia of the brain. *AJNR Am J Neuroradiol.* 2012 Apr;33(4):715-720.

Huddle DC, Chaloupka JC, Sehgal V. Clinically aggressive diffuse capillary telangiectasia of the brain stem: a clinical radiologic-pathologic case study. *AJNR Am J Neuroradiol.* 1999 Oct;20(9):1674-1677.

Lee RR, Becher MW, Benson ML, Rigamonti D. Brain capillary telangiectasia: MR imaging appearance and clinicohistopathologic findings. *Radiology.* 1997 Dec;205(3):797-805.

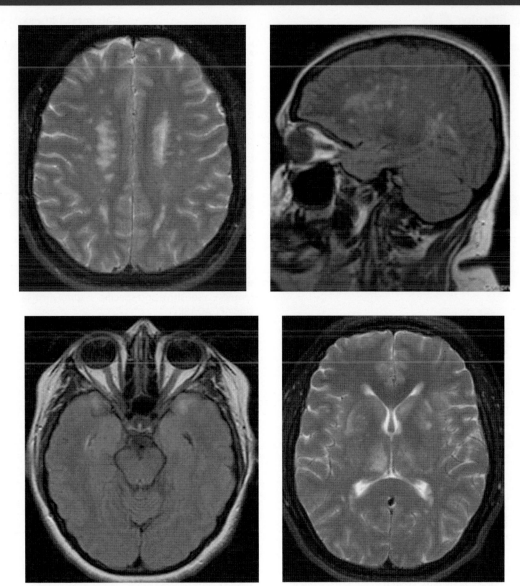

1. What is the differential diagnosis?

2. What is the typical clinical profile in this disease?

3. What are commonly involved brain structures?

4. What is a sensitive and specific sign for this disease?

5. What is the prognosis of this disease?

Case ranking/difficulty:

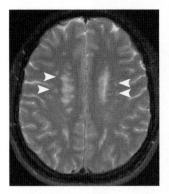

Axial T2 image shows multiple hyperintense lesions in the centrum semiovale (*arrowheads*).

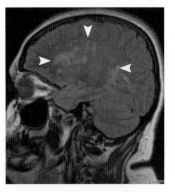

Off-midline sagittal FLAIR image shows multiple periventricular and subcortical hyperintensities (*arrowheads*).

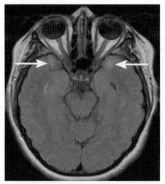

Axial FLAIR image shows bilateral subcortical white matter hyperintensity of the anterior temporal lobes (*arrows*), a sensitive and specific sign of CADASIL.

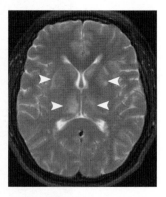

Axial T2 image through the basal ganglia also shows focal and patchy T2 hyperintensity in the deep gray nuclei (*arrowheads*).

Answers

1. Patchy periventricular white matter areas of gliosis are typical of small vessel vasculopathy, with subcortical arteriosclerosis from hypertension as the most common cause. CNS vasculitis and CADASIL are rare causes of this imaging finding.

2. The typical clinical profile is a young adult presenting with TIA, stroke-like symptoms, or migraines often without the traditional risk factors for stroke.

3. Involved areas of stroke in CADASIL are similar to those affected by hypertension with small vessel distribution, including periventricular and subcortical white matter, basal ganglia, and capsular white matter. The cerebral cortex is usually spared.

4. A sensitive and specific sign for CADASIL is T2 hyperintense involvement of the bilateral anterior temporal subcortical white matter, not commonly seen in small vessel disease from hypertension.

5. No specific treatment exists for CADASIL. Most patient progress to cognitive decline and behavioral changes, with men demonstrating a shorter lifespan.

Pearls

- Cerebral autosomal dominant arteriopathy with subcortical infarcts and leukoencephalopathy (CADASIL) is a hereditary disease of small vessels with mutation of NOTCH3.
- Transient ischemic attacks, stroke-like symptoms, and migraines are the typical initial presentation with progression to neurologic disability, including cognitive deficits and behavioral disturbances.
- Patients may have absence of traditional stroke risk factors and present at a younger age.
- Distribution of lacunar infarcts is similar to subcortical arteriosclerotic encephalopathy seen with hypertension.
- Involvement of the anterior temporal subcortical white matter is a highly sensitive and specific sign of CADASIL not typically seen in hypertensive arteriosclerosis.

Suggested Readings

De Guio F, Reyes S, Duering M, Pirpamer L, Chabriat H, Jouvent E. Decreased T1 contrast between gray matter and normal-appearing white matter in CADASIL. *AJNR Am J Neuroradiol.* 2014 Jan;35(1):72-76.

Liem MK, Lesnik Oberstein SA, Haan J, et al. Cerebrovascular reactivity is a main determinant of white matter hyperintensity progression in CADASIL. *AJNR Am J Neuroradiol.* 2009 Jun;30(6):1244-1247.

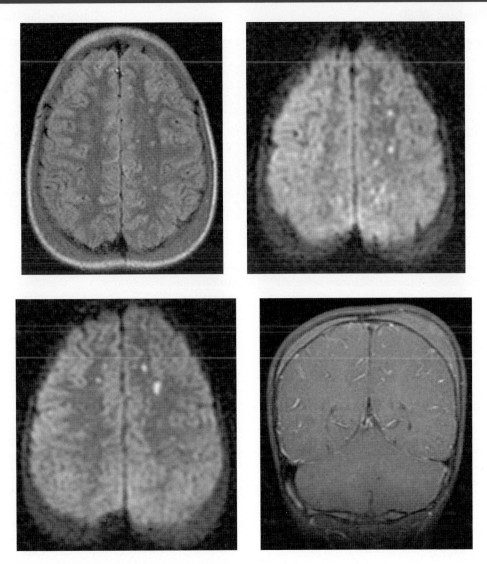

1. What is the differential diagnosis?

2. What are associated vasculopathies with this disease?

3. What abnormality can be seen on intracranial arteriography with this disease?

4. What therapy induces fetal hemoglobin as a treatment for this disease?

5. Where is the typical location of cerebral infarcts on imaging in this disease?

Case ranking/difficulty:

Category: Intra-axial supratentorial

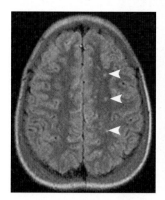

Axial FLAIR image shows punctate subcortical white matter hyperintensities of the left frontal lobe (*arrowheads*).

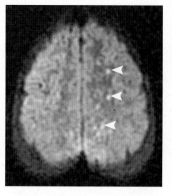

Axial DWI b = 1000 image shows bright punctate signal of the left frontal subcortical white matter (*arrowheads*) from restricted diffusion from acute infarct.

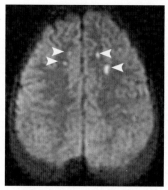

Axial DWI b = 1000 image shows bilateral frontal subcortical white matter areas of diffusion restriction (*arrowheads*) from acute infarct.

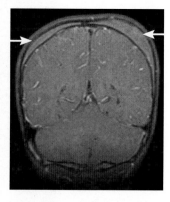

Coronal postcontrast with fat-sat image shows calvarial thickening and expansion of the diploic space from marrow expansion (*arrows*).

Answers

1. The differential of small punctate or patchy white matter infarcts includes CADASIL, CNS vasculitis, hypertensive arteriosclerosis, and sickle cell disease. Of this list, only sickle cell disease causes red marrow expansion of the calvarium.

2. Vasculopathies associated with sickle cell disease includes vaso-occlusive crises from red cell sickling, large vessel vasculopathy and aneurysm, and moyamoya.

3. Distal internal carotid stenosis with lenticulostriate collaterals in a moyamoya pattern can be seen with sickle cell disease. Arterial aneurysms, venous thrombosis, and arterial dissection have also been described.

4. Hydroxyurea induces fetal hemoglobin and lessens the number of painful vaso-occlusive crises in sickle cell disease.

5. Watershed locations and small vessel locations are most common such as the parasagittal white matter and between the ACA and MCA distributions.

Pearls

- Sickle cell disease is an autosomal recessive disease with mutation of the hemoglobin beta gene on chromosome 11p15.5.
- The sickling of deoxygenated RBCs causes clumping and vascular occlusion of capillaries as well as larger vessel vasculopathy from adherence to the endothelium.
- Patients typically present in childhood with stroke and is the primary cause of stroke in African American children.
- MR brain imaging may show predominantly small vessel distribution infarcts: ACA, MCA watershed distribution including the parasagittal white matter.
- Angiography can show associated moyamoya vasculopathy with severe stenosis of the distal internal carotid artery with prominent lenticulostriate collaterals.
- Expanded diploic space of the calvarium is typical from red marrow hyperplasia from anemia.

Suggested Readings

Sun B, Brown RC, Hayes L, et al. White matter damage in asymptomatic patients with sickle cell anemia: screening with diffusion tensor imaging. *AJNR Am J Neuroradiol.* 2012 Dec;33(11):2043-2049.

Winchell AM, Taylor BA, Song R, et al. Evaluation of SWI in children with sickle cell disease. *AJNR Am J Neuroradiol.* 2014 May;35(5):1016-1021.

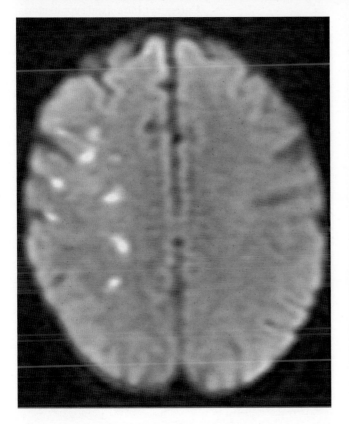 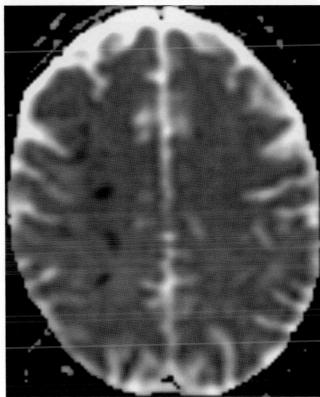

1. Where is the abnormality located?

2. What are the classic imaging findings for this entity?

3. What is the differential diagnosis?

4. What is the etiology of this entity?

5. What is the treatment for this entity?

Case ranking/difficulty:

Category: Intra-axial supratentorial

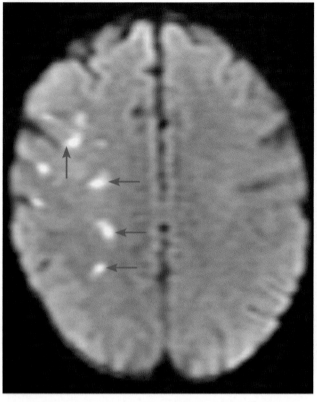

Axial DWI b-1000 image shows multiple punctate foci of abnormal high signal involving the right frontal and parietal white matter, as well as the overlying cortex in the MCA distribution and deep watershed distribution (*arrows*).

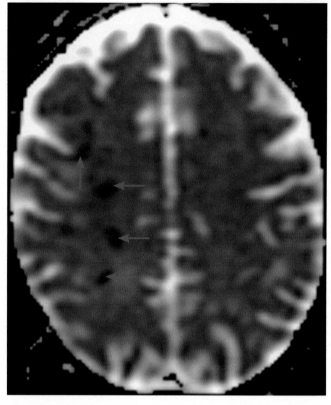

ADC map shows corresponding decreased signal consistent with cytotoxic edema from acute infarction (*arrows*).

Answers

1. The abnormality is located within the deep white matter and overlying cortex of the frontal lobe.

2. Embolic infarcts are usually multiple and can be variable in size and timing. Cortical end branches and perforating arteries are usually involved depending on the size of the embolus. Acute infarcts will show restricted diffusion on DWI.

3. The differential diagnosis includes metastasis, embolic infarction, septic emboli, and demyelinating disease.

4. Embolic infarcts are commonly from a cardiogenic source, either from valvular vegetations or from atrial fibrillation. Internal carotid atheromas are also a source of emboli.

5. The treatment for this entity is supportive care with consideration to antithrombotic therapy with atherosclerotic disease. Cardiac workup for source of emboli is indicated.

Pearls

- Involve terminal cortical branches and perforating arteries, depending on size of embolus.
- Within the perforating arteries in the deep white matter this can have a classic "string of pearls" or "rosary"-like appearance and typically have three or more of foci in a linear distribution.
- These so-called "pearls" are usually defined as foci of signal less than 2 cm.
- Multiple strokes in different vascular distributions of varying ages.
- Cardiac echo may be helpful to show vegetations.

Suggested Reading

Mangla R, Kolar B, Almast J, Ekholm SE. Border zone infarcts: pathophysiologic and imaging characteristics. *Radiographics*. 2011;31(5):1201-1214.

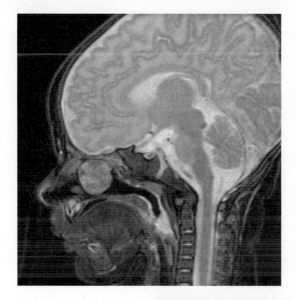
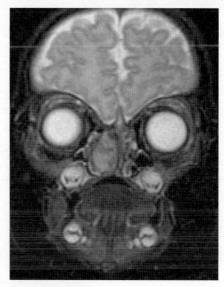
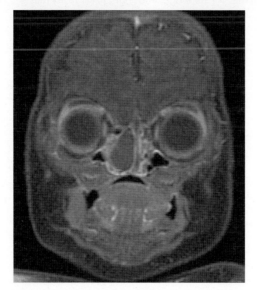

1. What is the differential diagnosis of this finding?

2. What is the pathophysiology of this lesion?

3. What is the treatment for this lesion?

4. What is the recurrence rate of this lesion?

5. What are potential complications of this lesion?

Case ranking/difficulty:

Category: Meninges, skull and scalp

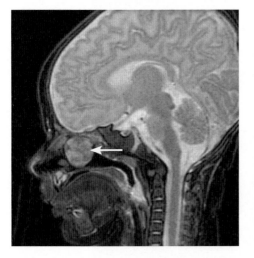

Sagittal T2 image of the midline shows a heterogeneous well-circumscribed mass in the nasal cavity (*arrow*).

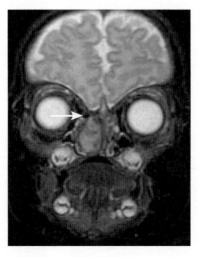

Coronal T2 image shows a heterogeneous right nasal cavity mass that is well circumscribed and points toward the cribriform plate (*arrow*).

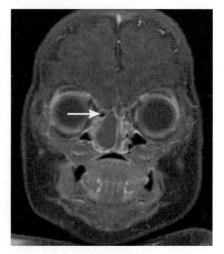

Coronal T1 postcontrast image shows the iso- to hypointense right nasal mass that points toward the cribriform plate (*arrow*). There is peripheral enhancement from nasal mucosa.

Answers

1. The differential diagnosis for pediatric midline nasal masses includes nasal glioma, epidermoid or dermoid cyst, hairy polyp, and sarcomas. Hemangioma is also usually considered, but is excluded in this case due to the lack of intense enhancement.

2. This intranasal glioma is thought to be from sequestered brain tissue in the prenasal space through the foramen cecum prior to fusion of the nasal bones.

3. The treatment for nasal gliomas is surgical excision. If an intracranial communication exists, a combined intra- and extracranial approach may be necessary.

4. While the term glioma is considered a misnomer due to a lack of a true neoplasm within nasal gliomas, there is a 10% recurrence rate of nasal glioma after resection. Recurrent nasal gliomas can demonstrate contrast enhancement not previously seen in the original lesion. Histologically, there are fibrous tissue, astrocytes, and rare neurons without mitotic features or bizarre nuclear forms.

5. Nasal obstruction and respiratory difficulties can be seen with intranasal gliomas of significant size. In the minority with a persistent communication to the intracranial space, meningitis is a potential complication.

Pearls

- Nasal gliomas (glial heterotopias) are congenital sequestered dysplastic brain matter presenting within the nasal cavity or anterior to the nasal bones at the bridge of the nose.
- Only 15% have small persistent intracranial communication primarily through the cribriform plate.
- MRI imaging shows T1 mixed to low intensity, T2 iso- to hyperintense, nonenhancing circumscribed mass.
- Peripheral enhancement can be seen from surrounding nasal mucosa.
- 10% recurrence rate after surgical resection is seen with possible enhancement of the recurrent lesion.

Suggested Readings

Barkovich AJ, Vandermarck P, Edwards MS, Cogen PH. Congenital nasal masses: CT and MR imaging features in 16 cases. *AJNR Am J Neuroradiol.* 1992;12(1):105-116.

Braun M, Boman F, Hascoet JM, Chastagner P, Brunet A, Simon C. Brain tissue heterotopia in the nasopharynx. Contribution of MRI to assessment of extension. *J Neuroradiol.* 1992;19(1):68-74.

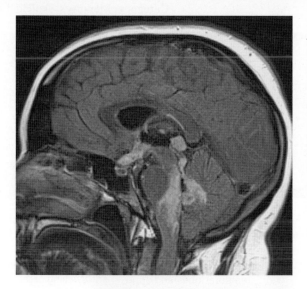
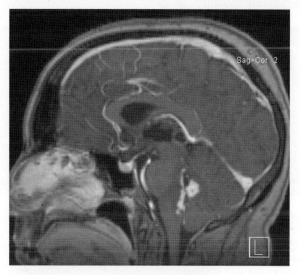
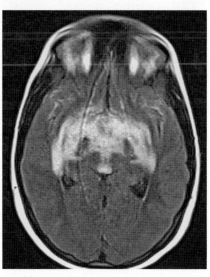
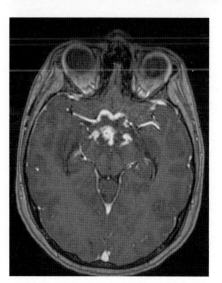

1. What are the described MRI findings for this disease?

2. What can be seen with imaging of the spine in this disease?

3. What are the differential diagnoses for this finding?

4. What are microscopic features of this disease?

5. What are relative risk factors for this disease?

Case ranking/difficulty:

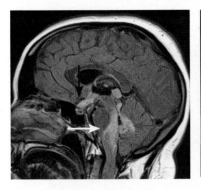

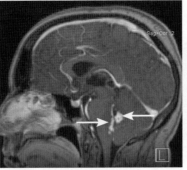

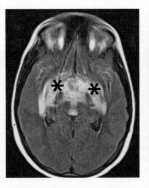

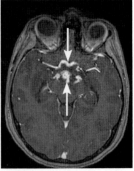

Sagittal FLAIR image through the midline shows vasogenic edema of the dorsal brainstem (*white arrow*) and vermis (*red arrow*). There is also increased T2 signal of the optic nerves (*blue arrow*).

Sagittal postcontrast images show the predominantly pial and ependymal enhancement within the fourth ventricle (*white arrows*).

Axial FLAIR image of the same patient from a prior study shows diffuse edema of the midbrain, medial temporal lobes, and optic pathways (*asterisks*).

Axial T1 postcontrast image of the same patient from a prior study shows nodular and pial enhancement and swelling of the optic chiasm, infundibulum, and hypothalamus (*white arrows*).

Answers

1. Neurosarcoidosis can have heterogeneous imaging findings, with the classic leptomeningeal basilar nodular enhancement being most often described. Isolated enhancing lesions in the extraaxial structures such as infundibulum, dural mass, or cranial nerves are not uncommon. Solitary or multiple enhancing parenchymal masses have also been described. Nonenhancing T2 hyperintense lesions can also be seen.

2. Spine and spinal cord involvement can be challenging from a differential diagnostic standpoint with multiple enhancing or nonenhancing lesions within the spinal cord, pial enhancement, and vertebral body involvement. While disk enhancement can be seen, isolated involvement of the disk without other vertebral body lesions has not been described. Disk spaces are usually spared.

3. Basilar meningitis, leptomeningeal carcinomatosis, and neurosarcoidosis can be indistinguishable and are the typical differentials for basilar leptomeningeal enhancement. Given the lack of mass or significant mass effect fourth ventricular neoplasms such as ependymoma or medulloblastoma are unlikely.

4. Noncaseating granulomas, with large multinucleated cells, arterial wall invasion, perivascular and lymphocytic invasion of cranial nerves, and granulomas within the perivascular space extending to the parenchyma, have been described with neurosarcoidosis, giving rise to the heterogeneous imaging appearance.

5. Nonsmokers, temperate over tropical climates, African Americans over Caucasian Americans, women, and Swedish and Danish populations all have a relatively higher incidence of sarcoidosis.

Pearls

- Neurosarcoidosis has heterogeneous imaging features, most of which demonstrates some form of enhancement due to granulomatous inflammation.
- Classically, basilar thick/nodular leptomeningeal enhancement with associated vasogenic edema is described.
- Parenchymal enhancement can be single or multiple, with vasculitic pattern also described.
- Nearly half of patients have T2 hyperintense lesions in the periventricular white matter.
- Spinal cord involvement, dural enhancement, as well as skull and spine lesions have also been described.

Suggested Readings

Nozaki K, Judson MA. Neurosarcoidosis. *Curr Treat Options Neurol.* 2013 Aug;15(4):492-504.

Nozaki K, Scott TF, Sohn M, Judson MA. Isolated neurosarcoidosis: case series in 2 sarcoidosis centers. *Neurologist.* 2012 Nov;18(6):373-377.

Wengert O, Rothenfusser-Korber E, Vollrath B, et al. Neurosarcoidosis: correlation of cerebrospinal fluid findings with diffuse leptomeningeal gadolinium enhancement on MRI and clinical disease activity. *J Neurol Sci.* 2013 Dec;335(1-2):124-130.

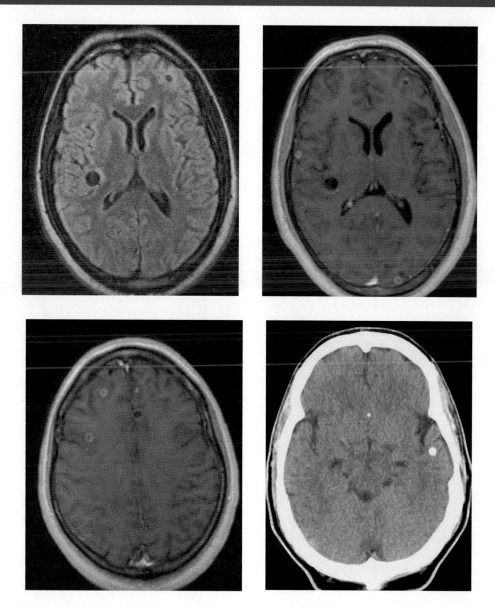

1. What is the etiology of this disease?

2. What are the differential diagnoses for this finding?

3. What are the four stages of this disease?

4. What is the treatment for this disease?

5. What is the typical clinical presentation for this disease?

Case ranking/difficulty:

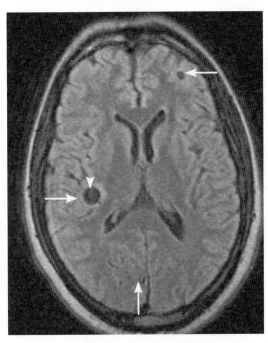

Axial FLAIR image demonstrate CSF suppression of these cysts with some internal signal and mild surrounding inflammation suggesting late vesicular or early colloidal vesicular phase of neurocysticercosis (*arrows*). Note the internal signal within the larger cyst likely represents a scolex (*arrowhead*).

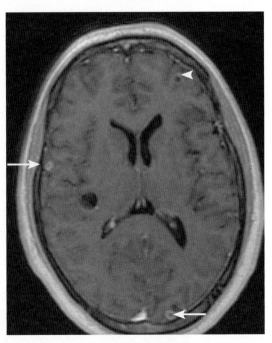

Axial postcontrast T1 shows signet ring enhancement of the left frontal lesion consistent with early colloidal vesicular phase (*arrowhead*). The peripheral nodular focus likely represents the degenerating scolex. Multiple ring-enhancing lesions without central fluid are seen representing the granular nodular phase (*arrows*).

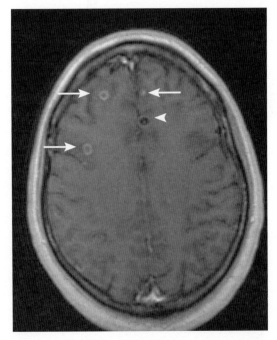

Axial postcontrast T1 demonstrates multiple ring-enhancing and solid nodules in the granular nodular phase (*arrows*), and a cyst with mild ring enhancement and central nodular enhancement representing the scolex in the colloidal vesicular phase (*arrowhead*).

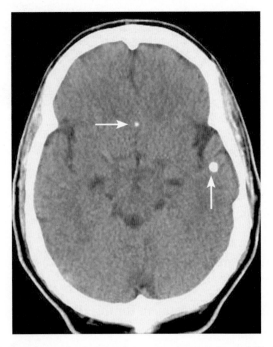

Axial CT of the same patient after treatment showing calcified nodules without edema in the nodular calcified stage (*arrows*).

Answers

1. This is a classic case of multiple lesions that demonstrate differing stages of CNS infection from cysticerci of neurocysticercosis.

2. Neurocysticercosis (this case), bacterial abscess, fungal abscess, metastatic disease, and toxoplasmosis in AIDS are the differential for multiple ring-enhancing lesions.

3. Four stages of neurocysticercosis can be seen at one time especially with repeated ingestion and multiple lesions. Time course of progression through the stages can take 1-9 years.

   The vesicular stage includes a clear cyst that suppresses on FLAIR, and little to no surrounding edema and enhancement.

   The colloidal vesicular stage shows early degeneration of the scolex, which may appear as central enhancement within the cyst, and increasing turbidity of the cyst fluid, causing increased FLAIR signal and surrounding inflammation and enhancement.

   The granular nodular stage shows coalescing cyst with ring-like or nodular enhancement with decreasing surrounding edema.

   The nodular calcified stage is a nodule of calcification without surrounding edema or enhancement, representing old granulomatous calcification.

4. Antiparasitics such as albendazole can decrease parasitic burden and treat primary GI disease in human carriers, as well as lessen seizures. Antiparasitics may be contraindicated with significant edema from the encephalitic form common in children. Corticosteroids can help decrease inflammation. Surgical drainage or resection of cyst due to mass effect or on more sensitive structures may be indicated.

5. Patients commonly present with headache and seizures. Neurocysticercosis is the most common etiology of seizures in endemic regions.

Pearls

- Neurocysticercosis is a CNS infection from the ingestion of the eggs of *T soli*, a pig tapeworm.
- Four stages of disease can be seen especially with repeated ingestion and multiple lesions.
- Racemose forms with grapelike cyst clusters can be seen in the basilar cisterns.
- Children may have more associated edema in the encephalitic form, which may be a contraindication for antiparasitic therapy.

Suggested Readings

Lerner A, Shiroishi MS, Zee CS, Law M, Go JL. Imaging of neurocysticercosis. *Neuroimaging Clin N Am.* 2012 Nov;22(4):659-676.

Lucato LT, Guedes MS, Sato JR, Bacheschi LA, Machado LR, Leite CC. The role of conventional MR imaging sequences in the evaluation of neurocysticercosis: impact on characterization of the scolex and lesion burden. *AJNR Am J Neuroradiol.* 2007 Sep;28(8):1501-1504.

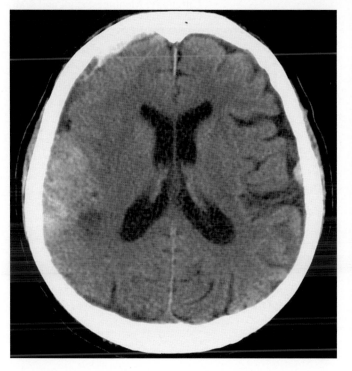
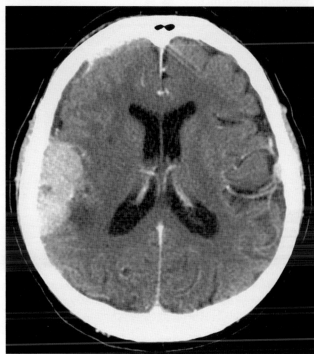

1. Where is the abnormality located?

2. What are the classic imaging findings for this entity?

3. What is the differential diagnosis?

4. What are common etiologies of this finding?

5. What is the most common location of intracranial metastasis?

Case ranking/difficulty: 🧠🧠

Category: Meninges, skull and scalp

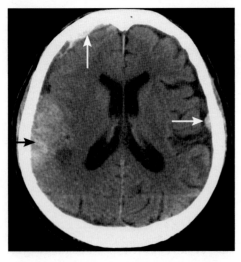

Axial CT noncontrast image shows high-density extraaxial lesions bilaterally (*white arrows*). The larger lesion on the right creates mass effect on the right hemisphere (*black arrow*).

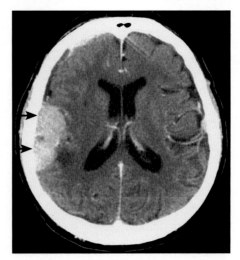

Axial CT postcontrast image shows contrast enhancement, especially of the larger right extraaxial mass (*arrows*).

Answers

1. The abnormality is located within the meninges.

2. The classic imaging findings for this entity include an extraaxial mass with contrast enhancement.

3. The differential diagnosis includes meningioma, metastasis, and extraaxial hematomas (epidural and subdural).

4. Causes of dural metastasis include breast, melanoma, prostate, lymphoma, and renal carcinoma. Direct spread to the dura may also be caused by carcinomas of the sinuses.

5. Intracranial metastasis is seen in approximately one in five patients with systemic malignant neoplasms at autopsy. Parenchymal brain metastases are more common than meningeal involvement. Leptomeningeal (pia and arachnoid) involvement is twice as common as pachymeningeal (dura and arachnoid) involvement.

- Leptomeningeal (pia and arachnoid) involvement is twice as common as pachymeningeal (dura and arachnoid) spread.
- Causes of dural metastasis include breast, melanoma, prostate, lymphoma, and renal carcinoma.
- If dural metastasis is suspected, search for other lesions within the skull and brain.
- Multiple dural lesions with hyperostosis consider NF-2 (multiple meningiomas).
- If a skull fracture or trauma history is present, do not forget extraaxial hematoma.
- Leptomeningeal metastasis usually follows sulci or surrounds brainstem or cranial nerves.

Suggested Readings

Maroldi R, Ambrosi C, Farina D. Metastatic disease of the brain: extra-axial metastases (skull, dura, leptomeningeal) and tumour spread. *Eur Radiol*. 2005 Mar;15(3):617-626.

Smirniotopoulos JG, Murphy FM, Rushing EJ, Rees JH, Schroeder JW. Patterns of contrast enhancement in the brain and meninges. *Radiographics*. 2010 Nov;27(2):525-551.

Yu WL, Sitt CM, Cheung TC. Dural metastases from prostate cancer mimicking acute sub-dural hematoma. *Emerg Radiol*. 2012 Dec;19(6):549-552.

Pearls

- Intracranial metastasis is seen in approximately one in five patients with systemic malignant neoplasms at autopsy.
- Parenchymal brain masses are more common than meningeal involvement.

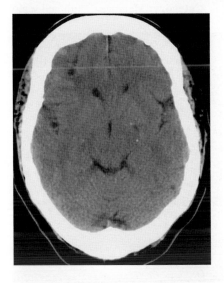 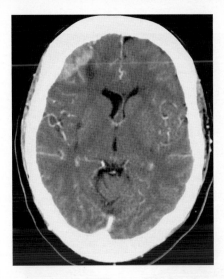 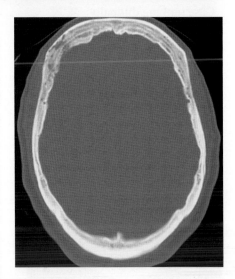

1. Where is the abnormality located?

2. What are the classic imaging findings for this entity?

3. What is the differential diagnosis?

4. What structure does this mass arise from?

5. What is the treatment for this entity?

Case ranking/difficulty:

Category: Meninges, skull and scalp

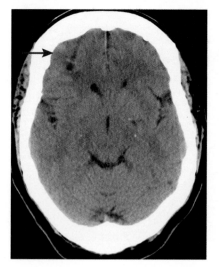

Axial CT shows an oval-shaped, heterogeneous extraaxial lesion (*arrow*) overlying the right frontal lobe with associated vasogenic edema.

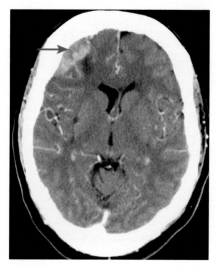

Axial CT with contrast shows heterogeneous enhancement of the extraaxial lesion (*arrow*).

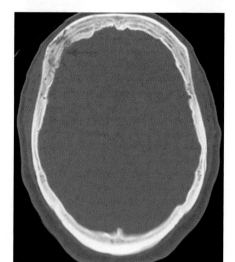

Axial CT bone window demonstrates erosion of the frontal bone with loss of the inner table (*arrow*).

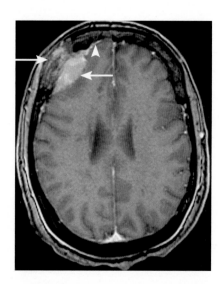

Axial T1 postcontrast demonstrates enhancing extraaxial lesion with invasion of the skull (*white arrows*) and a dural tail (*arrowhead*).

Answers

1. The abnormality is located adjacent to the right frontal lobe.

2. Hemangiopericytomas are not associated with calcifications. These lesions are associated with bone erosion, heterogeneous enhancement, and necrosis.

3. The differential diagnosis includes meningioma, metastasis, and hemangiopericytoma.

4. Hemangiopericytomas are neoplasms of the meninges.

5. The treatment for this entity is surgical removal. Chemotherapy may improve survival in recurrent tumors.

Pearls

- Hemangiopericytomas are neoplasms of the meninges that originate from pericytes.
- The most common sites are sphenoid/parasellar, lateral convexity, and superior parasellar.
- Look for bone erosion.
- Calcifications and hyperostosis consider meningioma.
- If the patient has a primary carcinoma, consider metastasis.
- Consider hemangiopericytomas in aggressive or atypical appearances of a meningioma.

Suggested Reading

Chiechi MV, Smirniotopoulos JG, Mena H. Intracranial hemangiopericytomas: MR and CT features. *AJNR Am J Neuroradiol*. 1996 Aug;17(7):1365-1371.

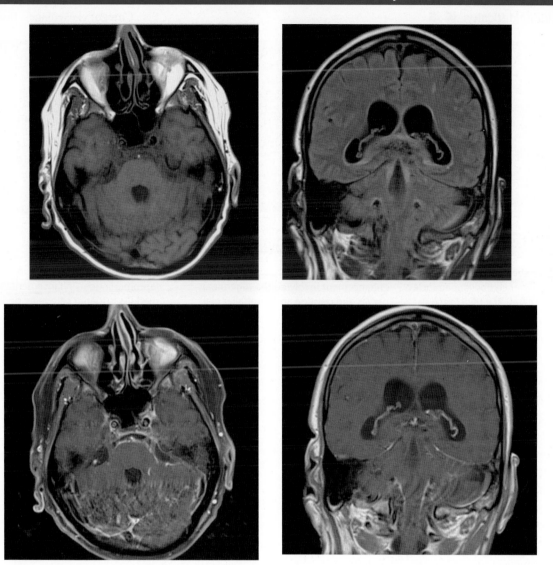

1. Where is the abnormality located?

2. What are the classic imaging findings for this entity?

3. What is the differential diagnosis?

4. Which malignant etiologies are most commonly associated with this type of contrast-enhancing pattern?

5. What is the treatment for this entity?

Case ranking/difficulty:

Category: Meninges, skull and scalp

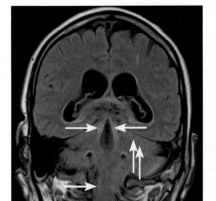

Coronal FLAIR shows linear high signal along the superior cerebellar peduncles, medulla, and cerebellar folia (*arrows*).

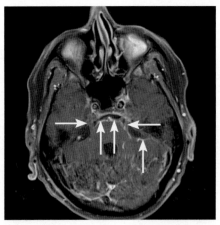

Axial T1 postcontrast shows leptomeningeal enhancement involving the trigeminal nerves and pontine and cerebellar pial surfaces (*arrows*).

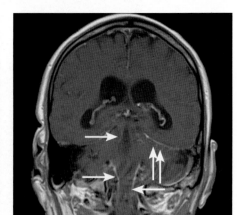

Coronal T1 postcontrast shows leptomeningeal enhancement involving the medulla, superior cerebellar peduncles, and cerebellar folia (*arrows*).

Answers

1. The abnormality involves the infratentorial leptomeninges.

2. On imaging, leptomeningeal metastases usually have a curvilinear or gyriform appearance and typically outline the brain anatomy along the pial surface. In general, meningeal enhancement is easier to identify on contrast-enhanced MRI when compared to CT.

3. The differential diagnosis includes metastasis, meningitis (bacterial and viral), and granulomatous disease (sarcoid and TB).

4. Leptomeningeal (pia and arachnoid) metastasis is most commonly caused by breast carcinoma, acute lymphocytic leukemia, non-Hodgkin lymphoma, small cell lung carcinoma, and renal carcinoma. Primary CNS tumors may also cause leptomeningeal metastasis; these include medulloblastoma, ependymoma, glioblastoma, and oligodendroglioma.

5. The treatment for leptomeningeal metastasis includes radiation and chemotherapy (usually intrathecal).

Pearls

- Leptomeningeal metastasis is most commonly the result of hematogenous dissemination.
- Causes of leptomeningeal metastasis include breast, acute lymphocytic leukemia, non-Hodgkin lymphoma, small cell lung carcinoma, and renal carcinoma.
- Primary CNS tumors causing leptomeningeal metastasis include medulloblastoma, ependymoma, glioblastoma, and oligodendroglioma.
- If pachymeningeal or leptomeningeal metastasis is suspected, search for other lesions within the skull and brain.
- If a history of infection is present, consider meningitis.
- Leptomeningeal metastasis usually follows sulci or surrounds brainstem or cranial nerves.
- CSF analysis can be confirmatory.

Suggested Readings

Maroldi R, Ambrosi C, Farina D. Metastatic disease of the brain: extra-axial metastases (skull, dura, leptomeningeal) and tumour spread. *Eur Radiol.* 2005 Mar;15(3):617-626.

Smirniotopoulos JG, Murphy FM, Rushing EJ, Rees JH, Schroeder JW. Patterns of contrast enhancement in the brain and meninges. *Radiographics.* 2010 Nov;27(2):525-551.

68-year-old female with progressive left eye swelling and pain. Additional history of sinusitis

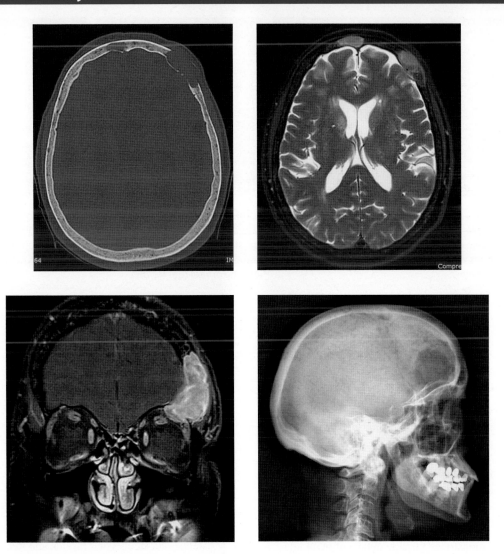

1. What is the differential diagnosis?

2. What is the best imaging modality in diagnosis?

3. What is the limitation of bone scintigraphy in this disease?

4. What is the typical radiographic finding?

5. What is the most common clinical presentation?

Case ranking/difficulty: 🌰🌰

Category: Meninges, skull and scalp

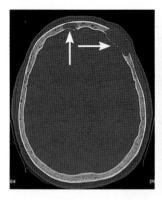

Axial CT image (*bone window*) demonstrates multiple lytic calvarial lesions in the bilateral frontal bones with irregular margins (*arrows*).

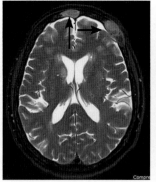

Axial T2 image with fat saturation shows T2 iso- to hyperintensity of the lytic lesions (*arrows*).

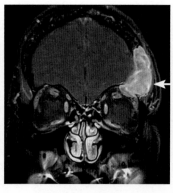

Coronal T1 postcontrast with fat saturation shows the extent of the enhancing left frontal calvarial lesion extending and protruding into the orbital roof (*arrow*).

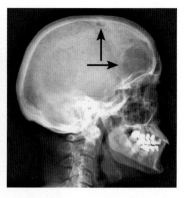

Lateral radiograph of the skull shows the punched out calvarial lesions (*arrows*).

Answers

1. Lytic metastasis, iatrogenic bony defect, hemangioma, and venous lakes are all part of the differential in lucent calvarial lesions. Langerhans cell histocytosis is in the differential diagnosis for lytic skull lesion in children.

2. Skeletal survey used to be the modality of choice in diagnosis, assessing treatment response and detecting potential complication. However, it can identify only lesions with minimum of 30% destruction of trabecular bone. FDG PET/CT is now used for staging and monitoring after treatment. Decreased FDG uptake represents decreased bone marrow activity after successful treatment.

3. Bone scan demonstrates variable uptake of myeloma lesions, most showing cold defect due to lack of osteoblastic activity.

4. Radiographic features include punched-out lytic lesions (90%) and diffuse osteopenia/osteoporosis (10%). Sclerotic lesions are rare except in posttreatment. Diffuse osteopenia/osteoporosis can be seen in the disseminated form.

5. The most common clinical presentation of multiple myeloma is bone pain. Symptomatic multiple myeloma is characterized by one or more of the following clinical manifestations with the mnemonic "CRAB": calcium elevation, renal insufficiency related to multiple myeloma, anemia, and bone abnormalities.

Pearls

- Plasma cell malignancy. Solitary lesions are termed plasmacytoma.
- Most common primary malignant neoplasm of the bone in adults, second most common blood cancer after non-Hodgkin lymphoma.
- Unknown etiology, with multiple reported associated chromosomal anomalies.
- Radiology plays an important role in diagnosis, treatment response, and detecting potential complications (pathological fractures).
- Skeletal survey used to be a modality of choice in detecting punched-out lesions (90%), diffuse osteopenia/osteoporosis (10%), and treatment response (sclerotic lesions).
- FDG PET/CT is now an important tool for staging and prognosis in multiple myeloma because of the ability to depict metabolic activity, extramedullary disease, and secondary lesions.
- CT is helpful to depict the extent of lesions.
- MRI can be helpful in identifying uncommon diffuse meningeal involvement, but serves as an adjunct to FDG PET and/or CT.

Suggested Reading

Hanrahan CJ, Christensen CR, Crim JR. Current concepts in the evaluation of multiple myeloma with MR imaging and FDG PET/CT. *Radiographics.* 2010 Jan;30(1):127-142.

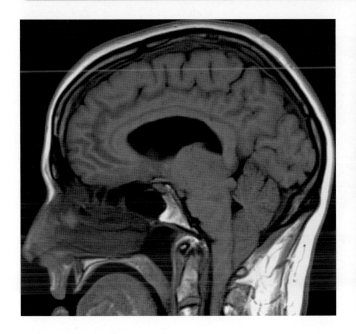
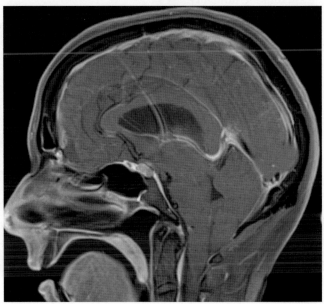

1. Where is the abnormality located?

2. What are the classic imaging findings?

3. What is the differential diagnosis?

4. What are etiologies for this finding?

5. What is the treatment for this entity?

Case ranking/difficulty:

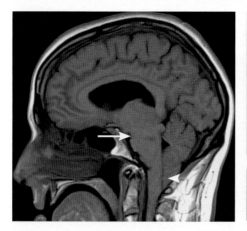

Sagittal T1 noncontrast image shows "sagging midbrain" displaced below the level of the sella with the pons compressed against the clivus. There is a closed pons-midbrain angle (*arrow*). Also noted is inferior displacement of the cerebellar tonsils through the foramen magnum (*arrowhead*).

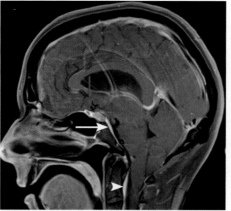

Sagittal T1 postcontrast image shows diffuse dural (*pachymeningeal*) enhancement present with distension of the upper vertebral plexus (*arrowhead*), basilar venous plexus (*white arrow*), and intercavernous sinus (*red arrow*).

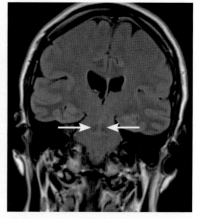

Coronal FLAIR image shows the red nuclei displaced inferiorly below the tentorium (*arrows*). These should be located above the level of the uncus.

Answers

1. The abnormality is located within the posterior cranial fossa involving the midbrain and cerebellar tonsils.

2. The classic imaging findings include "sagging midbrain"—downward displacement of the midbrain with effacement of the prepontine cistern, diffuse dural thickening with enhancement, and subdural hematoma. Displacement of the cerebellar tonsils is also commonly seen. After contrast, diffuse pachymeningeal enhancement is seen with distension of spinal epidural venous plexi.

3. The differential diagnosis includes intracranial hypotension, meningitis, traumatic subdural collections, and dural venous sinus thrombosis.

4. Intracranial hypotension may be secondary to iatrogenic injury during spinal tap, brain or spine trauma, spontaneous, severe dehydration, CSF overshunting, and vigorous exercise.

5. The treatment for this entity includes restoring CSF volume with fluid replacement, blood patch, or surgical repair with blood patch failure (when a large dural rent is present).

Pearls

- Intracranial hypotension may be secondary to CSF leakage from lumbar puncture, brain or spine trauma, spontaneous rupture, severe dehydration, CSF overshunting, and vigorous exercise.
- Look for "sagging midbrain" and tonsillar herniation.
- Diffuse smooth dural enhancement.
- Subdural fluid collections.
- Red nuclei may be below the tentorium and sella.
- Elongated pons and midbrain on axial images (fat midbrain, appearance).
- Prepontine and suprasellar cistern effaced.
- Not all these findings are necessary for diagnosis.

Suggested Readings

Sell JJ, Rupp FW, Orrison WW. Iatrogenically induced intracranial hypotension syndrome. *AJR Am J Roentgenol.* 1995 Dec;165(6):1513-1515.

Shah LM, McLean LA, Heilbrun ME, Salzman KL. Intracranial hypotension: improved MRI detection with diagnostic intracranial angles. *AJR Am J Roentgenol.* 2013 Feb;200(2):400-407.

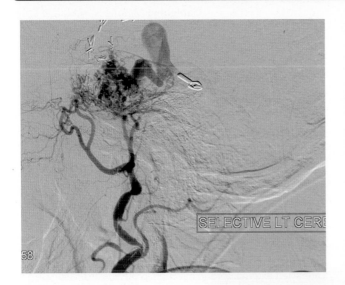 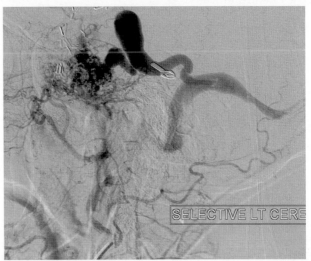

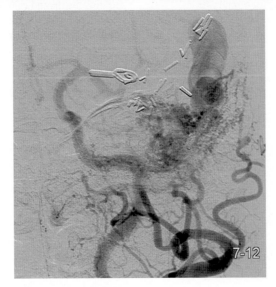

1. Where is the abnormality located?

2. What are the classic MR imaging findings for this entity?

3. What is the differential diagnosis?

4. What are possible clinical presentations?

5. What is the treatment for this entity?

Case ranking/difficulty:

Category: Meninges, skull and scalp

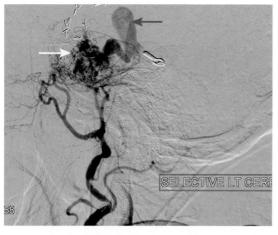

Lateral left external carotid injection DSA shows a tangle of vessels overlying the temporal lobe (*white arrow*) with early venous drainage into a large varix of the vein of Labbe (*green arrow*).

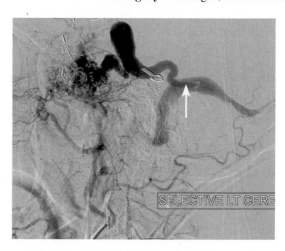

Lateral left external carotid injection in the late arterial phase confirms the dilated vein of Labbe draining into the transverse/sigmoid sinus junction (*arrow*). This is consistent with a grade 4 dural AVF with high risk of hemorrhage.

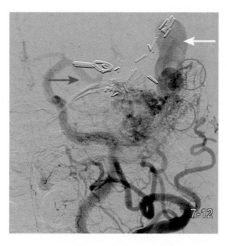

AP common carotid injection DSA during the arterial phase demonstrates multiple transosseous feeders (*green circles*) arising from the external carotid circulation. The left internal carotid artery is noted (*green arrow*). Again seen is early venous drainage into a large varix of the vein of Labbe (*white arrow*).

Answers

1. The abnormality involves supply from the external carotid artery.

2. The classic imaging MRI findings for this entity include a tangle of "flow voids" centered over the dura, with drainage into the intracerebral veins. Increased T2/FLAIR signal can be seen with venous congestion or infarct.

3. The differential diagnosis includes dural arteriovenous fistulas (dAVF), pial AVM, and dural venous sinus thrombosis with collateralization without fistula.

4. Patients usually present with pulsatile tinnitus, exophthalmos, cranial neuropathy, and rarely progressive dementia from venous hypertension.

5. The treatment for this entity includes surgical resection or catheter embolization.

Pearls

- Dural arteriovenous fistulas (dAVF) are high-flow vascular malformations with abnormal communication between arteries of the dura and intracranial veins.
- Dural AVFs are uncommon and account for 10%-15% of all intracranial AVMs.
- dAVF are usually a result of trauma, postoperative or venous sinus thrombosis in adults.
- DSA is the gold standard.
- Evaluate both internal and external carotid circulations as both can provide arterial feeders.
- Selective injections needed for ICA and ECA as both may have feeders to AVM or dAVF
- Evaluate the dural venous sinuses for thrombosis.
- Cortical and retrograde venous drainage is associated with higher grades and higher risk of hemorrhage.

Suggested Reading

Srinivasa RN, Burrows PE. Dural arteriovenous malformation in a child with Bannayan-Riley-Ruvalcaba syndrome. *AJNR Am J Neuroradiol.* 2006 Oct;27(9):1927-1929.

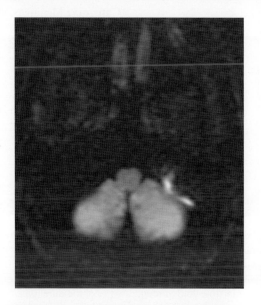
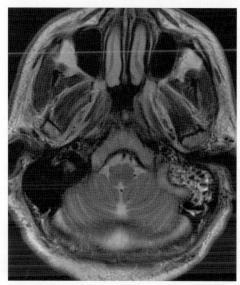
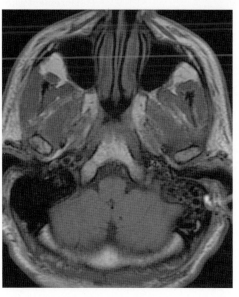
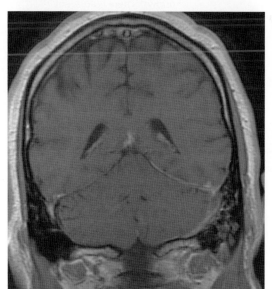

1. Where is the main finding located?

2. What are the classic imaging findings?

3. What is the significance of the empty delta sign?

4. What are associated etiologies for this entity?

5. What are MRI findings in acute lesions?

Case ranking/difficulty:

Category: Meninges, skull and scalp

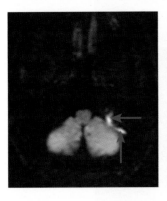

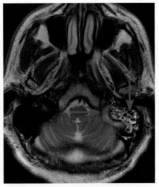

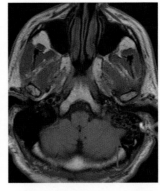

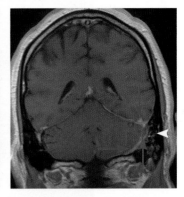

Axial DWI b-1000 image shows restricted diffusion within the left sigmoid sinus with lack of normal flow void (*arrows*).

Axial T2 image shows high signal intensity is present within the left sigmoid sinus with lack of visualization of the normal flow void (*green arrows*). There is adjacent mucosal thickening and air fluid levels within the left mastoid air cells (*red arrow*), suggesting mastoiditis.

Axial T1 image shows intermediate to high T1 signal within the left sigmoid sinus with lack of visualization of the normal flow void (*arrow*).

Coronal postcontrast image shows nonenhancing thrombus (*red arrow*). There is surrounding pachymeningeal enhancement of the dura (*green arrows*). Enhancement within the adjacent left mastoid air cells (*arrowhead*) suggests mastoiditis.

Answers

1. The main finding is located within the left sigmoid sinus.

2. Noncontrast CT will demonstrate high attenuation within the venous sinus. With administration of IV contrast an intravenous filling defect or "empty delta" sign may be seen. The most common finding on MRI imaging is loss of the normal flow void and altered signal within the dural sinus. Imaging findings can include parenchymal abnormalities with cytotoxic and vasogenic edema that do not conform to an arterial vascular territory. Hemorrhage may or may not be present.

3. The "empty delta" sign signifies thrombus within the dural venous sinus on contrast-enhanced CT and appears as a filling defect with surrounding dural enhancement.

4. Risk factors are trauma, infection, malignancy, and any systemic pathology leading to a hypercoagulable state. There is an association with dural sinus thrombosis or stenosis with idiopathic intracranial hypertension.

5. Isointensity on T1 and hypointensity on T2 can be seen with acute thrombus. Errors of perception most often occur in cases of acute thrombus because the signal characteristics of the blood breakdown products most resemble the normal venous sinus.

Pearls

- Cerebral venous thrombosis patients present with headache, nausea, and vomiting, possibly with neurologic deficit.
- Risk factors include trauma, infection, malignancy, and hypercoagulable state.
- Classically, noncontrast CT will demonstrate high attenuation within the venous sinus.
- In CT with contrast, the key finding is a filling defect in the sinus, usually triangular in shape—the "empty delta" sign.
- When imaging with MRI, time of flight, contrast-enhanced venography techniques, and gradient echo sequences should be used.
- Parenchymal abnormalities include both cytotoxic and vasogenic edema with or without hemorrhage and may be reversible.
- Pachymeningeal enhancement may be seen.

Suggested Readings

Leach JL, Fortuna RB, Jones BV, Gaskill-Shipley MF. Imaging of cerebral venous thrombosis: current techniques, spectrum of findings, and diagnostic pitfalls. *Radiographics*. 2006 Oct;26(suppl 1):S19-S41; discussion S42-3.

Provenzale JM, Kranz PG. Dural sinus thrombosis: sources of error in image interpretation. *AJR Am J Roentgenol*. 2011 Jan;196(1):23-31.

6-year-old female with gelastic seizures and precocious puberty

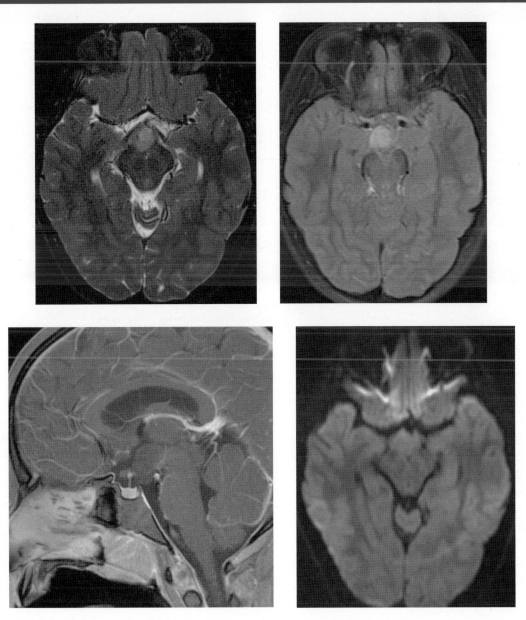

1. Where is the abnormality located?

2. What are typical imaging findings for this entity?

3. What is the differential diagnosis?

4. What is the etiology of this entity?

5. What are the classic symptoms in this entity?

Case ranking/difficulty: **Category:** Sellar/suprasellar

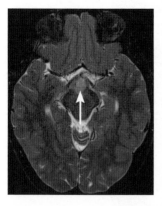

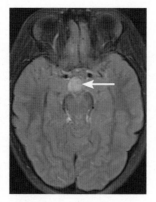

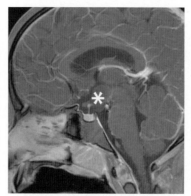

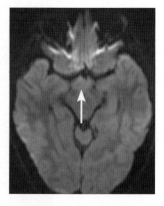

Axial T2 image shows a mass in the hypothalamus that is well circumscribed and slightly hyperintense to gray matter (*arrow*).

Axial FLAIR image shows the suprasellar mass with hyperintensity to gray matter (*arrow*).

Sagittal T1 postcontrast image demonstrates no enhancement of the suprasellar mass, which is pedunculated off of the tuber cinereum (*asterisk*) located posterior to the infundibulum and anterior to the mammillary bodies (*not seen*). The mass is iso- to hypointense to gray matter.

Axial DWI b = 1000 image demonstrates no restricted diffusion with isointense signal to gray matter (*arrow*).

Answers

1. The mass is located in the tuber cinereum of the hypothalamus.

2. Tuber cinereum hamartomas (TCH) are well-circumscribed masses either sessile or pedunculated from the tuber cinereum. They generally follow gray matter on MR imaging but may be slightly hyperintense on T2 and hypointense on T1 from fibrillary gliosis. No enhancement is typical.

3. The differential diagnosis for a suprasellar mass includes tuber cinereum hamartoma, Langerhans cell histiocytosis (in a child), and suprasellar neoplasms such as germinoma and astrocytoma.

4. TCH is considered a neuronal migrational anomaly, as the histopathology primarily includes well-differentiated neurons.

5. The classic presenting symptoms of TCH include both gelastic seizures and precocious puberty. Gelastic seizures are sudden bursts of uncontrollable laughing or crying. While any seizure can be seen with TCH, gelastic seizures are specific to the hypothalamus.

Pearls

- Neuronal migrational anomaly to the tuber cinereum.
- Hypothalamus located between infundibulum and mammillary bodies.
- Follows gray matter on all sequences, with slight hyperintensity on T2/FLAIR secondary to fibrillary gliosis.
- No enhancement.
- With enhancing suprasellar masses, consider astrocytoma, germinoma, or Langerhans cell histiocytosis.

Suggested Readings

Boyko OB, Curnes JT, Oakes WJ, Burger PC. Hamartomas of the tuber cinereum: CT, MR, and pathologic findings. *AJNR Am J Neuroradiol.* 1991;12(2):309-314.

Martin DD, Seeger U, Ranke MB, Grodd W. MR imaging and spectroscopy of a tuber cinereum hamartoma in a patient with growth hormone deficiency and hypogonadotropic hypogonadism. *AJNR Am J Neuroradiol.* 2003;24(6):1177-1180.

23-year-old male with weight loss, cough, low-grade fevers, headache, blurry vision

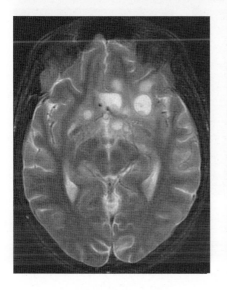
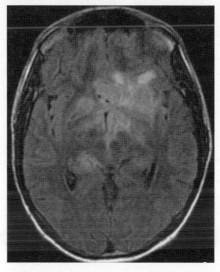
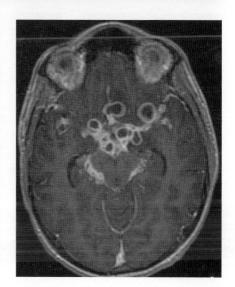

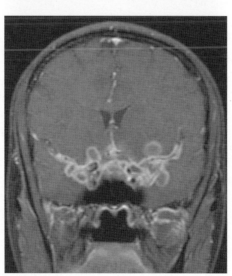

1. What is the differential diagnosis?

2. What are two CNS lesions that often coexist in this disease?

3. What are common associated morbidities in this disease?

4. Which patients are at risk for this disease?

5. What is the prognosis of this CNS disease?

Case ranking/difficulty:

Category: Sellar/suprasellar

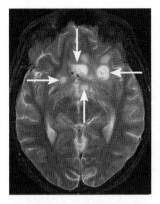

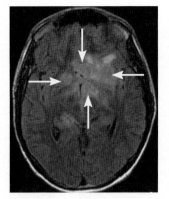

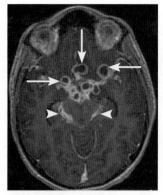

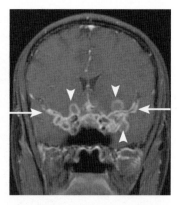

Axial T2 image shows cystic lesions (*arrows*) in the inferior frontal lobes and hypothalamus centered on the suprasellar cistern.

Axial FLAIR image shows cystic lesions (*arrows*) in the inferior frontal lobes and hypothalamus centered on the suprasellar cistern with associated edema.

Axial T1 post contrast image shows the cysts to be ring enhancing (*arrows*) with basilar meningeal enhancement (*arrowheads*).

Coronal T1 postcontrast image shows diffuse enhancement of the basilar meninges (*arrows*) with associated adjacent parenchymal ring-enhancing lesions (*arrowheads*).

Answers

1. The differential of leptomeningeal enhancement in the basilar cisterns includes basilar meningitis from bacterial, fungal, or tuberculous etiology, neurosarcoid, and leptomeningeal carcinomatosis.

2. Two tuberculous lesions occurring in the CNS are tuberculomas, which are coalescent tubercles that can be caseating or solid, and TB meningitis, which occurs with inflammation of the leptomeninges from rupture of tubercles into the subarachnoid space.

3. Associated morbidity of TB meningitis includes arteritis, leading to potential end artery infarction (up to 40% of patients). Meningitis and tuberculomas may cause hydrocephalus from mass effect or ventriculitis.

4. Both immunocompetent and immunocompromised individuals are at risk for TB, although immunocompromised individuals (HIV, transplantation) are more susceptible. Immunocompetent individuals may have sick contacts or live in an endemic area.

5. Up to 80% morbidity with long-term neurologic sequelae can be seen with treated CNS TB. Significant mortality in up to 1/3 of immunocompetent patients is seen, even higher for AIDS patients.

Pearls

- CNS tuberculosis in the intracranial space can be subdivided into two categories: tuberculoma and meningitis.

- Coalescing tubercles form larger granulomatous tuberculomas.
- TB meningitis is the dominant form of the disease, especially in children. Both forms can coexist.
- Tuberculomas may show a ring-enhancing hypodense lesion with surrounding edema on contrast-enhanced CT.
- Tuberculomas with caseating necrotic center: T1 hypointensity and T2 hyperintensity and ring enhancement.
- Tuberculomas with solid center: isointense T1 and hypointense T2 and central enhancement.
- TB meningitis: Classically in the basilar cisterns.
- TB meningitis: T1 iso- to hyperintense to CSF, T2 iso- or hyperintense to CSF and FLAIR hyperintensity; shaggy nodular leptomeningeal enhancement.
- Punctate enhancement within the basal ganglia.
- DWI may show central restricted diffusion in a tuberculoma.

Suggested Readings

Nair PP, Kalita J, Kumar S, Misra UK. MRI pattern of infarcts in basal ganglia region in patients with tuberculous meningitis. *Neuroradiology.* 2009 Apr;51(4):221-225.

Patkar D, Narang J, Yanamandala R, Lawande M, Shah GV. Central nervous system tuberculosis: pathophysiology and imaging findings. *Neuroimaging Clin N Am.* 2012 Nov;22(4):677-705.

5-year-old boy with history of decreased vision and optic nerve atrophy bilaterally

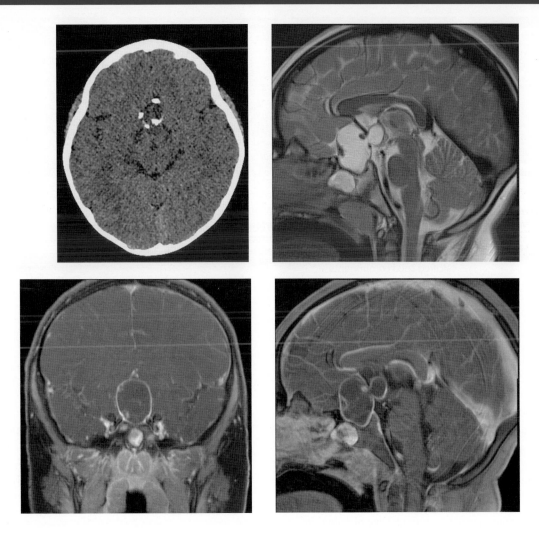

1. What is the differential diagnosis?

2. What is the embryological structure of origin for this tumor?

3. What age groups have the greatest incidence of this tumor?

4. What are typical neuroimaging findings for this tumor in children?

5. What is the prognosis for this disease?

Case ranking/difficulty:

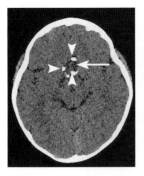

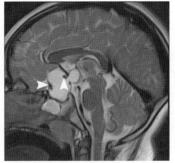

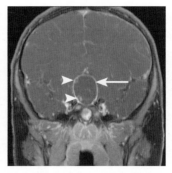

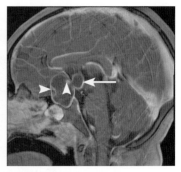

Axial CT image shows a cystic mass (*arrow*) in the suprasellar cistern with coarse dystrophic calcifications (*arrowheads*).

Sagittal T2 image shows a bilobed cystic lesion with T2 hyperintensity involving the sella and suprasellar cistern. Focal hypointensity likely represents calcified solid components (*arrowheads*).

Coronal T1 postcontrast shows enhancement of the cyst wall (*arrow*) and solid components (*arrowheads*).

Sagittal postcontrast image shows enhancement of the cyst wall (*arrow*) and solid nodular components (*arrowheads*).

Answers

1. The differential diagnosis for a cystic suprasellar mass includes craniopharyngioma, Rathke cleft cyst, epidermoid cyst, and arachnoid cyst. Germinoma is in the differential for a suprasellar neoplasm but does not demonstrate predominantly cystic changes.

2. Rathke pouch (craniopharyngeal duct), which arises from the oral ectoderm, migrates into the intracranial sella forming the anterior pituitary gland. Epithelial cells from Rathke pouch remnants in the stalk form the basis of craniopharyngiomas.

3. Craniopharyngiomas have a bimodal age distribution with adamantinomatous tumors in children between 5 and 15 years of age and papillary tumors in adults 50-75 years of age.

4. Adamantinomatous craniopharyngiomas are most common in children and are typically mixed multicystic with enhancing solid components and calcification in the suprasellar space.

5. Craniopharyngiomas are WHO grade I tumors with 90% 10-year survival. However, significant morbidity from hypothalamic, pituitary, and optic nerve dysfunction is common with 22% mortality from treatment complications beyond 10 years.

Pearls

- Craniopharyngiomas (CP) are WHO grade I epithelial tumors arising from Rathke pouch remnants most commonly in the suprasellar cistern.
- Craniopharyngioma have a bimodal distribution with adamantinomatous histological type in children and papillary type in adults.
- Adamantinomatous craniopharyngiomas are the most common intracranial nonglial tumor in children and greater than 50% of suprasellar tumors in children.
- Adamantinomatous CP are typically multicystic, with enhancing solid components and cyst walls.
- 90% of adamantinomatous CP have dystrophic coarse calcification.

Suggested Readings

Hamamoto Y, Niino K, Adachi M, Hosoya T. MR and CT findings of craniopharyngioma during and after radiation therapy. *Neuroradiology*. 2002 Feb;44(2):118-122.

Pisaneschi M, Kapoor G. Imaging the sella and parasellar region. *Neuroimaging Clin N Am*. 2005 Feb;15(1):203-219.

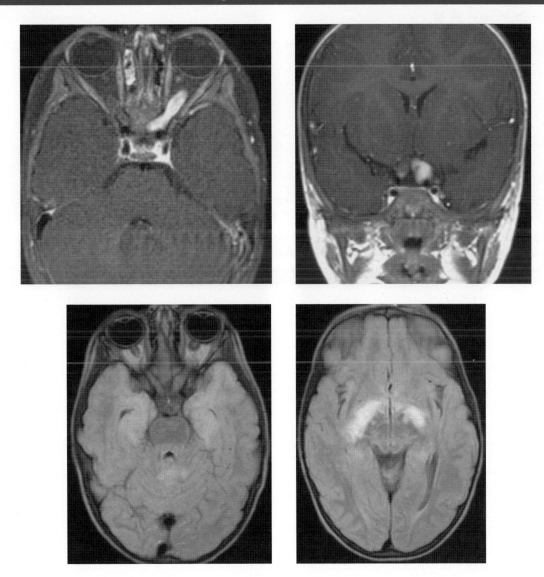

1. Where is the abnormality located?

2. What are the classic imaging findings for this entity?

3. What is the differential diagnosis?

4. What are findings for neurofibromatosis type 1?

5. What is the treatment for this entity?

Case ranking/difficulty:

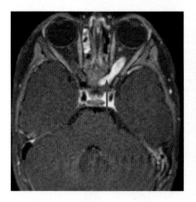

Axial postcontrast T1 shows enlarged enhancing left optic nerve (*green arrow*).

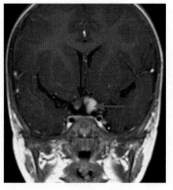

Coronal postcontrast T1 shows enlarged enhancing left optic nerve (*green arrow*) and optic chiasm (*blue arrow*).

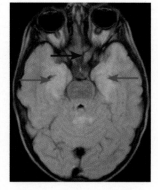

Axial FLAIR shows multiple hyperintense signal areas in bilateral mesial temporal lobes (*green arrows*). These are a typical location for focal areas of signal intensity in NF1. Enlarged left optic nerve (*blue arrow*) shows hyperintense signal.

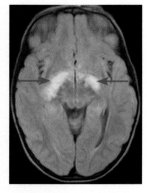

Axial FLAIR image 27 months later, showing multiple hyperintense signal areas in the basal ganglia and optic pathway (*green arrow*).

Answers

1. The abnormality is located within the enlarged, enhancing left optic nerve.

2. The classic imaging findings for this entity are an enlarged optic nerve with enhancement.

3. The differential diagnosis includes optic nerve glioma, optic neuritis, and optic nerve sheath meningioma.

4. Neurofibromatosis type 1 patients show other findings in multiple organ systems: cafe au lait spots, axillary freckling, Lisch nodules in the iris, subcutaneous neurofibromas, plexiform neurofibromas, sphenoid wing dysplasia, exophthalmos, buphthalmos, lambdoid suture defect, enlarged skull foramina, enlarged spinal neural foramina, scoliosis, dural ectasia, lateral meningocele, posterior vertebral scalloping, ribbon ribs, pseudoarthrosis of the tibia, multiple nonossifying fibromas, and unilateral hypertrophy of limbs.

5. Asymptomatic optic nerve gliomas can be observed unless it progresses toward the optic chiasm. Visual dysfunction, severe proptosis with exposure keratopathy, or growth toward optic chiasm requires treatment. Surgery is preferred if treatment is necessary. Chemotherapy and radiation are used only when unresectable or residual vision is desired.

Pearls

- Key to diagnosis of ONG is optic nerve enlargement and enhancement.
- Size of optic nerve gliomas does not correlate with symptoms.
- Optic nerve neuritis does not typically cause mass-like enlargement.
- Consider neurofibromatosis with history of cafe au lait spots or axillary freckling.

Suggested Readings

Parsa CF. Why visual function does not correlate with optic glioma size or growth. *Arch Ophthalmol.* 2012 Apr;130(4):521-522.

Shriver EM, Ragheb J, Tse DT. Combined transcranial-orbital approach for resection of optic nerve gliomas: a clinical and anatomical study. *Ophthal Plast Reconstr Surg.* 2012 May;28(3):184-191.

30-year-old female with headaches

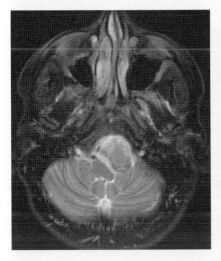
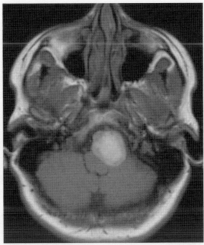
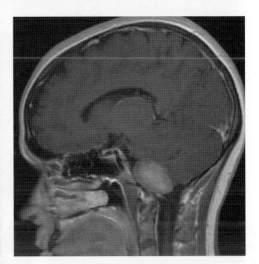
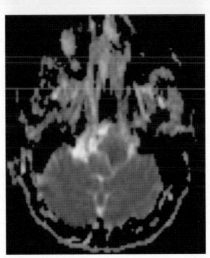

1. What is the differential diagnosis?

2. What causes the T1 hyperintensity and T2 hypointensity in this lesion?

3. What is the most common location for this lesion?

4. What is the embryological cell type of this lesion?

5. What is the treatment for this disease?

Case ranking/difficulty: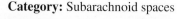

Category: Subarachnoid spaces

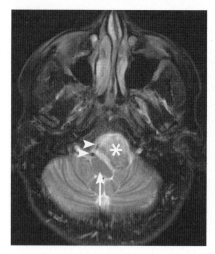

Axial T2 image shows an extraaxial mass (*asterisk*) with displacement of the vertebral arteries (*arrowhead*) and brainstem (*arrow*) to the right. The mass has heterogeneous signal with central T2 hypointensity.

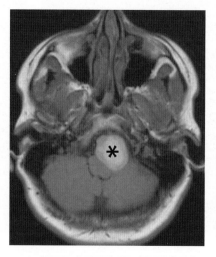

Axial T1 image shows the well-circumscribed mass with central T1 hyperintensity (*asterisk*).

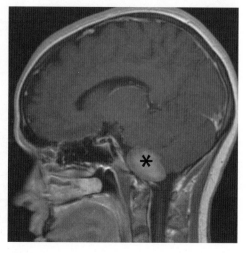

Sagittal T1 postcontrast image demonstrates no additional T1 shortening to suggest enhancement (*asterisk*).

4. Neurenteric cysts arise from endoderm.

5. Surgical resection or observation can be options depending on the size of the lesion and associated clinical history.

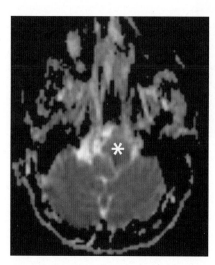

Axial DWI ADC image shows restricted diffusion within the mass (*asterisk*).

Pearls

- Neurenteric cysts are congenital endodermal cysts that likely arise from the neurenteric canal failing to separate from the notochord.
- 3/4 of reported lesions are seen anterior or lateral to the pontomedullary junction in an extraaxial location.
- On CT, T1, and T2 imaging the cysts can have variable internal density and hypointensity due to viscous mucoid fluid.
- The majority tend to be bright on T2.
- Restricted diffusion may be seen but is variable.
- No internal enhancement is seen, but may have thin rim enhancement.
- Neurenteric cysts can be a reported cause of chemical meningitis from content leakage.

Answers

1. The differential for an extraaxial cystic lesion with heterogeneous internal signal, no enhancement, and restricted diffusion includes dermoid or epidermoid cyst and neurenteric cyst.

2. Viscous mucoid material can cause T1 hyperintense and T2 hypointense signal in a neurenteric cyst.

3. 3/4 of reported intracranial cases of neurenteric cyst are within the posterior fossa.

Suggested Readings

Preece MT, Osborn AG, Chin SS, Smirniotopoulos JG. Intracranial neurenteric cysts: imaging and pathology spectrum. *AJNR Am J Neuroradiol.* 2006;27(6): 1211-1216.

Shin JH, Byun BJ, Kim DW, Choi DL. Neurenteric cyst in the cerebellopontine angle with xanthogranulomatous changes: serial MR findings with pathologic correlation. *AJNR Am J Neuroradiol.* 2002 Apr;23(4):663-665.

55-year-old male with retroorbitial headache

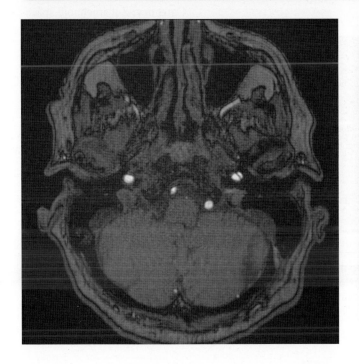 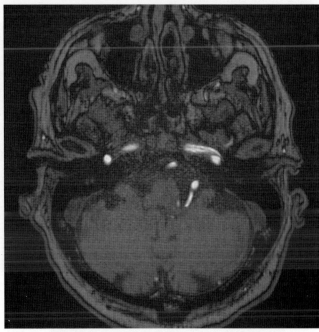

1. Where is the abnormality located?

2. What are the classic imaging findings for this entity?

3. What is the differential diagnosis?

4. What are the most common etiologies of this finding?

5. What is the treatment for this entity?

Case ranking/difficulty:

Category: Subarachnoid spaces

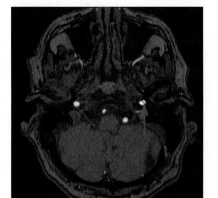

Axial 3D time of flight image shows irregular appearance of the left internal carotid artery within the petrous carotid canal (*arrow*).

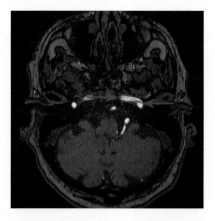

Axial 3D time of flight image shows irregular appearance to the left petrous internal carotid artery. Note the internal linear structure representing an intimal flap (*arrows*).

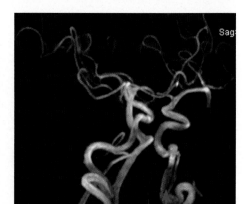

Maximum intensity projection MRA image demonstrates the classic "dual lumen" appearance to the distal left internal carotid artery (*arrow*).

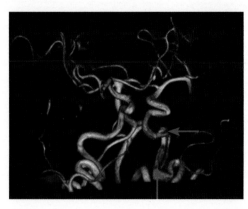

CTA volume rendered 3D image demonstrates the classic "dual lumen" appearance of the distal left internal carotid artery (*arrows*).

Pearls

- Dissection is an injury resulting in hemorrhage within the wall of the artery.
- Dissections are usually spontaneous or traumatic.
- T1 with fat saturation may help visualize intraluminal thrombus of the false or true lumen.
- When in doubt on CTA and MRA, catheter angiography may confirm.
- If multiple vessels involved in the region of subarachnoid hemorrhage, consider vasospasm.
- Look for "double lumen" and "flame" (tapered cut off) appearances.
- MIP and volume-rendered images may be helpful.

Answers

1. The abnormality involves the internal carotid artery.

2. Dissection classically will have a double-lumen appearance created by an intimal flap.

3. The differential diagnosis includes dissection, vasospasm, and atherosclerosis.

4. Dissection etiologies are usually spontaneous or traumatic. Spontaneous dissections are related to hypertension, cystic medial necrosis, fibromuscular dysplasia, and connective tissue disorders (Marfan and Ehlers-Danlos).

5. Typical treatement involves medical therapy with anticoagulation, but interventions may be performed including occlusion, wrapping, bypass, and stenting.

Suggested Readings

Provenzale JM. Dissection of the internal carotid and vertebral arteries: imaging features. *AJR Am J Roentgenol.* 1995 Nov;165(5):1099-1104.

Provenzale JM, Sarikaya B. Comparison of test performance characteristics of MRI, MR angiography, and CT angiography in the diagnosis of carotid and vertebral artery dissection: a review of the medical literature. *AJR Am J Roentgenol.* 2009 Oct;193(4):1167-1174.

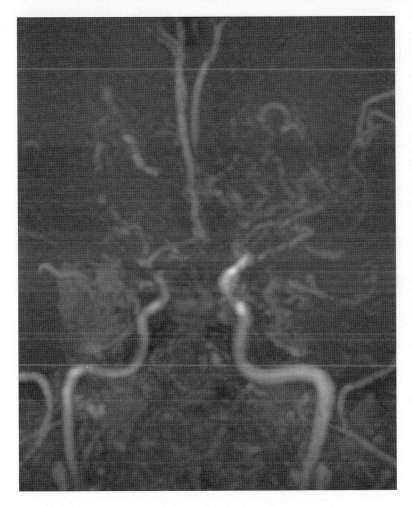 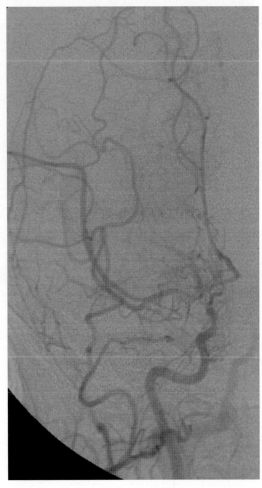

1. Where is the abnormality located?

2. What are the classic imaging findings for this entity?

3. What is the differential diagnosis?

4. What syndromes are associated with this finding?

5. What is the treatment for this entity?

Case ranking/difficulty:

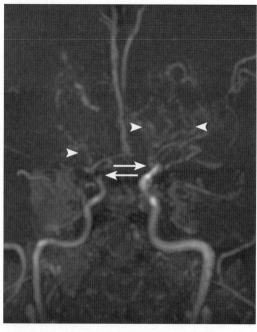

Frontal maximum intensity projection image taken from time of flight imaging technique shows an irregular circle of Willis with bilateral distal ICA occlusion (*arrows*) and prominent lenticulostriate collaterals (*arrowheads*).

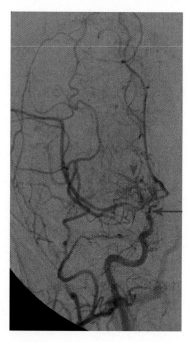

Frontal view of right internal carotid DSA demonstrates severe stenosis of the supraclinoid segment of the ICA (*red arrow*) with prominent lenticulate collaterals (*arrowhead*) resembling a "puff of smoke." The collaterals help reconstitute the MCA and ACA.

Answers

1. The abnormality is located in the distal intracranial internal carotid artery.

2. On MR, prominent flow voids and leptomeningeal contrast enhancement may be seen in the basal ganglia. On angiogram, typically the distal internal carotid arteries and proximal MCA and ACA demonstrate severe stenosis resulting in prominent lenticulostriate collaterals.

3. The differential diagnosis includes vasculitis, moyamoya, and atherosclerosis.

4. Moyamoya may be associated with sickle cell disease, Down syndrome, NF 1, and tuberous sclerosis.

5. Antithrombotic therapy may be helpful to prevent strokes. Surgical bypass, either direct (superficial temporal artery [STA] and MCA anastomosis) or indirect (STA pial synangiosis), may be performed.

Pearls

- Vasculopathy characteristically involving the internal carotid artery (ICA) bifurcation.

- The key to diagnosis is noting severe ICA stenosis or occlusion resulting in multiple lenticulostriate collaterals.
- Primary idiopathic form most commonly seen in the Asian population.
- Secondary forms associated with Down syndrome, sickle cell, NF1, vasculitis, and radiation vasculopathy.
- The term moyamoya is Japanese and translates to "puff of smoke," which was the name given secondary to its characteristic appearance on angiogram.

Suggested Readings

Jang DK, Lee KS, Rha HK, et al. Clinical and angiographic features and stroke types in adult moyamoya disease. *AJNR Am J Neuroradiol.* 2014 Jun;35(6):1124-1131.

Pereira PL, Farnsworth CT, Duda SH, Rose M, Reinbold WD, Claussen CD. Pediatric moyamoya syndrome: follow-up study with MR angiography. *AJR Am J Roentgenol.* 1996 Aug;167(2):526-528.

Yoon HK, Shin HJ, Lee M, Byun HS, Na DG, Han BK. MR angiography of moyamoya disease before and after encephaloduroarteriosynangiosis. *AJR Am J Roentgenol.* 2000 Jan;174(1):195-200.

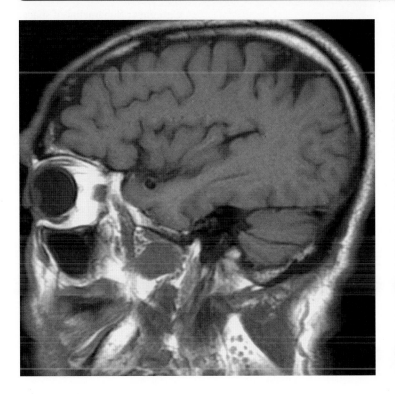
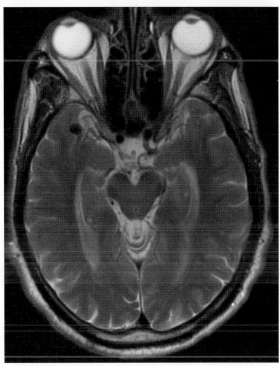

1. Where is the abnormality located?

2. What are the classic imaging findings for this entity on noncontrast MR?

3. What is the differential diagnosis?

4. What are associated risk factors for this entity?

5. What is the treatment for this entity?

Case ranking/difficulty: **Category:** Subarachnoid spaces

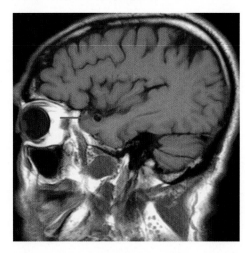

Sagittal T1 image shows a prominent hypointensity suggesting flow void of the MCA bifurcation just superior to temporal lobe (*arrow*).

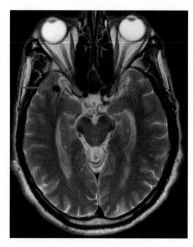

Axial T2 image shows a round extraaxial hypointensity at the expected location of the right MCA bifurcation (*arrow*).

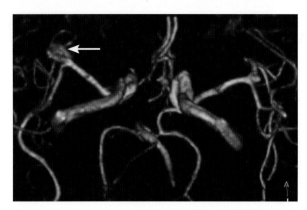

This 3D reconstructed image from time of flight MR angiography confirms the saccular aneurysm originating from the right MCA bifurcation (*arrow*).

Answers

1. The abnormality is located within the subarachnoid space just superior to the right temporal lobe, in the expected location of the MCA bifurcation.

2. On MRI the classic finding is an enlarged flow void that appears as low T1 and T2 signal.

3. The differential diagnosis includes aneurysm, meningioma, and aerated clinoid process mimicking vascular flow void.

4. Risk factors for intracranial aneurysms include family history, autosomal dominant polycystic kidney disease, Ehlers-Danlos, NF-1, fibromuscular dysplasia, AVM, cystic fibrosis, Klippel-Trenaunay-Weber, Osler-Weber-Rendu, and Kawasaki disease.

5. The treatment for this entity may be endovascular therapy (coiling, stents, or liquid embolic agents) or surgical clipping.

Pearls

- Intracranial aneurysms are most commonly saccular (berry type).
- Aneurysms commonly occur at bifurcations (stress points).
- Look for abnormal focal vascular dilatation (an enlarged flow void).
- Most aneurysms seen in clinical practice are less than 1.5 cm in size.
- Typically the larger the aneurysm, the more likely it will rupture.
- Reformatted images including MIPs and 3D may be helpful.
- When noncontrast imaging findings suspect aneurysm, confirm with CTA or MRA.

Suggested Readings

Hacein-Bey L, Provenzale JM. Current imaging assessment and treatment of intracranial aneurysms. *AJR Am J Roentgenol.* 2011 Jan;196(1):32-44.

Kemmling A, Noelte I, Gerigk L, Singer S, Groden C, Scharf J. A diagnostic pitfall for intracranial aneurysms in time-of-flight MR angiography: small intracranial lipomas. *AJR Am J Roentgenol.* 2008 Jan;190(1):W62-W67.

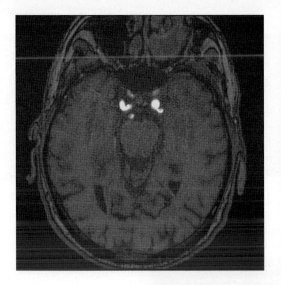 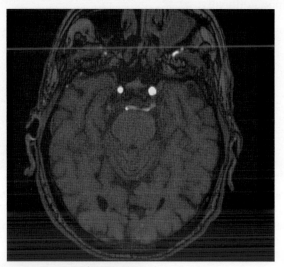

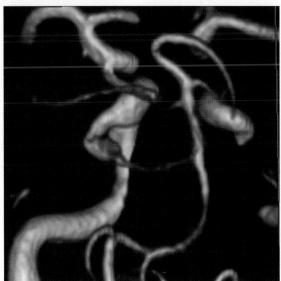

1. What structure does the abnormality involve?

2. What is the angiographic classification?

3. What is the differential diagnosis?

4. What are presenting symptoms?

5. What is the treatment for this entity?

Case ranking/difficulty:

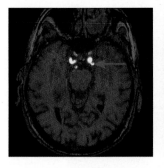

Axial 3D time of flight MRA shows an anomalous vessel projecting off the left cavernous internal carotid artery posteriorly (*arrow*).

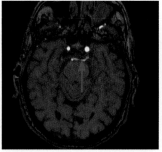

Axial 3D time of flight MRA shows a direct connection to the hypoplastic basilar artery (*arrow*).

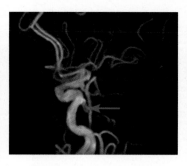

Maximum intensity projection image from time of flight data shows a direct connection between the left cavernous internal carotid artery and the basilar artery (*arrow*).

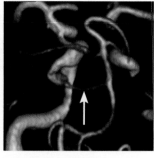

3D reconstructed image from time of flight data shows a direct connection is seen between the left cavernous internal carotid artery and the basilar artery (*arrow*).

Answers

1. Persistent trigeminal artery (PTA) is an embryonic anastomosis between the anterior and posterior circulation connecting the cavernous internal carotid artery and the basilar artery.

2. Saltzman characterized the persistent trigeminal artery into two main types. Type I is associated with a hypoplastic basilar and absent to hypoplastic posterior communicating arteries, with the PTA as the main supply of the superior cerebellar arteries (SCA) and posterior cerebral arteries. In Saltzman type II, the basilar is normal size and the PTA supplies the SCA and patent posterior communicating arteries supply the posterior cerebral arteries.

3. The differential diagnosis includes persistent trigeminal artery, persistent hypoglossal artery, and persistent otic artery.

4. PTA is usually asymptomatic but can rarely be associated with trigeminal neuralgia.

5. No treatment is necessary for this entity, unless for trigeminal neuralgia.

Pearls

- Persistent trigeminal artery (PTA) is an embryonic anastomosis between the anterior and posterior circulation.
- PTA is the most common persistent carotid basilar anastomosis followed by the persistent hypoglossal artery.
- PTA is usually asymptomatic but can rarely be associated with trigeminal neuralgia.
- PTA may follow trigeminal nerve path.
- Basilar artery commonly hypoplastic.

Suggested Readings

Patel AB, Gandhi CD, Bederson JB. Angiographic documentation of a persistent otic artery. *AJNR Am J Neuroradiol.* 2003 Jan;24(1):124-126.

Soens J, Vrabec M, Demaerel P, Wilms G. Persistent trigeminal artery variant: MR angiographic demonstration. A report of two cases. *Neuroradiol J.* 2010 Dec;23(6):696-699.

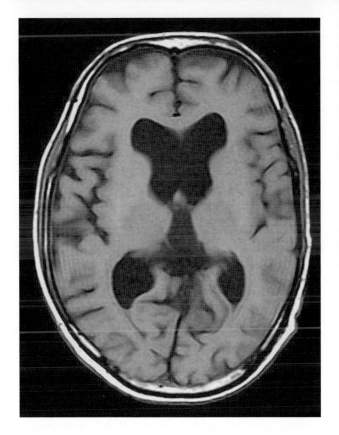 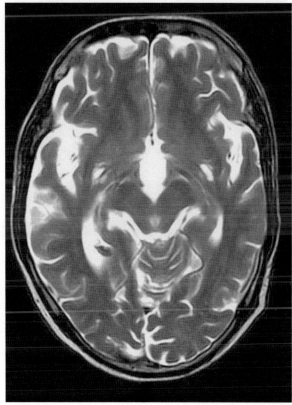

1. What is the most common cause of this entity?

2. What are the classic imaging findings for this entity?

3. What is the differential diagnosis?

4. What is the treatment for this entity?

5. What are the classic symptoms in this entity?

Case ranking/difficulty: **Category:** Ventricles and cisterns

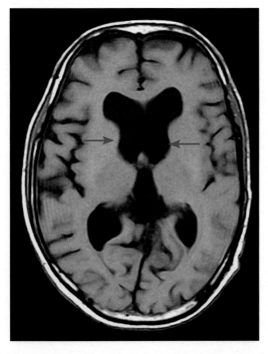

Axial T1 image shows dilated lateral ventricles (*green arrows*).

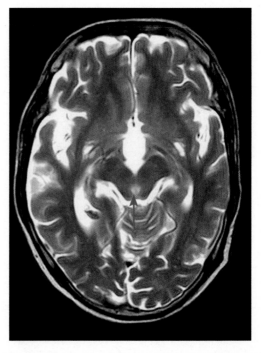

Axial T2 image shows exaggerated aqueductal CSF flow void (*green arrow*).

Answers

1. 50% of NPH is idiopathic. Other causes include trauma, hemorrhage, and infection.

2. On imaging, the ventricles will be dilated out of proportion to the sulcal enlargement. On MRI, the aqueduct and third ventricle may create "flow voids" signifying increased flow rate of CSF. CSF seepage into the periventricular white matter may be seen acutely, resulting in stretching of the fibers.

3. The differential diagnosis includes normal-pressure hydrocephalus, vascular dementia, and Alzheimer disease.

4. Mainstay of NPH treatment is to divert CSF; therefore, shunting is utilized.

5. The classic triad of NPH includes urinary incontinence, dementia, and gait apraxia ("wet, wacky, and wobbly").

Pearls

- Normal-pressure hydrocephalus (NPH) has a classic triad of gait disturbance, dementia, and urinary incontinence.
- Dilatation of ventricles is out of proportion to sulcal atrophy.
- "Flow voids" in aqueduct and third ventricle.
- Indium-labeled CSF may also be diagnostic with ventricular reflux at 24-48 hours.

Suggested Readings

Bradley WG, Safar FG, Furtado C, Ord J, Alksne JF. Increased intracranial volume: a clue to the etiology of idiopathic normal-pressure hydrocephalus? *AJNR Am J Neuroradiol*. 2004 Oct;25(9):1479-1484.

Kitagaki H, Mori E, Ishii K, Yamaji S, Hirono N, Imamura T. CSF spaces in idiopathic normal pressure hydrocephalus: morphology and volumetry. *AJNR Am J Neuroradiol*. 1998 Aug;19(7):1277-1284.

Tullberg M, Jensen C, Ekholm S, Wikkelsø C. Normal pressure hydrocephalus: vascular white matter changes on MR images must not exclude patients from shunt surgery. *AJNR Am J Neuroradiol*. 2001 Oct;22(9):1665-1673.

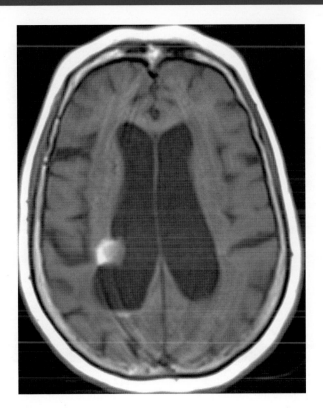

1. Where is the abnormality located?

2. What is the differential diagnosis?

3. What are common etiologies in adults for these lesions?

4. What are common etiologies for these lesions in children?

5. Which of these metastases are most commonly associated with hemorrhage?

Case ranking/difficulty:

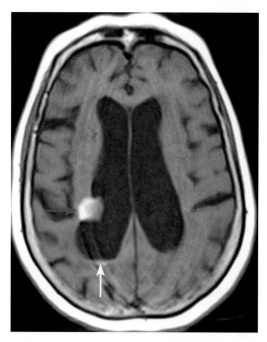

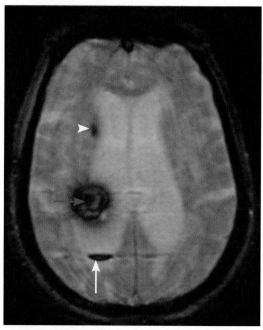

Axial T1 noncontrast image shows a lobulated, mixed signal lesion is seen along the ependymal margin of the right lateral ventricle (*green arrow*). There is an associated subtle fluid-fluid level dependently within the ventricle (*white arrow*). This high signal is secondary to methemoglobin.

Axial T2 gradient echo shows "blooming" involving the right lateral ventricle lesion (*green arrow*) and also dependently within the ventricle (*white arrow*). A third hemorrhagic lesion is noted with the right basal ganglia (*arrowhead*). This "blooming" artifact confirms hemorrhage.

Answers

1. The abnormality is located within the right lateral ventricle along the ependymal margin.

2. The differential diagnosis includes metastasis, choroid plexus neoplasm, and subependymoma.

3. Intraventricular metastasis is most commonly from renal, colon, and lung carcinomas in adults.

4. Intraventricular metastasis is most commonly from Wilms tumor, retinoblastoma, and neuroblastoma in the pediatric population.

5. The most common hemorrhagic brain metastases are melanoma, renal, choriocarcinoma, and thyroid (MR. CT).

Pearls

- Intraventricular metastasis account for 5% of cerebral neoplasms.
- The most common intraventricular metastases seen in adults are renal, colon, and lung.
- Multiplicity favors metastasis.
- If the lesion is centered on the septum pellucidum consider central neurocytoma.
- Hemorrhagic metastasis differential consider melanoma, renal cell carcinoma, choriocarcinoma, and thyroid carcinoma ("Mr. CT")
- Hemorrhage favors metastasis as it is rarely seen with other intraventricular tumors.

Suggested Reading

Smith AB, Smirniotopoulos JG, Horkanyne-Szakaly I. From the radiologic pathology archives: intraventricular neoplasms: radiologic-pathologic correlation. *Radiographics*. 2013 Aug;33(1):21-43.

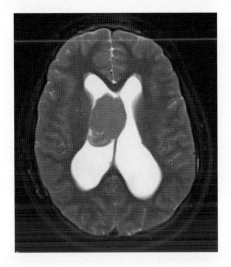
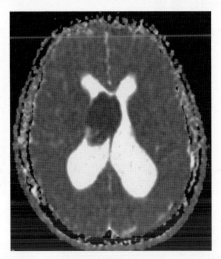
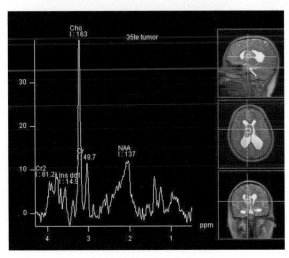
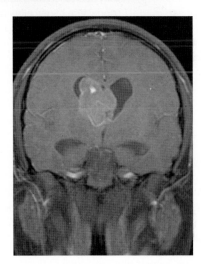

1. What is the differential diagnosis?

2. What are the typical MRI findings for this tumor?

3. What histopathologic labeling index correlates with prognosis?

4. What is the most common intraventricular tumor in adults?

5. What are the most common presentation symptoms for this entity?

Case ranking/difficulty:

Category: Ventricles and cisterns

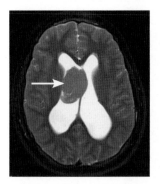

Axial T2 image through the lateral ventricles shows a lobular T2 hypointense tumor in the right lateral ventricle, which appears to arise from the septum pellucidum (*arrow*). The lateral ventricles are enlarged from hydrocephalus.

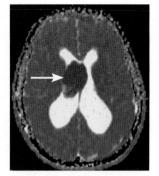

Axial DWI ADC image shows the hypointensity of the tumor corresponding with decreased diffusion, suggesting hypercellularity (*arrow*).

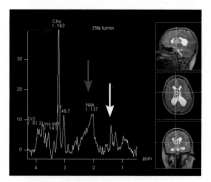

MR spectroscopy shows the presence of lactate (*white arrow*), decreased NAA (*red arrow*), and elevated choline (*blue arrow*). This is the "malignant" tumor profile that can be seen in higher-grade tumors.

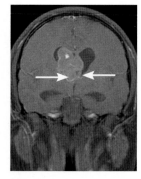

Coronal T1 postcontrast image shows a heterogeneously enhancing ventricular mass that obstructs the bilateral foramina of Monro (*arrows*).

Answers

1. The appearance of an intraventricular tumor associated with the septum pellucidum is classic for a central neurocytoma. Other differentials include intraventricular meningioma, choroid plexus tumor, and subependymoma. Ependymomas in the supratentorial space are rarely intraventricular.

2. A bubbly, cystic lobular mass attached to the septum pellucidum causing hydrocephalus is a classic appearance for central neurocytoma. Diffusion restriction is uncommon but may be seen in atypical cases.

3. Most central neurocytomas show little mitotic activity with a MIB-1 labeling index less than 2% with 90% 5-year survival. MIB-1 labeling index greater than 2% is associated with the atypical central neurocytoma with higher recurrence rates and poorer prognosis.

4. Central neurocytomas account for nearly half of all intraventricular tumors in adults, and are the most common.

5. Signs of hydrocephalus are the most common presentation of central neurocytoma including headache, vomiting, and visual changes.

Pearls

- Central neurocytomas are the most common intraventricular tumors in adults but are overall rare tumors.
- The classic appearance is a lobular, bubbly heterogeneous tumor associated with the septum pellucidum in the lateral ventricles.
- Involvement of third and fourth ventricles and extraventricular locations are rare.
- Outcome is generally good with 90% 5-year survival.
- MIB-1 index of greater than 2% is associated with atypia and correlates with a worse outcome.

Suggested Readings

Ramsahye H, He H, Feng X, Li S, Xiong J. Central neurocytoma: radiological and clinico-pathological findings in 18 patients and one additional MRS case. *J Neuroradiol.* 2013 May;40(2):101-111.

Tlili-Graiess K, Mama N, Arifa N, et al. Diffusion weighted MR imaging and proton MR spectroscopy findings of central neurocytoma with pathological correlation. *J Neuroradiol.* 2014 Oct;41(4):243-250.

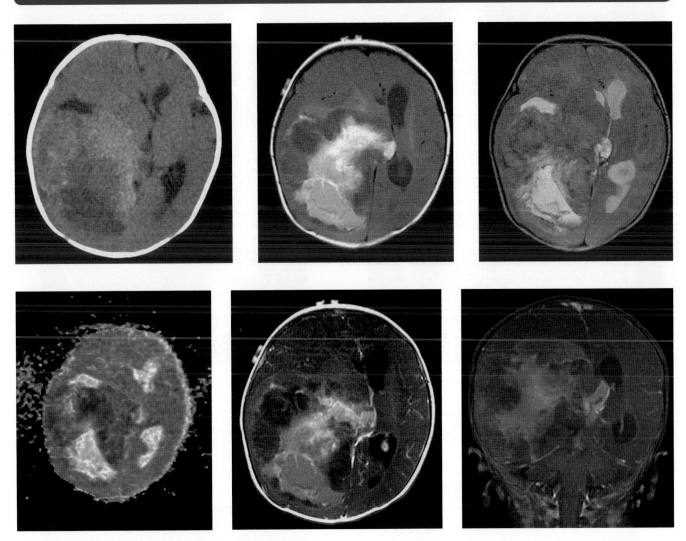

1. What is the differential diagnosis in a child?

2. What is the clinical presentation?

3. What imaging findings affect the prognosis for this disease?

4. What are typical radiographic features of this disease?

5. What is the most common location of this tumor?

Case ranking/difficulty:

Category: Ventricles and cisterns

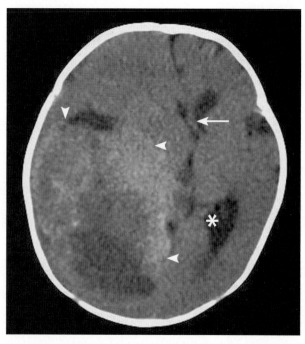

Axial CT image demonstrates a large mass (*white arrowheads*) in the right hemisphere involving the frontal, temporal, and parietal lobes, likely centered at the atrium of the right lateral ventricle. This mass shows mixed hyper/hypodensity, corresponding with calcification and hemorrhage. Also noted is right to left midline shift, subfalcine herniation (*white arrow*), and hydrocephalus (*white asterisk*).

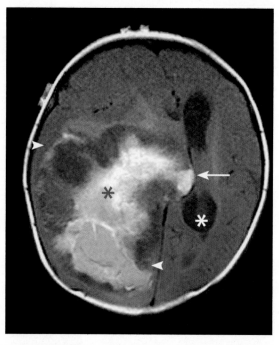

Axial T1 image demonstrates a large mixed T1 hypo/hyperintensity mass (*white arrowheads*) in the right hemisphere, likely centered at the atrium of the right lateral ventricle. A large area of T1 shortening is suggestive of hemorrhage and calcification (*red asterisk*), corresponding with areas of hyperdensity seen on prior CT. Also noted is right to left midline shift, subfalcine herniation (*white arrow*), and hydrocephalus (*white asterisk*).

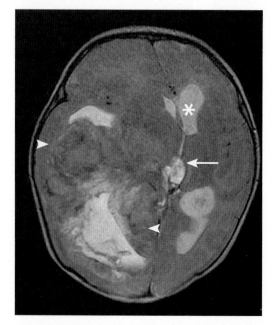

Axial T2 image demonstrates a large mixed T2 hypo/hyperintensity mass (*white arrowheads*) in the right hemisphere, likely centered at the atrium of the right lateral ventricle, causing right to left midline shift, subfalcine herniation (*white arrow*), and hydrocephalus (*white asterisk*).

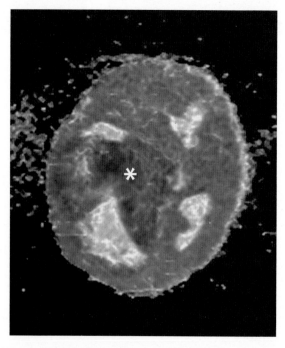

ADC image demonstrates restricted diffusion of the right cerebral hemisphere mass (*white asterisk*).

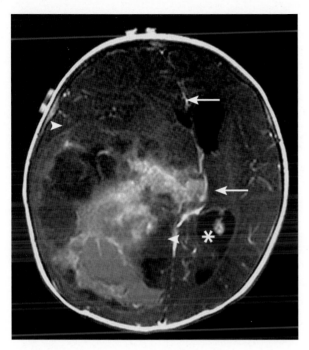

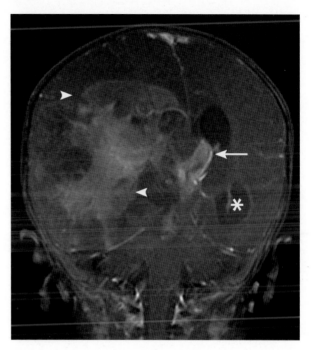

Axial T1 postcontrast image demonstrates a large mass in the right hemisphere (*white arrowheads*), likely centered in the atrium of the right lateral ventricle with faint contrast enhancement. Also noted are right to left midline shift and subfalcine herniation (*white arrows*), and hydrocephalus (*white asterisk*).

Coronal T1 postcontrast image demonstrate a large mass in the right hemisphere (*white arrowheads*), likely centered in the atrium of the right lateral ventricle, involving the frontal, temporal, and parietal lobes. This mass shows T1 shortening with heterogeneous enhancement. Also noted is right to left midline shift (*white arrow*), subfalcine herniation (*white arrow*), and hydrocephalus (*white asterisk*).

Answers

1. Differential diagnosis of a large heterogeneous intra- or periventricular mass in a child includes choroid plexus tumor, supratentorial ependymoma, and subependymal giant cell astrocytoma. Central neurocytoma does not typically occur in young children.

2. Clinical presentations include sign of increased intracranial pressure and hydrocephalus.

3. Poor prognostic factors include extraventricular extension, large tumor, CSF seeding, as well as association with Li-Fraumeni syndrome (p53 tumor suppressor gene mutation).

4. Typical radiographic features of choroid plexus carcinoma include heterogeneous enhancing lobular intraventricular mass with heterogenous signal intensity secondary to necrosis, hemorrhage, or cystic component, associated with periventricular white matter edema in some cases. DWI usually demonstrates restricted diffusion in the solid portion of mass, suggestive of high-grade tumor. However, imaging is not a reliable differentiator of between choroid plexus carcinoma and lower-grade variants.

5. CPC usually arises in the lateral ventricles (50%), followed by the fourth (40%) and third ventricles (5%).

Pearls

- Rare malignant intraventricular tumor (WHO grade III).
- Overlapping imaging characteristics with choroid plexus papilloma, histology necessary to confirm diagnosis.
- Lateral ventricles are the most common location.
- Typical radiographic features include a large heterogeneously enhancing intraventricular mass with central necrosis/cystic or hemorrhagic components, often with extraventricular extension.
- Spinal imaging is necessary to exclude distal CSF dissemination.
- Surgery is the main treatment option, plus adjuvant chemoradiation.
- Poor prognosis in cases of CSF dissemination and extraventricular invasion.

Suggested Readings

Coates TL, Hinshaw DB, Peckman N, Thompson JR, Hasso AN, Holshouser BA, Knierim DS. Pediatric choroid plexus neoplasms: MR, CT, and pathologic correlation. *Radiology*. 1989 Oct;173(1):81-88.

Koeller KK, Sandberg GD, Sandberg GD. From the archives of the AFIP. Cerebral intraventricular neoplasms: radiologic-pathologic correlation. *Radiographics*. 2002;22(6):1473-1505.

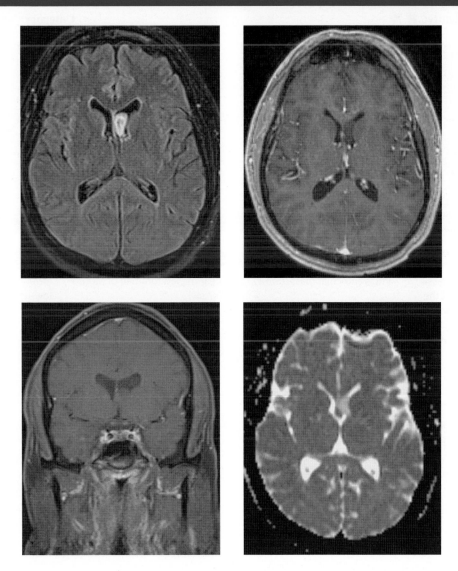

1. What is the differential diagnosis?

2. What is the most common location for this tumor?

3. What is the most common clinical presentation?

4. What are the typical imaging characteristics of this tumor?

5. Which age groups have a higher incidence of this lesion?

Case ranking/difficulty:

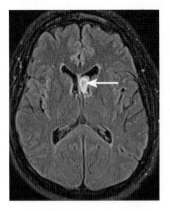

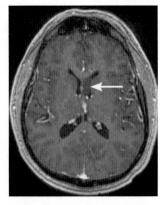

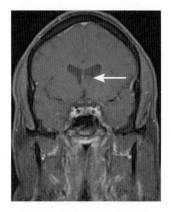

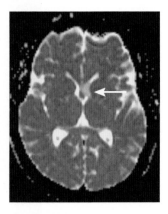

Axial FLAIR image shows a T2 hyperintense well-circumscribed lobular mass in the left frontal horn at the foramen of Monro. There is a central hypointensity that is associated with calcification (*arrow*).

Axial T1 postcontrast image shows no enhancement of the intraventricular mass (*arrow*).

Coronal T1 postcontrast image shows the nonenhancing mass near the left foramen of Monro (*arrow*).

Axial DWI ADC image shows increased diffusion of the mass (*arrow*) corresponding with the low-grade nature of this lesion.

Answers

1. The differential for an intraventricular tumor includes subependymoma and central neurocytoma. Subependymal giant cell astrocytomas also occur in this location, although commonly seen with tuberous sclerosis.

2. The fourth ventricle is the most common location for subependymomas (40%). The next most common location is in the lateral ventricles.

3. Most cases of subependymoma are found incidentally as the most common presentation is asymptomatic in regard to the tumor.

4. Subependymomas are typically well-circumscribed, intraventricular, T2 hyperintense tumors. They usually have no enhancement, although hemorrhage and calcification can be seen when the tumors are larger.

5. Subependymomas tend to present in the fifth to sixth decades of life, with earlier presentation due to obstructive hydrocephalus.

Pearls

- Subependymomas are slow-growing WHO grade I tumors typically firmly attached to a ventricular margin.
- The fourth ventricle is the most common location followed by the lateral ventricles.
- The mass is usually well-circumscribed, T2 hyperintense with typically no enhancement.
- Subependymomas are usually found in middle-aged to older adults, with a slight male predilection.
- The majority are asymptomatic with diagnosis made incidentally.
- Tumors causing obstructive hydrocephalus may present earlier.

Suggested Readings

Hoeffel C, Boukobza M, Polivka M, et al. MR manifestations of subependymomas. *AJNR Am J Neuroradiol.* 1997 Mar;16(10):2121-2129.

Rath TJ, Sundgren PC, Brahma B, Lieberman AP, Chandler WF, Gebarski SS. Massive symptomatic subependymoma of the lateral ventricles: case report and review of the literature. *Neuroradiology.* 2005 Mar;47(3):183-188.

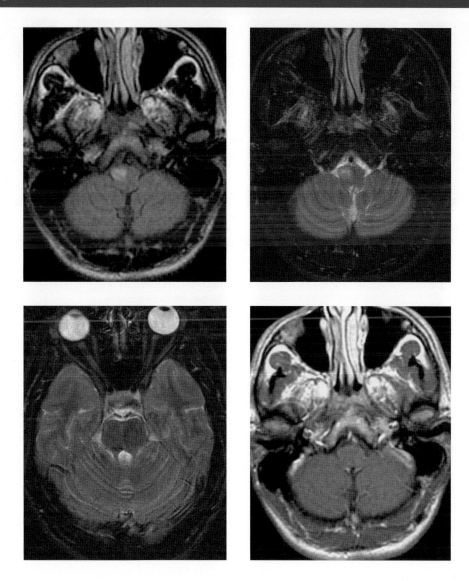

1. What is the differential diagnosis?

2. What are the classic imaging findings for this entity?

3. What is the etiology of this disease?

4. What is the time course of this appearance?

5. What is the typical clinical presentation for this lesion?

Case ranking/difficulty: **Category:** Intra-axial infratentorial

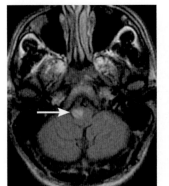

Axial FLAIR image shows T2 hyperintensity and enlargement of the right medullary olive *(arrow)*.

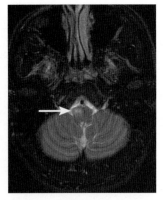

Axial T2 image again shows hyperintensity and enlargement of the right olivary nucleus *(arrow)*.

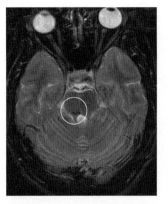

Axial T2 image shows a lesion at the base of the superior cerebellar peduncle of the right dorsal pons *(circle)* in the expected pathway of the Guillain-Mollaret triangle.

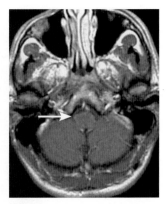

Axial T1 image postcontrast shows no enhancement of the right olive *(arrow)*.

Answers

1. The differential for a T2 hyperintense lesion in the inferior olive with enlargement includes astrocytoma, demyelination in MS, hypertrophic olivary degeneration (HOD), and lateral medullary infarct.

2. HOD typically presents with T2 hyperintensity and T1 hypointensity with enlargement of the inferior olivary nucleus without enhancement.

3. HOD is a paradoxical enlargement of the inferior olivary nucleus from transsynaptic degeneration due to interruption of the pathway of the Guillain-Mollaret triangle involving the ipsilateral red nucleus and contralateral dentate nucleus.

4. The three stages of HOD on MRI show T2 hyperintensity without hypertrophy as early as 4 weeks after injury, T2 hyperintensity with hypertrophy as early as 4 months that resolves after 2-3 years, and T2 hyperintensity with resolved hypertrophy that may last indefinitely.

5. Palatal myoclonus is a characteristic finding in patients with HOD, although not all HOD patients will have palatal myoclonus.

Pearls

- Paradoxical enlargement of the inferior olivary nucleus from injury to the dentato-rubro-olivary pathway.
- Guillain-Mollaret triangle connects the inferior olive to the ipsilateral red nucleus through the central tegmental tracts, from the red nucleus to the contralateral dentate nucleus through the superior cerebellar peduncle, and from the contralateral dentate nucleus back to the olivary nucleus through the inferior cerebellar peduncle.
- Any insult to the pathway can lead to HOD.
- Increased T2 hyperintensity can persist from 4 weeks to years.
- Hypertrophy begins at 4 months and can last 3-4 years.
- Look for lesion involving the pathway.

Suggested Readings

Goyal M, Versnick E, Tuite P, et al. Hypertrophic olivary degeneration: metaanalysis of the temporal evolution of MR findings. *AJNR Am J Neuroradiol.* 2010 Oct;21(6):1073-1077.

Patay Z, Enterkin J, Harreld JH, et al. MR imaging evaluation of inferior olivary nuclei: comparison of postoperative subjects with and without posterior fossa syndrome. AJNR *Am J Neuroradiol.* 2014;35(4):797-802.

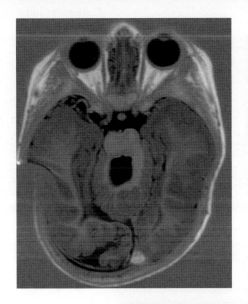
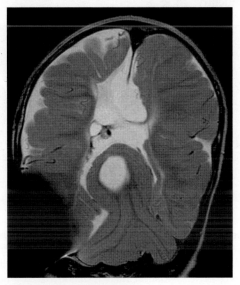
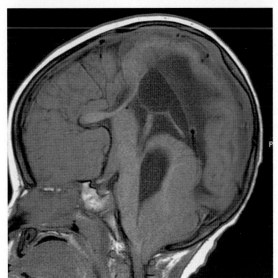

1. What is the diagnosis, with respect to the cerebellum?

2. What are the findings in this entity?

3. What are the findings on DTI?

4. What are the associated anomalies?

5. What are clinical symptoms associated with this condition?

Case ranking/difficulty:

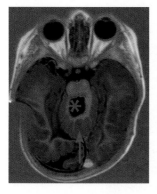

Axial T1 image shows cerebellar hemisphere fusion (*green arrow*), and absent vermis with dilated fourth ventricle (*red asterisk*).

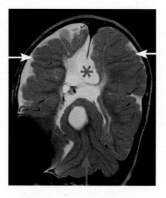

Coronal T2 image shows cerebellar hemisphere fusion (*green arrow*) and absent septum pellucidum (*red asterisk*). There is stenogyria (*white arrows*), seen with Chiari II malformation.

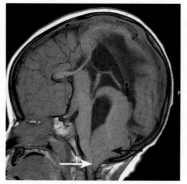

Sagittal T1 image shows dysgenesis of the corpus callosum (*green arrow*) and cerebellum (*blue arrow*). Note the tonsillar herniation associated with Chiari malformation (*white arrow*).

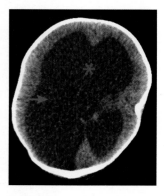

Axial CT shows hydrocephalus (*green arrow*) at birth with absent septum pellucidum (*red asterisk*).

Answers

1. Rhombencephalosynapsis shows continuity of cerebellar folia across the midline. It is due to dorsoventral patterning defect. In this case, rhombencephalosynapsis is associated with Chiari II malformation.

2. Rhombencephalosynapsis shows continuity of cerebellar folia and deep cerebellar nuclei across the midline, absent (80%) or severely hypoplastic (20%) vermis, absent septum pellucidum, ventriculomegaly, dysgenesis of corpus callosum, and posterior pointing of the fourth ventricle.

3. DTI would show axons running in the supero-inferior direction at midline instead of the normal left to right transverse direction.

4. Associated anomalies include bilateral lambdoid synostosis, cortical malformations, VACTERL (vertebral, anorectal, cardiac, tracheoesophageal fistula, renal, limb), and Chiari II malformation.

5. Patients may have hydrocephalus, seizures, cerebral palsy, mental retardation, and may show cerebellar signs like ataxia.

Pearls

- Rhombencephalosynapsis (RES) is due to dorsoventral patterning defect during midbrain/hindbrain development and results in fusion of the cerebellar hemispheres.
- Key to the diagnosis of RES is the continuation of the cerebellar folia and fissure across midline.
- Absent septum pellucidum.
- Posterior pointing of the fourth ventricle.
- Cerebellar vermis is absent (80%).
- Chiari II malformation may be associated with RES.
- DTI would show axons running in supero-inferior direction in the midline instead of the normal left to right direction.

Suggested Readings

Guntur Ramkumar P, Kanodia AK, Ananthakrishnan G, Roberts R. Chiari II malformation mimicking partial rhombencephalosynapsis? a case report. *Cerebellum*. 2010 Mar;9(1):111-114.

Merlini L, Fluss J, Korff C, Hanquinet S. Partial rhombencephalosynapsis and Chiari type II malformation in a child: a true association supported by DTI tractography. *Cerebellum*. 2012 Mar;11(1):227-232.

Wan SM, Khong PL, Ip P, Ooi GC. Partial rhombencephalosynapsis and Chiari II malformation. *Hong Kong Med J*. 2005 Aug;11(4):299-302.

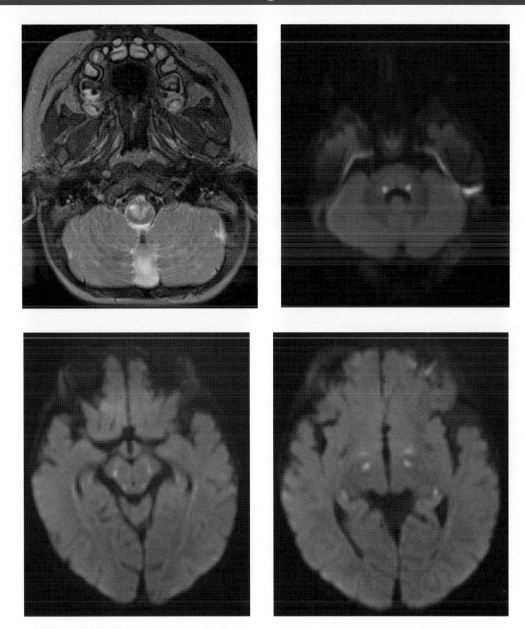

1. What is the differential diagnosis?

2. What is the mode of genetic inheritance?

3. What is the prognosis of this disease?

4. What is the treatment for this disease?

5. What is the pathophysiology of this disease?

Case ranking/difficulty:

Category: Intra-axial infratentorial

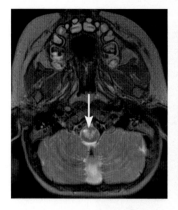

Axial T2 image at the level of the lower medulla shows abnormal T2 hyperintensity of the central gray structures (*white arrow*).

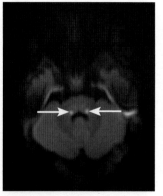

Axial DWI b = 1000 shows focal symmetric bilateral diffusion restriction of the pontine tegmentum (*white arrows*).

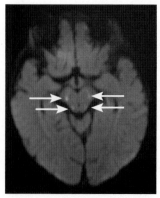

Axial DWI b = 1000 shows focal symmetric restricted diffusion of the midbrain tegmentum (*white arrows*).

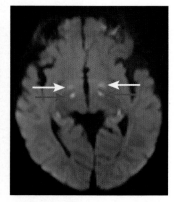

Axial DWI b = 1000 shows focal symmetric restricted diffusion of the subthalamic nuclei (*white arrows*), and cerebral peduncles (*red arrows*).

MRI spectroscopy of the basal ganglia shows lactate doublet (*white arrow*), even with no involvement from anatomic MRI images. This is typical due to lactic acidosis seen in Leigh syndrome.

Answers

1. Surf1 Leigh syndrome, maple syrup urine disease, and hypermethioninemia can cause brainstem edema and diffusion restriction. The focal involvement of gray matter nuclei and subthalamic nuclei is more consistent with SURF1 Leigh syndrome, which is this patient's diagnosis. Hypermethioninemia and maple syrup urine disease have a white matter predominance, involving the brainstem and central and cerebellar white matter, which may show diffusion restriction during acute phases.

2. While Leigh syndrome also includes mitochondrial and x-linked inheritance, SURF1 mutations, which are the most common of the causes of Leigh syndrome, are autosomal recessive.

3. SURF1 mutation Leigh syndrome has earlier onset in infancy and typically a dismal prognosis with rapid

deterioration to death in early childhood. No treatment is available.

4. No cure is available for Leigh syndrome with treatment focused on vitamin supplementation and buffering of lactic acid buildup.

5. SURF1 Leigh syndrome has a deficiency of cytochrome C oxidase, involved in the electron transport chain, which normally synthesizes ATP in the mitochondria.

Pearls

- Leigh syndrome is a genetically heterogeneous group of metabolic neurodegenerative disorders with abnormality of mitochondrial respiration.
- SURF1 mutations are the most common of the Leigh syndromes that show characteristic symmetric involvement of the subthalamic nuclei, cerebellum, and lower brainstem. There is relative sparing of the basal ganglia, with worse prognosis and rapid deterioration to death.
- Acute areas of involvement typically show T2 hyperintensity from swelling and diffusion restriction without significant enhancement.

Suggested Readings

Farina L, Chiapparini L, Uziel G, Bugiani M, Zeviani M, Savoiardo M. MR findings in Leigh syndrome with COX deficiency and SURF-1 mutations. *AJNR Am J Neuroradiol*. 2002 Aug;23(7):1095-1100.

Rossi A, Biancheri R, Bruno C, Di Rocco M, Calvi A, Pessagno A, Tortori-Donati P. Leigh syndrome with COX deficiency and SURF1 gene mutations: MR imaging findings. *AJNR Am J Neuroradiol*. 2003 Sep;24(6):1188-1191.

4-year-old male with history of severe hypotonia, muscle weakness, ataxia, and poor visual tracking

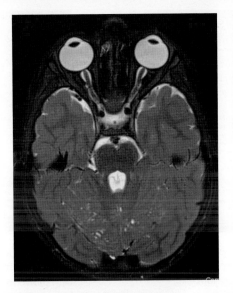
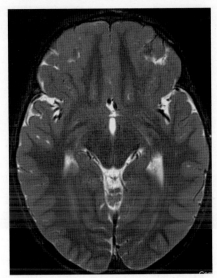
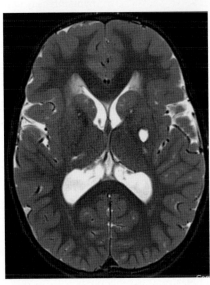
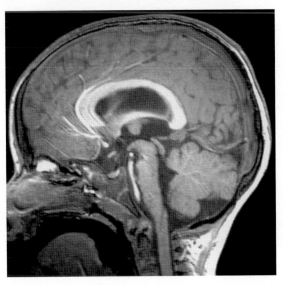

1. What are the abnormal findings on MRI?

2. What is the differential diagnosis?

3. What is the pathophysiology of this disease?

4. What are the characteristic clinical findings?

5. What are eye abnormalities associated with this disease?

Case ranking/difficulty:

Category: Intra-axial infratentorial

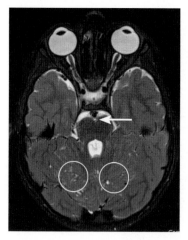

Axial T2 image shows multiple cysts in the cerebellum (*circles*). There is hypoplasia of the pons with clefting (*arrow*).

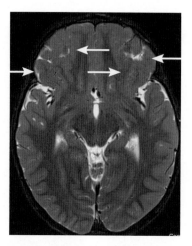

Axial T2 image shows bilateral frontal polymicrogyria in a cobblestone lissencephaly pattern (*arrows*).

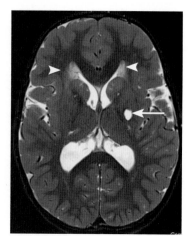

Axial T2 image shows a prominent cyst in the left putamen (*arrow*), with periventricular white matter T2 hyperintensity (*arrowheads*).

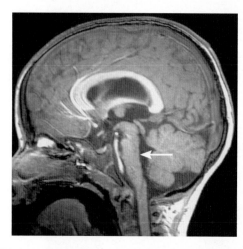

Sagittal T1 image shows hypoplasia of the pons and brainstem (*arrow*).

Answers

1. There is frontal lobe cobblestone polymicrogyria, periventricular white matter hypomyelination/leukomalacia, multiple cysts in the cerebellum and bilateral basal ganglia, and brainstem atrophy with pontine clefting.

2. With findings of gray matter migration anomalies, pathologies such as TORCH infections should be considered. With cobblestone lissencephaly, lissencephaly type II diseases are in the differential, which includes the congenital muscular dystrophies such as Muscle-eye-brain, Walker-Warburg syndrome, and Fukuyama congenital muscular dystrophy.

3. Hypoglycosylation of dystroglycan leads to neuronal migrational anomalies and muscle dysfunction.

4. Clinical history includes characteristic eye abnormalities with muscular dystrophy. Hypotonia, muscle weakness, mental retardation, developmental delay, and seizures have also been reported in groups of patients with the disease.

5. Eye abnormalities described with muscle-eye-brain disease include congenital glaucoma, optic nerve hypoplasia, and congenital myopia.

Pearls

- Muscle-eye-brain disease is an inherited disorder of alpha-dystroglycan, resulting in brain migrational anomalies, eye abnormalities, and muscular dystrophy.
- Related to Walker-Warburg and Fukuyama congenital muscular dystrophy; all three diseases have type II (cobblestone) lissencephaly.
- Migrational anomalies include cobblestone lissencephaly, polymicrogyria, and pachygyria.
- Multiple cysts in the cerebellum have been described.
- Brainstem hypoplasia and pontine clefting.
- White matter hypomyelination and abnormal T2 hyperintensity.

Suggested Readings

Barkovich AJ. Neuroimaging manifestations and classification of congenital muscular dystrophies. *AJNR Am J Neuroradiol.* 1998 Sep;19(8):1389-1396.

Yiş U, Uyanik G, Rosendahl DM, et al. Clinical, radiological, and genetic survey of patients with muscle-eye-brain disease caused by mutations in POMGNT1. *Pediatr Neurol.* 2014 May;50(5):491-497.

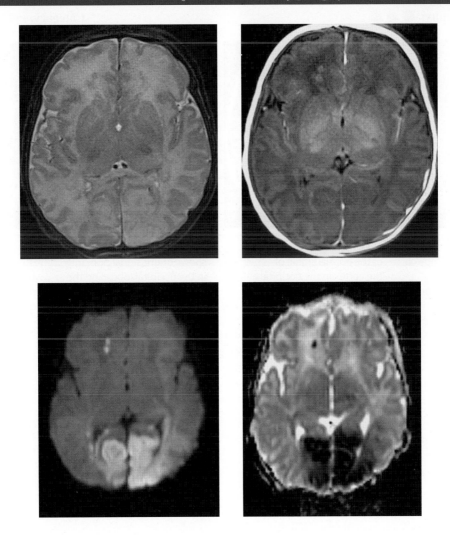

1. What is the differential diagnosis?

2. What are the more common locations of parenchymal injury for this disease in a term infant?

3. What is the most common location of parenchymal injury in preterm neonates for this disease?

4. What are common etiologies of this disease in infants?

5. What clinical symptoms do patients with this disease present with?

Case ranking/difficulty:

Category: Intra-axial supratentorial

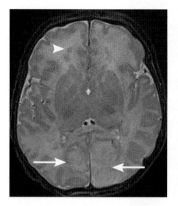

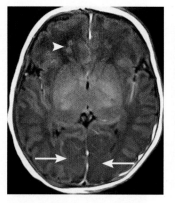

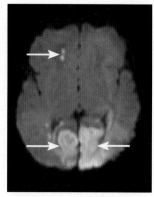

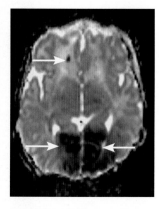

Axial T2 image shows increased T2 signal with loss of the normal signal of the cortex in the occipital lobes (*arrows*). There is also punctate hypointensity in the right frontal white matter (*arrowhead*).

Axial T1 image shows loss of the normal signal of the cortex in the occipital lobes (*arrows*). There is also punctate hyperintensity in the right frontal white matter (*arrowhead*). There are incidental T1 hyperintense subdural blood products from birth trauma (*red arrowhead*).

Axial DWI b = 1000 image shows bright signal primarily in the occipital lobes and the right frontal white matter (*arrows*).

Axial DWI ADC image shows restricted diffusion consistent with cytotoxic edema in the occipital lobes and the right frontal white matter (*arrows*).

Answers

1. The differential for diffuse bilateral cortical restricted diffusion includes hypoglycemia, hypoxic ischemic injury, metabolic disease, and status epilepticus.

2. While any structure can be involved in hypoglycemia injury, a bilateral posterior pattern involving the occipital and parietal lobes is more common in term infants.

3. The periventricular white matter is more sensitive to metabolic injury in preterm neonates and is a common area of injury in hypoglycemia.

4. Uncontrolled maternal diabetes, IUGR, prematurity, fetal stress, and preeclampsia can all cause neonatal hypoglycemia.

5. Neonates with hypoglycemia may have no appreciable symptoms but can present with seizures, stupor, jitteriness, and hypotonia.

Pearls

- Neonatal hypoglycemia results from inadequate glucose stores from preeclampsia, IUGR, maternal hypoglycemia or prematurity, increased utilization from hypoxia and stress, increased insulin in uncontrolled maternal diabetes, familial hyperinsulinemia, or other endocrinopathies.

- Involvement does not conform to a typical vascular distribution and may affect predominantly cortex within term neonates and periventricular white matter in premature infants.
- Typically there is a bilateral posterior (occipital and parietal) distribution compared to frontal and temporal lobes.
- The deep gray nuclei and brainstem may also be involved.
- Decreased T1, increased T2, and diffusion restriction are seen in acute injury.

Suggested Readings

Menezes MP, Nowland T, Onikul E. Diffusion-weighted imaging changes caused by acute hypoglycemia and prolonged febrile convulsion in childhood. *AJNR Am J Neuroradiol*. 2013 Apr;34(4):E43-E44.

Wong DS, Poskitt KJ, Chau V, et al. Brain injury patterns in hypoglycemia in neonatal encephalopathy. *AJNR Am J Neuroradiol*. 2013 Jul;34(7):1456-1461.

19-month-old male with history of short gut syndrome, and new-onset seizures, found to have hypernatremia

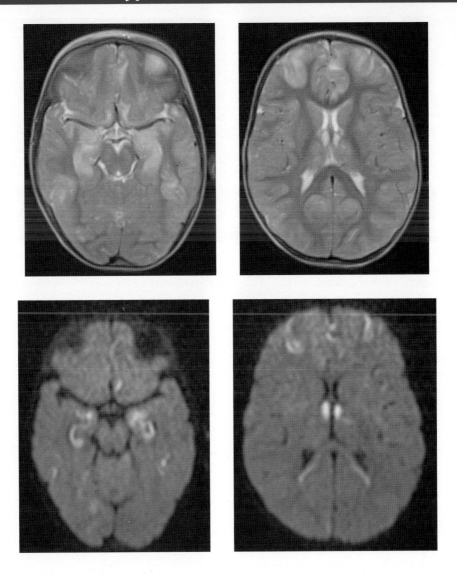

1. What is the differential diagnosis?

2. What osmotic derangements can cause this disease?

3. What is the classic location for this disease?

4. What can be seen on MRI in the acute phase of this disease?

5. What are associated conditions that increase the likelihood of this disease?

Case ranking/difficulty:

Category: Intra-axial supratentorial

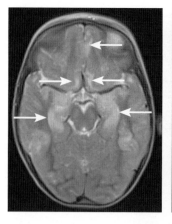 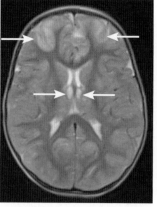 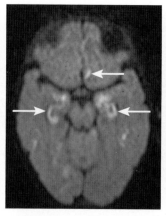 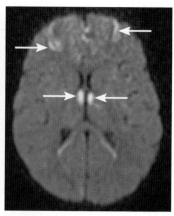

Axial T2 image shows symmetric hyperintensity and swelling of the bilateral medial temporal lobes and frontal lobes (*arrows*).

Axial T2 image shows symmetric involvement of the thalami and frontal cortical subcortical white matter (*arrows*).

Axial DWI b = 1000 image shows cortical diffusion restriction of the hippocampi and left frontal lobe (*arrows*).

Axial DWI b = 1000 image shows symmetric diffusion restriction of the thalami and frontal cortex (*arrows*).

Answers

1. The differential diagnosis of bilateral cortical, symmetric diffusion restriction includes status epilepticus, ischemia, Creutzfeldt-Jakob disease, and viral encephalitis. Osmotic demyelination in an extrapontine location can uncommonly occur with this distribution.

2. While rapid correction of hypernatremia is the most common etiology, osmotic demyelination has been reported with other osmotic derangement such as azotemia, hyperglycemia, hypokalemia, and ketoacidosis.

3. The classic location for osmotic demyelination is the central pontine fibers, which occurs in half of cases. Extrapontine locations include basal ganglia and white matter, and less commonly cortex and hippocampi in a bilateral symmetric distribution.

4. Hypointense T1, hyperintense T2/FLAIR, and diffusion restriction can be seen in the acute phase, with enhancement being atypical.

5. Patients with malnutrition such as alcoholism or chronic vomiting are at risk of osmotic demyelination. Other risk factors include organ transplantation, renal failure, endocrinopathies, and burn patients.

Pearls

- Osmotic demyelination is formerly categorized as central pontine myelinolysis or extrapontine myelinolysis.

- While rapid correction of hypernatremia is the most common etiology, osmotic demyelination has been reported with other osmotic derangement such as azotemia, hyperglycemia, hypokalemia, and ketoacidosis.
- Patients typically present with seizures and altered mental status, usually 2-4 days after rapid correction of sodium.
- Half of cases demonstrate the classic central pontine location.
- Extrapontine sites are typically symmetric and include the basal ganglia, white matter, and less commonly the cortex, and hippocampi can also be involved with or without pontine lesions.
- Hypointense T1, hyperintense T2, and diffusion restriction in the acute phase.
- Enhancement is atypical.
- Depending on the severity of osmolar injury, lesions may resolve.

Suggested Readings

Ismail FY, Szóllics A, Szólics M, Nagelkerke N, Ljubisavljevic M. Clinical semiology and neuroradiologic correlates of acute hypernatremic osmotic challenge in adults: a literature review. *AJNR Am J Neuroradiol.* 2013 Dec;34(12):2225-2232.

Roh JH, Kim JH, Oh K, Kim SG, Park KW, Kim BJ. Cortical laminar necrosis caused by rapidly corrected hyponatremia. *J Neuroimaging.* 2009 Apr;19(2):185-187.

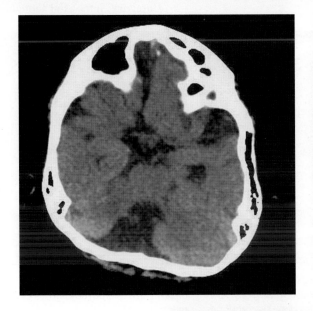
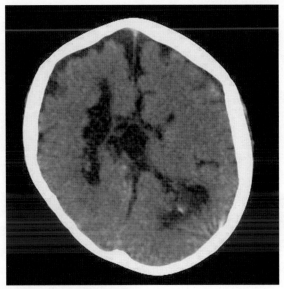
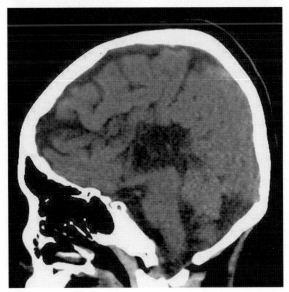

1. What is the differential diagnosis?

2. What is the genetic inheritance of this disease?

3. What is the classic triad in this disease?

4. What are the characteristic radiographic features?

5. What is the typical clinical presentation?

Case ranking/difficulty:

Category: Intra-axial supratentorial

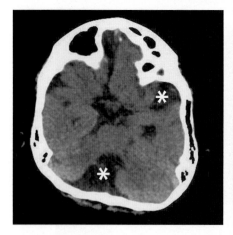

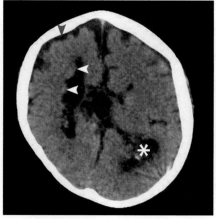

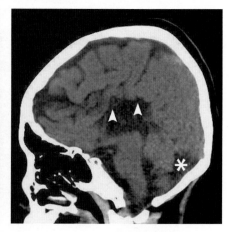

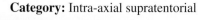

Axial CT image demonstrates midline posterior fossa and left middle cranial fossa cysts (*white asterisks*).

Axial CT image demonstrates nodularity along the lateral wall of the right lateral ventricle (*white arrowheads*), consistent with gray matter heterotropia. Also noted is corpus callosal agenesis with colpocephaly (*green arrowhead*). There is a cystic lesion in the left periatrial white matter, consistent with porencephalic cyst (*white asterisk*). Right frontal polymicrogyria is also noted (*red arrowhead*).

Sagittal CT image demonstrates complete agenesis of corpus callosum (*white arrowheads*) and posterior fossa cyst (*white asterisk*).

Answers

1. The differential of posterior fossa cyst with small vermis and corpus callosal agenesis includes Dandy-Walker malformation. The differential with the addition of multiple migrational anomalies include congenital CMV, Type II (cobblestone) lissencephaly, and the diagnosis in this patient, Aicardi syndrome.

2. Aicardi syndrome is a rare genetic disease, classified as x-linked dominant, although all reported cases are sporadic mutations. It may be lethal in males, with manifestation only in females and rare cases of males with Klinefelter syndrome (XXY).

3. Classic triad is corpus callosal agenesis, infantile spasm, and chorioretinal lacunae.

4. Classic radiographic features of Aicardi syndrome include corpus callosal dysgenesis (either partial or complete), colpocephaly, gray matter heterotropia, polymicrogyria, posterior fossa abnormalities/Dandy-Walker continuum, intracranial cyst (midline interhemispheric, intraventricular, parenchymal, or extraaxial), and widened operculum.

5. The typical clinical profile in Aicardi syndrome is a female infant presenting with spasms.

- Possibly lethal in males, manifests solely in females and in rare cases with Klinefelter syndrome (XXY).
- Classic triad includes callosal dysgenesis, infantile spasms, and chorioretinal lacunae.
- Classic clinical presentations: seizure, developmental delay, and mental retardation.
- Chorioretinal lacuna is a pathognomonic physical examination.
- Cleft lip and cleft palate occur with increased frequency.
- Typical radiographic features: corpus callosal dysgenesis (partial/complete), colpocephaly, gray matter heterotropia/poly microgyria, widening of the operculum, Dandy-Walker continuum, and intracranial cysts.

Pearls

- Rare genetic disease, x-linked dominant only reported in sporadic mutations.

Suggested Readings

Baierl P, Markl A, Thelen M, Laub MC. MR imaging in Aicardi syndrome. *AJNR Am J Neuroradiol*. 1990 May;9(4):805-806.

Hall-Craggs MA, Harbord MG, Finn JP, Brett E, Kendall BE. Aicardi syndrome: MR assessment of brain structure and myelination. *AJNR Am J Neuroradiol*. 1990 May;11(3):532-536.

Uggetti C, La Piana R, Orcesi S, Egitto MG, Crow YJ, Fazzi E. Aicardi-Goutieres syndrome: neuroradiologic findings and follow-up. *AJNR Am J Neuroradiol*. 2009 Nov;30(10):1971-1976.

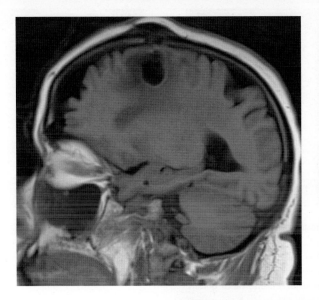
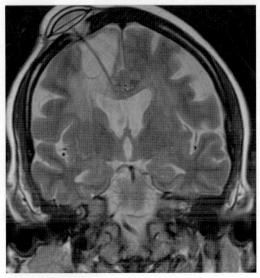

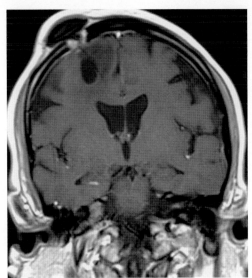

1. Where is the abnormality located?

2. What are the classic imaging findings for this entity?

3. What is the differential diagnosis?

4. What is the etiology of this entity?

5. What is the treatment for this entity?

Case ranking/difficulty: **Category:** Intra-axial supratentorial

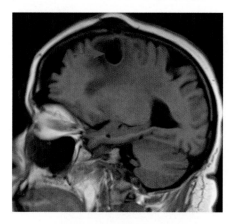

Sagittal T1 noncontrast shows a low-density cyst with CSF signal within the right frontal lobe subcortical white matter with associated vasogenic edema or gliosis (*arrow*).

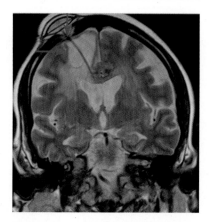

Coronal T2 image shows the cyst (*green arrow*) follows CSF and is adjacent to a ventriculostomy catheter (*red arrow*) with reservoir for chemotherapy in this patient. Again noted is adjacent edema or gliosis.

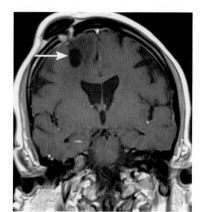

Coronal T1 postcontrast shows no contrast enhancement within the cyst (*arrow*).

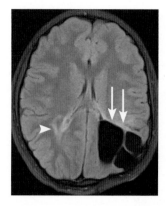

Axial FLAIR image in an 8-year-old female with long-standing history of hydrocephalus and perinatal intraventricular hemorrhage shows a multiloculated cystic lesion following CSF communicating the left lateral ventricle with the subarachnoid space. Note the mild gliosis and white matter lining the cyst cavity (*arrows*). There is periventricular gliosis in the right periatrial white matter from perinatal ischemic insult (*arrowhead*).

Answers

1. The abnormality is within the frontal lobe.

2. On MR imaging, the key finding is a cyst that follows CSF signal, which can communicate between the ventricle and subarachnoid space. Typically, no contrast enhancement is seen. Significant gliosis can be seen with acquired lesions. Congenital lesions are typically lined by white matter.

3. The differential diagnosis includes encephaloclastic porencephalic cyst, neoplastic cyst, arachnoid cyst, and abscess.

4. Acquired encephaloclastic porencephalic cysts can be from multiple etiologies that cause brain destruction and result in a CSF-filled cyst.

5. No treatment is typically necessary. If ongoing brain destruction, treatment of the offending agent is necessary. Rarely cysts may enlarge, requiring fenestration or shunting.

Pearls

- Encephaloclastic cysts are acquired porencephalic cysts that result from destruction of brain tissue from multiple etiologies including trauma, infarct, or infection.
- In this case, intraventricular chemotherapy (IVC) is postulated to reflux back along the catheter to cause brain destruction and cyst formation.
- When the etiology is related to IVC, the cyst will form around the catheter.
- Congenital porencephalic cysts are typically a result of in utero stroke or infection after gray matter migration is complete.
- Lined by white matter and/or gliosis.
- Cyst follows CSF on all pulse sequences.
- Communication with the ventricle and subarachnoid space is classic.

Suggested Readings

Chowdhary S, Chalmers LM, Chamberlain PA. Methotrexate-induced encephaloclastic cyst: a complication of intraventricular chemotherapy. *Neurology.* 2006 Jul;67(2):319.

Ho SS, Kuzniecky RI, Gilliam F, Faught E, Bebin M, Morawetz R. Congenital porencephaly: MR features and relationship to hippocampal sclerosis. *AJNR Am J Neuroradiol.* 1998 Jan;19(1):135-141.

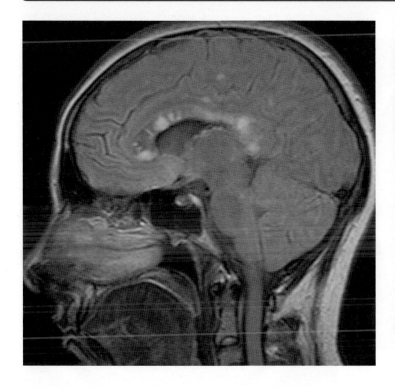 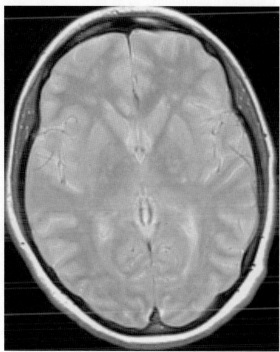

1. Where is the abnormality on the sagittal image located?

2. What are the classic imaging findings for this entity?

3. What is the differential diagnosis for corpus callosal lesions?

4. What is the classic clinical triad for this disease?

5. What is the treatment for this entity?

Case ranking/difficulty: 🌰🌰🌰

Category: Intra-axial supratentorial

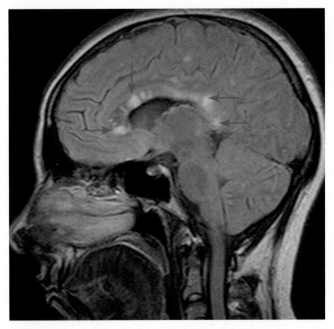

Sagittal FLAIR shows multiple high-signal lesions involving the corpus callosal central fibers from anterior to posterior (*arrows*).

Answers

1. The abnormality is located in the corpus callosum.

2. Susac syndrome (SS) typically demonstrates lesions of the central fibers of the corpus callosum.

3. The differential diagnosis includes Susac syndrome, multiple sclerosis, and Marchiafava-Bignami disease.

4. The classic clinical triad includes encephalopathy, visual changes, and sensorineural hearing loss. SS can affect any part of the brain, but has an affinity for the central fibers of the corpus callosum.

5. The treatment for this entity includes immunosuppressives and antithrombotic agents.

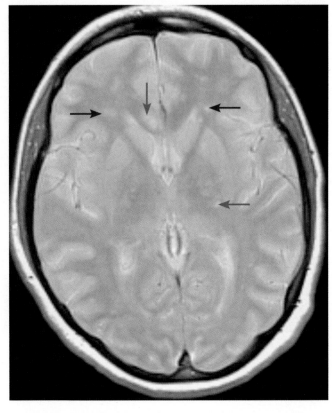

Axial proton density shows multiple high-signal lesions involving the anterior corpus callosum (*green arrow*), subcortical white matter of the frontal lobes (*blue arrows*), the lentiform nuclei (*red arrow*), and subcortical white matter of the occipital lobes.

Pearls

- Susac syndrome (SS) is a neurological microangiopathy, likely autoimmune.
- The classic clinical triad includes encephalopathy, visual changes, and sensorineural hearing loss.
- Key to diagnosis is the characteristic "snowball" corpus callosal lesions.
- Corpus involvement along the callosal septal interface favor multiple sclerosis.
- With corpus splenium, mammillary body, and/or periaqueductal gray involvement consider Marchiafava-Bignami disease.

Suggested Reading

Dörr J, Krautwald S, Wildemann B, et al. Characteristics of Susac syndrome: a review of all reported cases. *Nat Rev Neurol.* 2013 Jun;9(6):307-316.

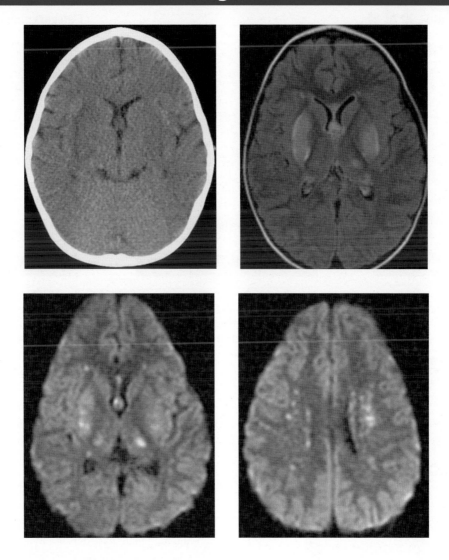

1. What is the differential diagnosis?

2. What are the different diseases with a common hematologic pathway of thrombocytopenia and coagulopathic consumption?

3. What hematologic characteristics are seen in this disease?

4. What is the typical pattern of CNS involvement in this disease?

5. Which imaging sequences are the most helpful in this diagnosis?

Case ranking/difficulty:

Category: Intra-axial supratentorial

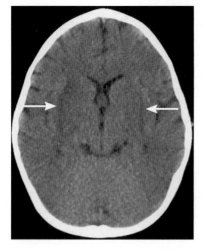

Axial CT image shows hypodensity of the bilateral basal ganglia (*arrows*).

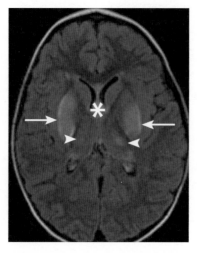

Axial FLAIR image demonstrates bilateral increased T2 signal of the putamen (*arrows*), thalami (*arrowheads*), and fornix (*asterisk*).

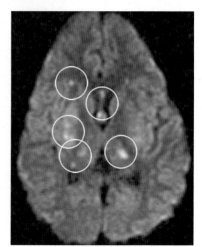

Axial DWI b = 1000 image shows only punctate areas of cytotoxic edema (*circles*) of the involved edematous areas in a microangiopathic pattern.

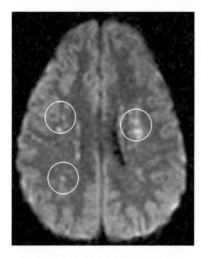

Axial DWI b = 1000 image shows further punctate areas of restricted diffusion in the periventricular and subcortical white matter (*circles*) from microangiopathy.

Answers

1. The differential for multiple white matter punctate lesions with diffusion restriction and basal ganglia edema includes small vessel disease such as thrombotic microangiopathy, CNS vasculitis, and CADASIL. Viral encephalitis may also affect this distribution of deep gray and white matter.

2. Causes of thrombotic microangiopathy are varied and commonly include hemolytic uremic syndrome, thrombocytopenic thrombotic purpura, disseminated intravascular coagulopathy, and malignant hypertension.

3. Hematologic abnormalities of thrombotic microangiopathy include thrombocytopenia, hemolytic anemia, and microvascular occlusion.

4. The typically described pattern of thrombotic microangiopathy is multifocal, often hemorrhagic infarcts of the cortex and subcortical white matter.

5. In thrombotic microangiopathy, multifocal small vessel hemorrhagic infarcts are best seen with DWI and susceptibility-weighted imaging.

Pearls

- HUS in children, thrombotic thrombocytopenic purpura and malignant hypertension in adults, and disseminated intravascular coagulation (DIC) in both age groups are grouped under the common pathology of thrombotic microangiopathy.
- Differing etiologies cause the common pathway of platelet aggregation and microcirculation occlusion.
- Imaging shows multifocal small hemorrhagic infarcts predominantly in the cortex and subcortical white matter.
- These lesions are typically bright on T2 imaging, with possible blooming artifact on susceptibility-weighted imaging and diffusion restriction.

Suggested Readings

Ellchuk TN, Shah LM, Hewlett RH, Osborn AG. Suspicious neuroimaging pattern of thrombotic microangiopathy. *AJNR Am J Neuroradiol*. 2011 Apr;32(4):734-738.

Nakamura H, Takaba H, Inoue T, Saku Y, Saito F, Ibayashi S, Fujishima M. MRI findings of hemolytic uremic syndrome with encephalopathy: widespread symmetrical distribution. *J Neuroimaging*. 2003 Jan;13(1):75-78.

3-year-old male presents with developmental delay, macrocephaly, and seizures

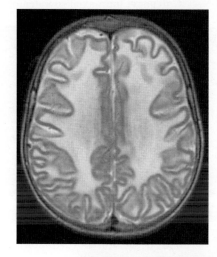
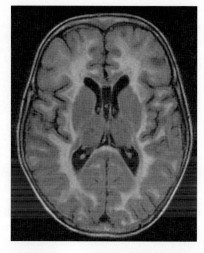
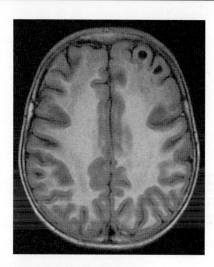

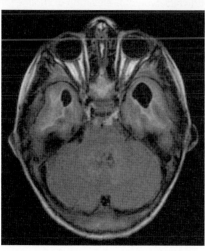
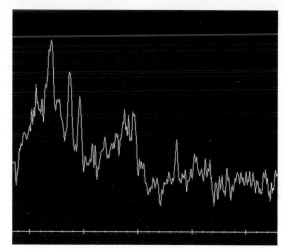

1. What are the usual clinical characteristics of this disease?

2. What are the typical imaging findings of this disease?

3. What is the method of inheritance of this disease?

4. What are synonyms for this disease that has been reported in the literature?

5. What are the differential diagnoses of these MR findings?

Case ranking/difficulty:

Category: Intra-axial supratentorial

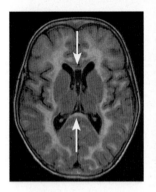 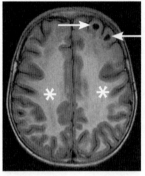 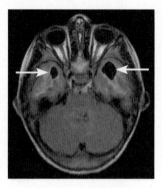 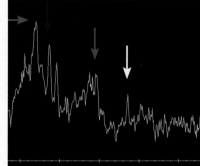

Axial FLAIR images show diffuse white matter hyperintensity, with relative sparing of the corpus callosum, including the genu and splenium (*white arrows*).

Axial FLAIR image shows left frontal subcortical cysts (*white arrows*), which follow CSF signal. There is diffuse T2 hyperintensity of the white matter (*asterisks*).

Axial FLAIR image through the cerebellum demonstrates bilateral anterior temporal subcortical cysts (*white arrows*). The cerebellum is typically spared in this disease.

MR spectroscopy of the involved white matter shows a small lactate peak (*white arrow*), decrease in NAA (*red arrow*), and elevation of choline (*blue arrow*) and myo-inositol (*green arrow*).

Answers

1. Megalencephalic leukoencephalopathy with subcortical cysts typically presents in the first year of life with macrocephaly, developmental delay, and seizures. Unlike most infantile onset leukoencephalopathies, progression is slow, with patients typically living for decades after presentation.

2. Typical imaging findings of megalencephalic leukoencephalopathy with subcortical cysts include diffuse involvement of the supratentorial white matter with early involvement of the U-fibers. There may be sparing of the central white matter tracts such as the corpus callosum. Sparing of the cerebellar white matter is typical. Subcortical cysts follow CSF in signal and occur primarily in the anterior temporal lobes and frontal parietal lobes. These cysts tend to enlarge in size and number over time.

3. Mutations in MLC1, MLC2A, and MLC2B have been identified to cause megalencephalic leukoencephalopathy with subcortical cysts. MLC1 and MLC2A mutations are inherited in an autosomal recessive manner while MLC2B mutations are autosomal dominant. In consanguineous populations, the carrier rate may be as high as 1/40.

4. Vacuolating megaloencephalic leukoencephalopathy, van der Knaap disease, and Indian Agarwal megaloencephalic leukodystrophy have all been reported within the literature referring to megalencephalic leukoencephalopathy with subcortical cysts. This disease has been described in the Agarwal surname population within India.

5. Metachromatic leukodystrophy usually spares subcortical white matter early and lacks subcortical cysts. Patients are not typically macrocephalic. Vanishing white matter disease will typically see rarefaction of white matter instead of focal subcortical cysts. Canavan disease can involve white matter disease but may also have basal ganglia involvement, which is atypical for megalencephalic leukoencephalopathy with subcortical cysts. MRS will also show elevated NAA. Pelizaeus-Merzbacher will have diffuse white matter hypomyelination without subcortical cysts.

Pearls

- Diffuse white matter T2 hyperintensity involving the subcortical U-fibers of the supratentorial hemispheres.
- Subcortical cysts following CSF signal primarily in the anterior temporal and frontal-parietal lobes.
- Clinical history of macrocephaly within the first year of life.

Suggested Readings

Bajaj SK, Misra R, Gupta R, Chandra R, Malik A. Megalencephalic leukoencephalopathy with sub cortical cysts: an inherited dysmyelinating disorder. *J Pediatr Neurosci.* 2013 Jan;8(1):77-80.

Tu YF, Chen CY, Huang CC, Lee CS. Vacuolating megalencephalic leukoencephalopathy with mild clinical course validated by diffusion tensor imaging and MR spectroscopy. *AJNR Am J Neuroradiol.* 2011 Dec;25(6):1041-1045.

3-month-old male with developmental delay, hypotonia, nystagmus, and stridor

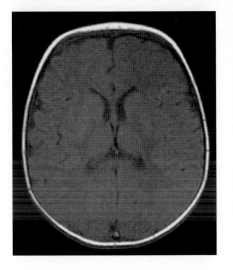 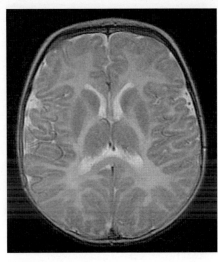 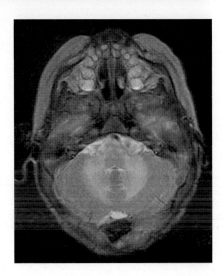

1. What are the normal patterns of myelination in infancy?

2. What does normal myelination look like on T1- and T2-weighted images?

3. What is the method of inheritance of this disease?

4. What is the pattern of white matter involvement of this disease?

5. What other syndromes are included in the hypomyelination disorders?

Case ranking/difficulty:

Category: Intra-axial supratentorial

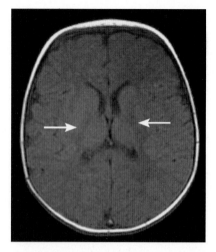

Axial T1 of the basal ganglia level shows lack of normal T1 hyperintensity of the posterior limb of the internal capsule (*white arrows*) in this 3-month-old, normally expected to be myelinated at birth.

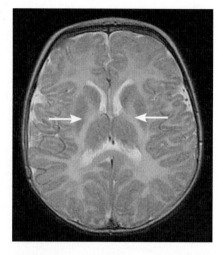

Axial T2 of the basal ganglia level shows a lack of T2 hypointensity from normal myelin compaction with some expansion of the posterior limb of the internal capsule from edematous change (*white arrows*).

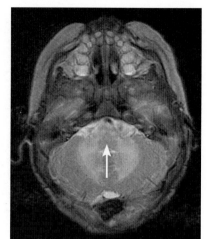

Axial T2 through the cerebellum shows diffuse T2 hyperintensity of the cerebellar white matter, normally expected to be myelinated with a decrease in T2 signal. There is only mild myelin compaction in the dorsal brainstem (*white arrow*).

Answers

1. At birth myelination can be seen in the corticospinal tracts and dorsal brainstem. The splenium of the corpus callosum can be bright on T1 by 3 months but almost always at 4 months.

   The anterior limb of the internal capsules is always bright on T1 by 6 months. Myelination progresses from posterior to anterior, inferior to superior, and central to peripheral.

2. Normal oligodendrocyte maturation first shows T1 hyperintensity followed by T2 hypointensity, reflecting myelin compaction. Due to the lag of T2 hypointensity, up to 6-8 months, T1 images are most helpful in assessing myelin maturation below 1 year of age. T2 images become more useful after 1 year of age. FLAIR images are not useful in distinguishing myelin maturation in the first year of life.

3. In Pelizaeus-Merzbacher, an x-linked disease of the proteolipid protein, hypomyelination results from apoptosis of normal oligodendrogliocytes. While only males demonstrate the full disease phenotype, carrier females can demonstrate mild neurologic symptoms and MRI imaging.

4. Pelizaeus-Merzbacher usually involves all of the white matter without significant gray matter involvement. As cell death of oligodendrogliocytes occurs, white matter atrophy usually results.

5. 18q syndrome, spastic paraplegia type 2, and hypomyelination with atrophy of the basal ganglia and cerebellum, along with Pelizaeus-Merzbacher, are associated with hypomyelination.

Pearls

- Hypomyelination syndromes can be diagnosed with the appropriate knowledge of normal myelination maturation in early infancy.
- T2 hypointensity corresponding to myelin compaction typically lags T1 hyperintensity, making T1 images more useful in assessing myelin maturation in the first year of life.
- Hypomyelination involves the white matter only, with abnormal T1 hypointensity and T2 hyperintensity in areas of expected myelination for age.

Suggested Readings

Barkovich AJ. Concepts of myelin and myelination in neuroradiology. *AJNR Am J Neuroradiol.* 2003 Sep;21(6):1099-1109.

Laukka JJ, Stanley JA, Garbern JY, et al. Neuroradiologic correlates of clinical disability and progression in the X-Linked leukodystrophy Pelizaeus-Merzbacher disease. *J Neurol Sci.* 2013 Dec;335(1-2):75-81.

20-month-old female with seizures, poor feeding, central hypotonia, and developmental delay

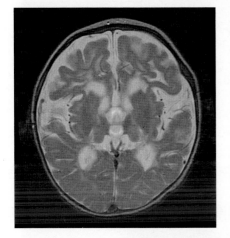
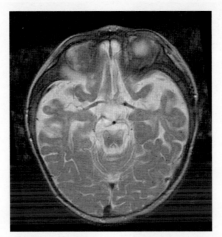
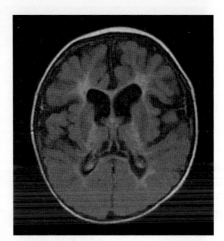
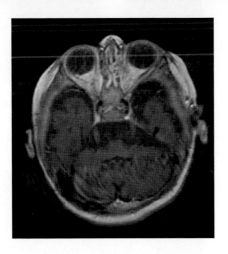
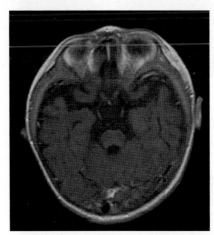

1. What are the typical patterns of white matter involvement in this disease?

2. Can CT be helpful in the diagnosis of this disease?

3. What findings can be seen outside of the brain parenchyma in this disease?

4. What is the biochemical abnormality in this disease?

5. What are clinical subtypes and associated prognosis of this disease?

Case ranking/difficulty: 🥜🥜🥜

Category: Intra-axial supratentorial

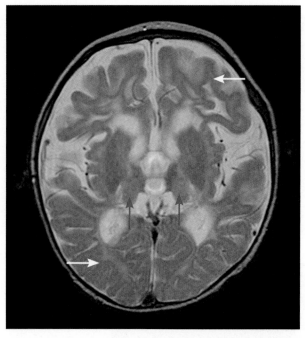

Axial T2 images at the ganglionic level shows diffuse confluent white matter T2 hyperintensity and atrophy with some sparing of subcortical U-fibers (*white arrow*). Note the atrophy of the involved bilateral thalami (*red arrows*).

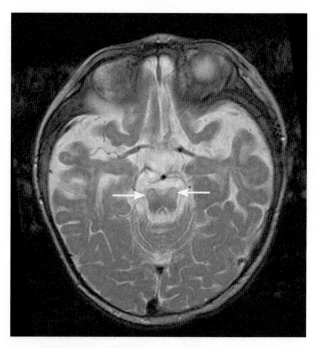

Axial T2 at the level of the midbrain shows brainstem atrophy, especially with T2 hyperintensity of the corticalspinal tracts in the cerebral peduncles (*white arrows*).

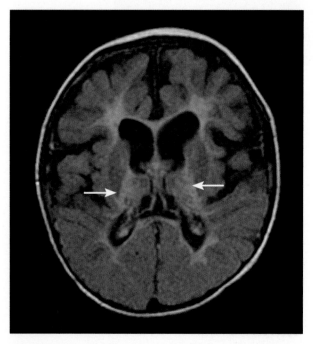

Axial FLAIR of the ganglionic level demonstrates symmetric, confluent T2 hyperintensity of the central white matter with involvement of the corticospinal tract (posterior limb of the internal capsule) (*white arrows*) and sparing of the subcortical white matter (*red arrows*).

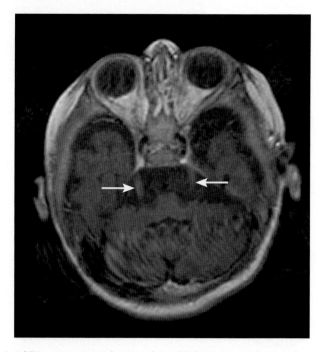

Axial T1 postcontrast shows enlarged bilateral cranial nerve V (*white arrows*), a hallmark of metabolite deposition in Krabbe disease.

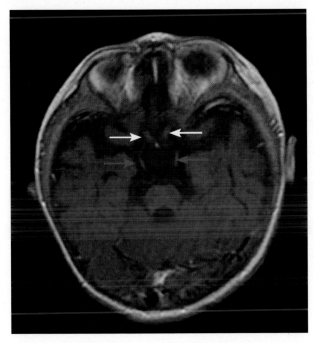

Axial T1 postcontrast at the suprasellar cistern shows enlargement and mild enhancement of the optic nerves (*white arrows*) and cranial nerve III (*red arrows*) consistent with galactosylceramide and psychosine in Krabbe disease.

Answers

1. Krabbe disease typically involves the central white matter including the corpus callosum, paraventricular, and corticospinal tracts in a symmetric, confluent distribution. Sparing of subcortical U-fibers can be seen late into the disease.

2. CT can show early hyperdensity of the corticospinal tract and thalami on CT in Krabbe disease. CT can be a useful screening tool; however, in infants, the cost of radiation and high likelihood of a follow-up MRI exam make MRI as the initial exam more safe and efficacious.

3. In Krabbe disease, deposition of metabolites in oligodendroglia and Schwann cells can cause enlargement and enhancement of the cranial nerves and peripheral nerves.

4. A lysosomal storage disorder, galactosylceramide and psychosine are typically broken down by galactocerebroside beta-galactosidase (GALC). Mutations of this gene on chromosome 14 lead to deposition of these toxic metabolites within the oligodendrogliocytes and Schwann cells, leading to white matter, cranial and peripheral nerve disease. Globoid cells refer to galactocerebroside-containing macrophages, which can be seen in tissues of patients with Krabbe disease.

5. Four clinical subtypes of Krabbe disease are associated with their age of onset. The classic infantile type is usually diagnosed in the first year of life with typically progression to death in a few years. As with many metabolic leukodystrophies, the later the onset as in the late infantile, juvenile, and adult types, the slower the disease progression. Due to some benefits with early stem cell transplant, newborn screening for Krabbe disease can be helpful in at least delaying the CNS deterioration and improving quality of life.

Pearls

- Bilateral central white matter involvement in a confluent pattern, especially including the corticalspinal tracts, which may show hyperdensity on CT.
- Basal ganglia and thalamic involvement.
- Cranial nerve and peripheral nerve enlargement and enhancement.

Suggested Readings

Beslow LA, Schwartz ES, Bönnemann CG. Thickening and enhancement of multiple cranial nerves in conjunction with cystic white matter lesions in early infantile Krabbe disease. *Pediatr Radiol.* 2008 Jun;38(6):694-696.

Farina L, Bizzi A, Finocchiaro G, et al. MR imaging and proton MR spectroscopy in adult Krabbe disease. *AJNR Am J Neuroradiol.* 2000 Sep;21(8):1478-1482.

Patel B, Gimi B, Vachha B, Agadi S, Koral K. Optic nerve and chiasm enlargement in a case of infantile Krabbe disease: quantitative comparison with 26 age-matched controls. *Pediatr Radiol.* 2008 Jun;38(6):697-699.

413

5-month-old female with seizures, poor feeding, central hypotonia, and apnea

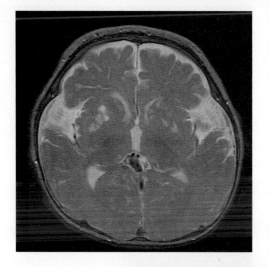
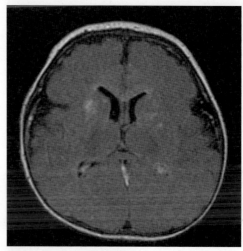

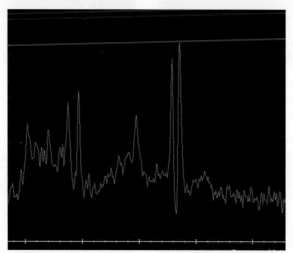

1. What are imaging findings that are hallmarks for this classification of diseases?

2. What differential diagnosis must the pediatric radiologist be aware of with these diseases?

3. What is the method of inheritance of this disease?

4. What are clinical symptoms of this disease?

5. What abnormal metabolites are seen with this disease?

Case ranking/difficulty: 🐾🐾🐾

Category: Intra-axial supratentorial

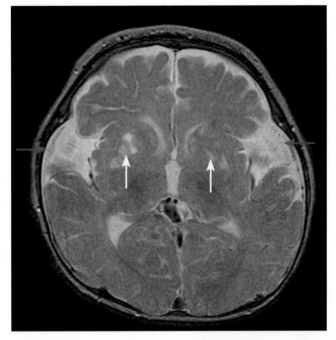

Axial T2 through the ganglionic level shows patchy T2 hyperintensities in the bilateral basal ganglia (*white arrows*). Note the widened sylvian fissures (*red arrows*).

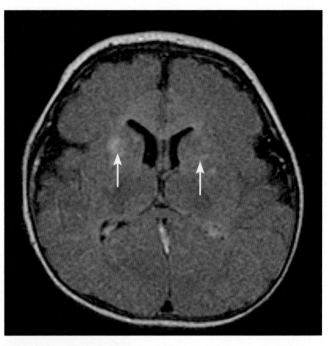

Axial FLAIR images show patchy T2 hyperintensity of the basal ganglia (*white arrows*) and involvement of the genu of the corpus callosum (*red arrow*).

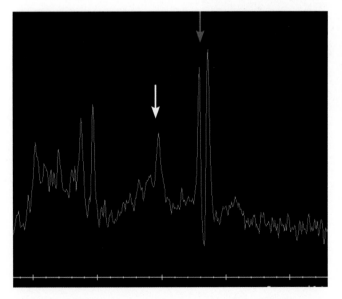

MR spectroscopy of the basal ganglia shows a diminished NAA (*white arrow*) and a large characteristic lactate doublet (*red arrow*).

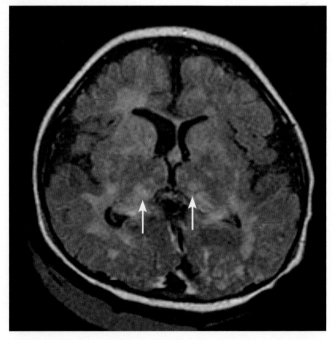

1-year follow-up axial FLAIR image at the ganglionic level shows progression of disease to involve the thalami (*white arrows*) and central white matter (*red arrows*) with progressive atrophy.

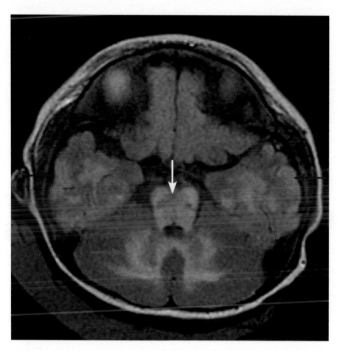

1-year follow-up axial FLAIR images of the cerebellum show brainstem T2 hyperintensity (*white arrow*) as well as deep cerebellar white matter involvement (*red arrows*). There is also involvement of the temporal white and gray matter (*blue arrows*).

Answers

1. Ethylmalonic encephalopathy is classified as an organic acidemia, with disruption of the normal mitochondrial respiration. Typical findings of organic acidemias include widened operculum (sylvian fissures), early basal ganglia involvement with diffusion restriction during the acute phase. Progression to involve the central white matter and atrophy is typical.

2. With progression to atrophy in organic acidemias and increased risk of injury to the bridging veins with minor head traumas, organic acidemias have been suggested as a differential to cases of suspected nonaccidental trauma. However, organic acidemias will not cause skull fractures or other findings of traumatic brain injury, such as contusions. In the acute phase, restricted diffusion in the basal ganglia can be seen commonly in hypoxic-anoxic injury without underlying metabolic disorder. Widened operculum with cystic spaces can also be seen in glycosaminoglycans in mucopolysaccharidoses.

3. Ethylmalonic encephalopathy is a rare autosomal recessive disease with defect of the ETHE1 gene. This has been only reported in 30 cases worldwide.

4. Ethylmalonic encephalopathy usually presents in infancy with neurologic symptoms such as encephalopathy, developmental delay, hypotonia, and seizures. Petechial rashes and chronic diarrhea are common features described in the Arab and Mediterranean populations.

5. In ethylmalonic encephalopathy, ethylmalonic and lactic acids are found in high concentrations. As brain toxicity occurs, NAA is decreased on MRI spectroscopy.

Pearls

- Ethylmalonic encephalopathy has MRI findings similar to other organic acidemias, such as early basal ganglia injury, which is bright on T2 imaging and can have restricted diffusion in the acute phase.
- Widening of the sylvian fissures is a hallmark of organic acidurias.
- Progressive disease leads to central white matter involvement with atrophy.
- In late stage atrophy, tearing of bridging veins with minimal head trauma may be a mimicker for nonaccidental trauma.
- Other organic acidurias include maple syrup urine disease, propionic aciduria, methylmalonic aciduria, homocystinuria, HMG-CoA lyase deficiency, and glutaric acidemia type I.

Suggested Readings

Brismar J, Ozand PT. CT and MR of the brain in the diagnosis of organic acidemias. Experiences from 107 patients. *Brain Dev.* 1994 Nov;16(suppl):104-124.

Jamroz E, Paprocka J, Adamek D, et al. Clinical and neuropathological picture of ethylmalonic aciduria – diagnostic dilemma. *Folia Neuropathol.* 2011 Nov;49(1):71-77.

Tiranti V, Zeviani M. Altered sulfide (H(2)S) metabolism in ethylmalonic encephalopathy. *Cold Spring Harb Perspect Biol.* 2013 Jan;5(1):a011437.

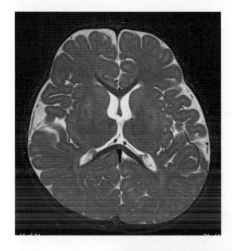
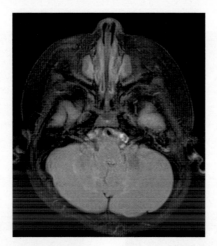
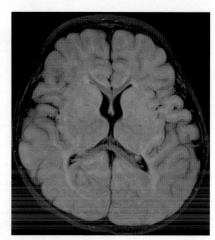
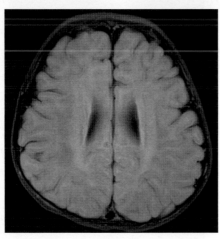
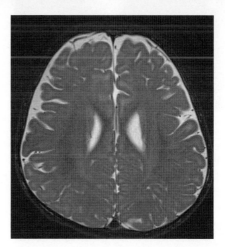

1. What are the typical MRI findings of the infantile form of this disease?

2. What are the typical MRI findings in the adult-onset form of the disease?

3. What are the clinical symptoms of adult-onset forms?

4. What are the pathophysiological characteristics of this disease?

5. What are the leukodystrophies with macrocephaly?

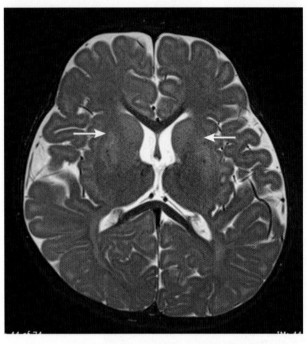

Axial T2 image at the ganglionic level shows increased T2 hyperintensity of the corpus striatum (*white arrows*) and lack of normal myelin compaction of the periatrial white matter within this 1-year-old patient (*red arrows*). There is sparing of the corpus callosum.

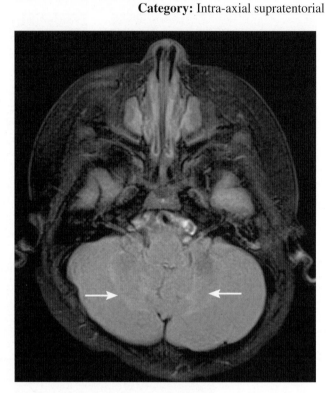

Axial T2 through the cerebellum shows mild involvement of the deep cerebellar white matter (*white arrows*).

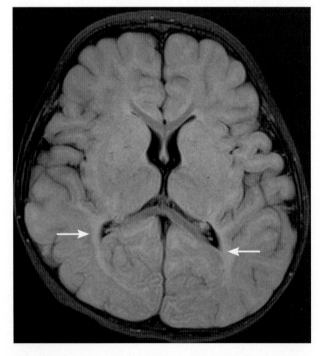

Axial FLAIR through the ganglionic level better demonstrates the posterior periventricular involvement of the white matter in this patient (*white arrows*).

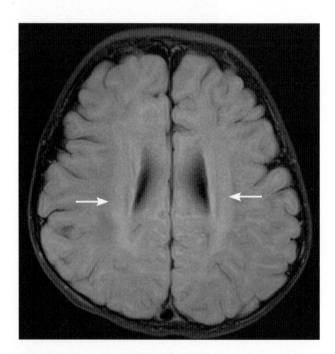

Axial FLAIR above the ganglionic level shows confluent periventricular white matter involvement (*white arrows*) beyond the periatrial region, greater than expected for terminal myelin zones.

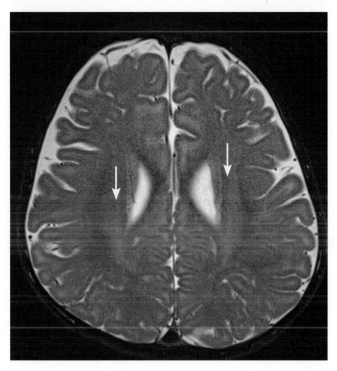

Axial T2 above the ganglionic level again shows periventricular white matter T2 hyperintensity (*white arrows*), which is expected to demonstrate normal T2 hypointensity from myelin compaction (*red arrows*).

Answers

1. Periventricular white matter involvement in a frontal to occipital gradient with enhancement is the "classic" MRI finding of Alexander disease. Basal ganglia and thalamic involvement is also common. Subcortical U-fibers are thought to be involved late in the disease process.

2. Adult-onset forms of Alexander disease have been described with cerebellar and brainstem predominance. Enhancement of the cerebellum and brainstem has also been described.

3. Given the cerebellar and brainstem predilection of the adult-onset form of Alexander disease, common presenting symptoms include bulbar signs such as dysarthria and palatal myoclonus as well as ataxia. Infantile forms present with macrocephaly, seizures, developmental delay, or arrest and spasticity.

4. Alexander disease is autosomal dominant, and while familial inheritance can occur with adult-onset types, most cases arrive from de novo mutations of GFAP. This mutation leads to Rosenthal fibers in the affected astrocytes and loss of normal function with oligodendrocytes.

5. Mucopolysaccharidoses, Alexander disease, Canavan disease, Tay-Sachs, and megalencephalic leukodystrophy with subcortical cysts can present with infantile macrocephaly.

Pearls

- Periventricular white matter involvement in a frontal to occipital gradient is classically described with Alexander disease.
- Basal ganglia involvement is seen in the infantile form.
- Enhancement of the periventricular white matter is characteristic, as enhancement of dysmyelinating leukodystrophies is usually associated with Alexander disease and x-linked adrenoleukodystrophy.

Suggested Readings

da Silva Pereira CC, Gattás GS, Lucato LT. Alexander disease: a novel mutation in the glial fibrillary acidic protein gene with initial uncommon clinical and magnetic resonance imaging findings. *J Comput Assist Tomogr.* 2013 Dec;37(5):698-700.

Farina L, Pareyson D, Minati L, et al. Can MR imaging diagnose adult-onset Alexander disease? *AJNR Am J Neuroradiol.* 2008 Jun;29(6):1190-1196.

Vázquez E, Macaya A, Mayolas N, Arévalo S, Poca MA, Enríquez G. Neonatal Alexander disease: MR imaging prenatal diagnosis. *AJNR Am J Neuroradiol.* 2008 Nov;29(10):1973-1975.

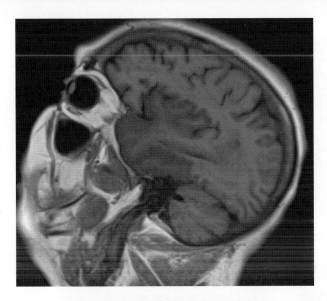
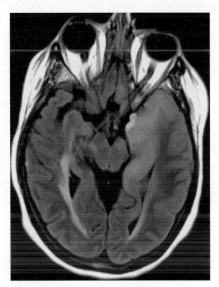
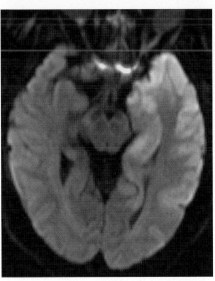
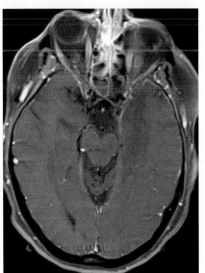

1. Where is the abnormality?

2. What is the differential diagnosis?

3. What are risk factors for status epilepticus?

4. What is the most common cause of chronic temporal lobe epilepsy?

5. In what condition are epileptic seizures, facial angiomata, and mental retardation found?

Case ranking/difficulty:

Category: Intra-axial supratentorial

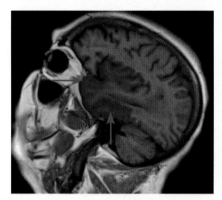

Abnormal low T1 signal (*arrows*) most pronounced in the left temporal lobe with local mass effect and effacement of the sulci.

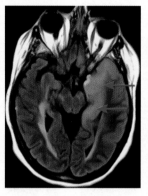

Axial FLAIR image shows abnormal high T2 signal (*arrows*) of the mesial left temporal lobe and hippocampus with enlargement of the gyri and effacement of the sulci.

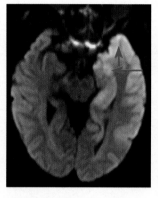

Axial DWI b-1000 image shows cortical restricted diffusion and abnormal high T2 signal involving the left hippocampus and temporal lobe (*arrows*).

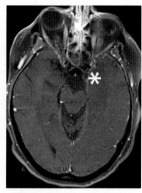

Axial T1 postcontrast shows no parenchymal enhancement of the left temporal lobe.

Answers

1. The main abnormality involves the left temporal lobe, primarily centered in the left hippocampus.

2. Status epilepticus, infarct, cerebritis, and HSV encephalitis are differential diagnoses for edema and restricted diffusion of the temporal lobe.

3. History of epilepsy, fever, stroke, prior brain insult, and tumors, such as dysembryoplastic neuroepithelial tumor (DNET).

4. Gangliogliomas are reported to be the most common cause of chronic temporal lobe seizures.

5. Tuberous sclerosis has the classic triad of seizures, facial angiomata, and mental retardation ("fits, zits, and nitwits").

Pearls

- Status epilepticus is a state in which a patient experiences greater than 30 minutes of continuous seizure activity or experiences two or more seizures without recovery between episodes.
- The findings on MR are transient and usually resolve in days to weeks after onset.

- Epilepsy history is helpful for the diagnosis.
- Imaging features include high T2 signal in the gray matter and subcortical white matter with associated mild mass effect (as in this case).
- Other structures reported to be involved are the cerebellum, thalami, and corpus callosum.
- Restricted diffusion may be seen acutely and there may be variable enhancement.
- Diffusion restriction may be reversible.
- If focal enhancement is seen, consider neoplasm

Suggested Readings

Cianfoni A, Caulo M, Cerase A, et al. Seizure-induced brain lesions: a wide spectrum of variably reversible MRI abnormalities. *Eur J Radiol*. 2013 Nov;82(11):1964-1972.

Chatzikonstantinou A, Gass A, Förster A, Hennerici MG, Szabo K. Features of acute DWI abnormalities related to status epilepticus. *Epilepsy Res*. 2011 Nov;97(1-2):45-51.

Fountain NB. Status epilepticus: risk factors and complications. *Epilepsia*. 2000 Jul;41(suppl 2):S23-S30.

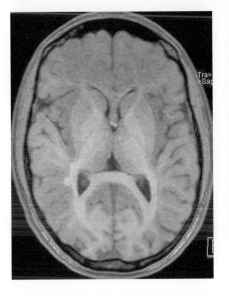
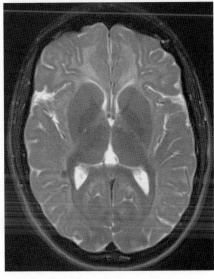
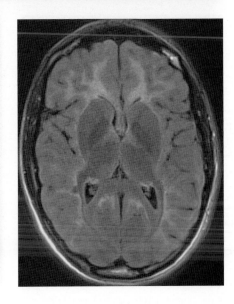

1. What are the clinical characteristics that give the disease its name?

2. What does normal myelination look like on T1- and T2-weighted images?

3. What are the normal patterns of myelination in infancy?

4. What is the genetic inheritance for this disease?

5. What neuroimaging findings are seen with this gene mutation?

Case ranking/difficulty:

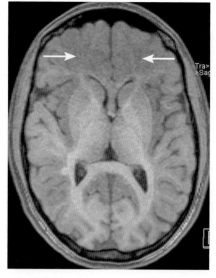

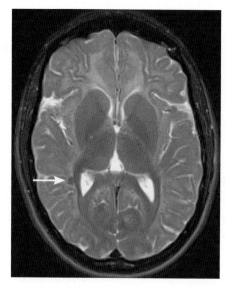

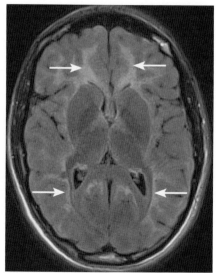

Axial T1 image through the ganglionic level shows appropriate T1 hyperintensity from myelination of the splenium, posterior periventricular white matter, and internal capsules. The frontal and peripheral white matter is abnormally hypointense (*white arrows*) and not myelinated in this 18-year-old.

Axial T2 image through the ganglionic level shows normal myelin compaction with T2 hypointensity only of the posterior capsular and periventricular white matter. Note the right periatrial nest of normal myelinated white matter (*white arrow*) within abnormal hypomyelination.

Axial FLAIR shows increased T2 signal of abnormal hypomyelination (*white arrows*).

Answers

1. 4H syndrome stands for hypomyelination, hypogonadotropic hypogonadism, and hypodontia.

2. Normal oligodendrocyte maturation first shows T1 hyperintensity followed by T2 hypointensity, reflecting myelin compaction. Due to the lag of T2 hypointensity, up to 6-8 months, T1 images are most helpful in assessing myelin maturation below 1 year of age. T2 images become more useful after 1 year of age. FLAIR images are not useful in distinguishing myelin maturation in the first year of life.

3. At birth myelination can be seen in the corticospinal tracts and dorsal brainstem.

   The splenium of the corpus callosum can be bright on T1 by 3 months but almost always at 4 months.

   The anterior limbs of the internal capsules are always bright on T1 by 6 months.

   Myelination progresses from posterior to anterior, inferior to superior, and central to peripheral.

4. 4H syndrome is categorized in the POL III–related leukodystrophy as these diseases involve mutation of the POLR3A or POLR3B gene with autosomal recessive inheritance.

5. POL III–related leukodystrophy has been described with hypomyelination, and cerebellar and callosal atrophy.

Pearls

- 4H syndrome (hypomyelination, hypogonadotropic hypogonadism, and hypodontia) is categorized within the POL III–related leukodystrophies which involves mutation of the POLR3A or 3B genes.
- Hypomyelination, with lack of normal T1 shortening and T2 hypointensity, is seen in white matter, which is expected to be myelinated for age.
- Cerebellar corpus callosal atrophy has also been described in this disease.

Suggested Readings

Synofzik M, Bernard G, Lindig T, Gburek-Augustat J. Teaching neuroimages: hypomyelinating leukodystrophy with hypodontia due to POLR3B: look into a leukodystrophy's mouth. *Neurology*. 2013 Nov;81(19):e145.

Takanashi J, Osaka H, Saitsu H. Different patterns of cerebellar abnormality and hypomyelination between POLR3A and POLR3B mutations. *Brain Dev*. 2014 Mar;36(3):259-263.

23-month-old male with seizures, loss of milestones, and feeding dysfunction

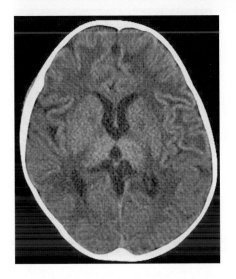 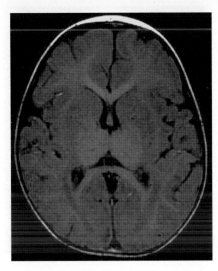 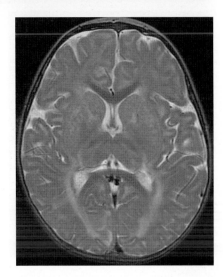

1. What are the typical MRI findings for this disease?

2. What is the typical finding on funduscopic exam?

3. What are the related diseases with a similar biochemical pathogenesis?

4. What is the prognosis for this disease?

5. Which population groups have a higher risk of this disease?

Case ranking/difficulty: 🐾🐾🐾

Category: Intra-axial supratentorial

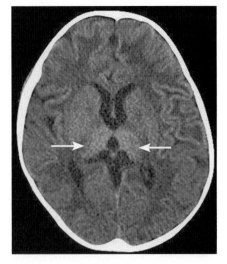

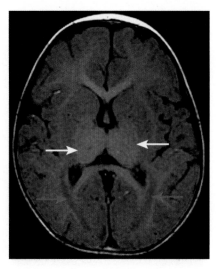

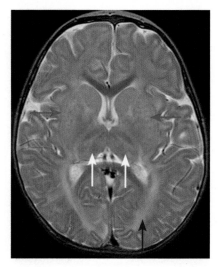

Axial CT through the ganglionic level shows bilateral diffuse symmetric hyperintensity of the thalami (*white arrows*).

Axial T1 image through the ganglionic level shows diffuse T1 hyperintensity of the thalami (*white arrows*), and lack of normal T1 bright myelination of the posterior periventricular white matter (*red arrows*). There is sparing of the corpus callosum.

Axial T2 image through the ganglionic level demonstrates heterogeneous signal of the thalami (*white arrows*) (more specific to Tay-Sachs) and increased T2 signal of the basal ganglia (*red arrows*). There is loss of normal T2 hypointense myelin compaction of the periventricular white matter (*blue arrow*) with sparing of the corpus callosum.

Answers

1. Typical findings for GM2 gangliosidosis and its subtypes, including Tay-Sachs disease, include T1 hyperintense and T2 hypointense thalami, T2 hyperintense basal ganglia, and hypomyelination with sparing of the corpus callosum.

2. The cherry-red spot macula can be seen in 90% of Tay-Sachs but is nonspecific as other metabolic storage disorders can have this finding.

3. GM2 gangliosidosis include a group of related lysosomal storage disorders all with failure of breaking down GM2 gangliosidosis due to defects in one of the two proteins responsible for this process. Tay Sachs, Sandhoff, and GM2 AB variant are all subtypes of GM2 gangliosidosis.

4. Infantile forms of Tay-Sachs typically progress to death in a few years. Juvenile forms have variable survival but most die within a decade. Adult-onset forms are rare but can have slow progression with potentially relatively normal life spans. No treatment currently exists with bone marrow transplant not particularly effective.

5. Higher incidence and carrier rates for Tay-Sachs are seen in Ashkenazi Jewish, French Canadian, and Cajun populations.

Pearls

- Tay-Sachs disease is a subtype of GM2 gangliosidosis, with failure to break down GM2 gangliosides.
- Toxic accumulation in the brain leads to deterioration and death in a few years in the classic infantile form.
- Cherry-red spot macula is a characteristic finding of the disease on funduscopic exam, but can be seen in other storage diseases.
- MRI shows characteristic increased density of the thalami diffusely on CT and increased T1 and decreased T2 signal on MRI.
- Hypomyelination with sparing of the corpus callosum is seen.
- Basal ganglia may also be edematous with increased T2 signal.

Suggested Readings

Autti T, Joensuu R, Aberg L. Decreased T2 signal in the thalami may be a sign of lysosomal storage disease. *Neuroradiology*. 2007 Jul;49(7):571-578.

Inglese M, Nusbaum AO, Pastores GM, Gianutsos J, Kolodny EH, Gonen O. MR imaging and proton spectroscopy of neuronal injury in late-onset GM2 gangliosidosis. *AJNR Am J Neuroradiol*. 2005 Sep;26(8):2037-2042.

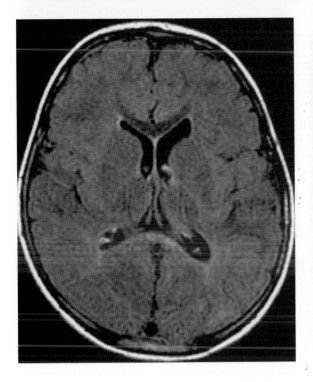
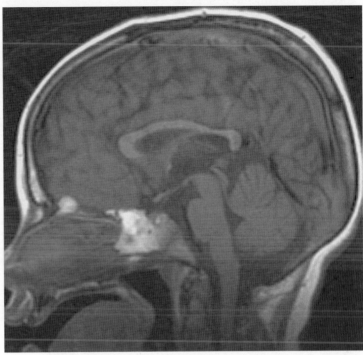

1. What are the differential diagnoses for these findings?

2. What is the deficient enzyme in this disease?

3. What is the inheritance of this disease?

4. What are the subtypes of this disease?

5. What is the prognosis for the disease?

Case ranking/difficulty:

Category: Intra-axial supratentorial

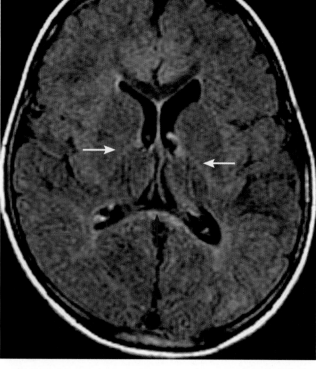

Axial FLAIR image at the ganglionic level shows increased signal involving the posterior limb of the internal capsule (*white arrows*), periatrial white matter (*red arrows*), and splenium of the corpus callosum (*blue arrow*) from dysmyelination in this patient with GM1 gangliosidosis.

Answers

1. This case with hypomyelination of the periventricular white matter with involvement of the posterior limb of the corticospinal tract is typical for hypomyelination syndromes such as Pelizaeus Merzbacher. Other diseases with dysmyelination include GM1 gangliosidosis and Krabbe disease, especially with involvement of the corticospinal tract. This patient had GM1 gangliosidosis.

2. GM1 gangliosidosis is caused by a deficiency of beta-galactosidase.

3. GM1 gangliosidosis is autosomal recessive.

4. Subtypes of GM1 gangliosidosis correlate with age of onset, with type 1 infantile, type 2 late infantile and juvenile, and type 3 adult.

5. Infantile-onset forms typically die within a few years; juvenile-onset forms have variable deterioration with most not living beyond early adulthood. Adult-onset types can have variable life expectancy with slow progression of extrapyramidal signs. No treatment exists.

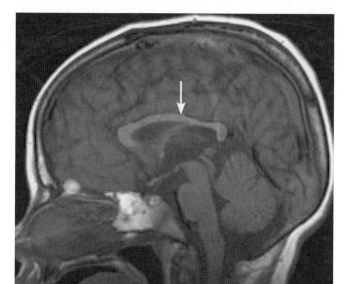

Sagittal T1 image shows a thinned corpus callosum (*white arrow*) from white matter atrophy.

Pearls

- GM1 gangliosidosis is an autosomal recessive lysosomal storage disorder with deficiency of beta-galactosidase.
- MRI findings typically involve white matter hypomyelination or demyelination.
- Globi pallidi hypointensity can be seen in juvenile forms.
- Adult-onset forms have putaminal T2 hyperintensity.
- Atrophy is typical later in the disease.

Suggested Readings

Chen CY, Zimmerman RA, Lee CC, Chen FH, Yuh YS, Hsiao HS. Neuroimaging findings in late infantile GM1 gangliosidosis. *AJNR Am J Neuroradiol.* 1998 Oct;19(9):1628-1630.

De Grandis E, Di Rocco M, Pessagno A, Veneselli E, Rossi A. MR imaging findings in 2 cases of late infantile GM1 gangliosidosis. *AJNR Am J Neuroradiol.* 2009 Aug;30(7):1325-1327.

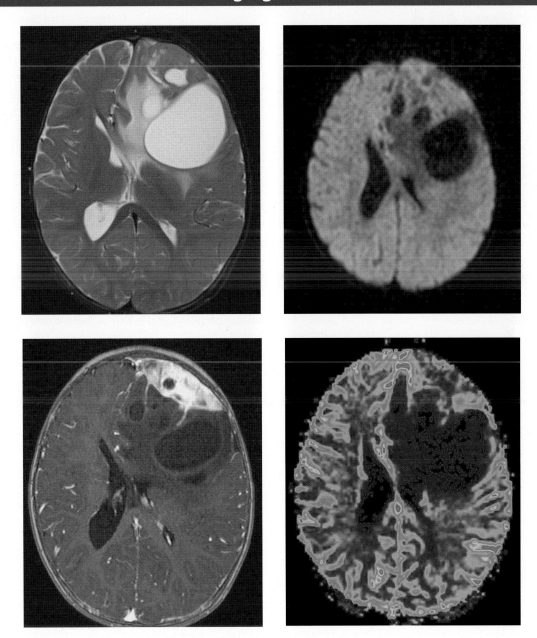

1. What is the differential diagnosis in this infant?

2. What are typical MRI findings for this entity?

3. What is the prognosis of this disease?

4. What are histologic findings in this tumor?

5. What is the treatment for this disease?

Case ranking/difficulty:

Category: Intra-axial supratentorial

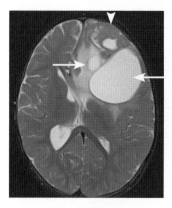

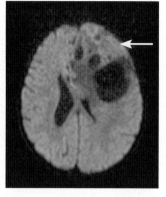

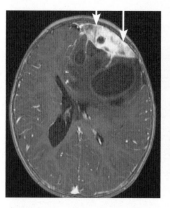

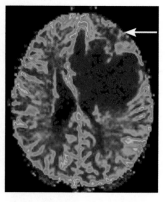

Axial T2 image shows a large heterogeneous mass with multiple cysts centrally (*arrows*) and a solid peripheral component with decreased T2 signal (*arrowhead*).

Axial DWI b = 1000 image shows the solid component of the tumor (*arrow*) with similar diffusion as the gray matter.

Axial T1 postcontrast shows the peripheral solid component with intense enhancement and broad dural base (*arrows*) consistent with a desmoplastic infantile ganglioglioma.

Axial color CBV map image from dynamic susceptibility contrast perfusion imaging shows the peripheral nodule with relatively less perfusion than the gray matter (*arrow*).

Answers

1. The differential for large heterogeneous CNS tumors in infants includes desmoplastic infantile tumors, supratentorial ependymoma, glioblastoma, primitive neuroectodermal tumor, and atypical teratoid rhabdoid tumor. Of this differential only the desmoplastic infantile tumors are considered WHO grade I with a generally benign course.

2. Intensely enhancing solid components with a broad dural attachment and central cysts are imaging hallmarks for desmoplastic infantile tumors.

3. The prognosis for desmoplastic infantile tumors is generally good with at least 75% survival at 15 years.

4. Desmoplastic infantile tumors have desmoplastic involvement of leptomeninges, typically the dura. The neoplastic neuroepithelial cells typically have a spindled or gemistocytic pattern. Neoplastic astrocytes are the only neuroepithelial cell type in desmoplastic infantile astrocytomas with the addition of small or large ganglion cells in the desmoplastic infantile ganglioglioma. Of note, nests of hypercellular poorly differentiated neuroepithelial cells can be found in these tumors, which can suggest the potential for poor prognosis, but with complete surgical resection, the outcome is typically positive.

5. Complete surgical resection is considered curative for desmoplastic infantile tumors with rare recurrence. Chemotherapy is indicated for unresectable tumor. As most of the tumors present in infancy, radiation is not indicated in children under 3 years of age due to devastating effects on the maturing brain.

Pearls

- Desmoplastic infantile gangliogliomas (DIG) and astrocytomas are WHO grade I tumors with generally good outcome despite their large heterogeneous appearance.
- These tumors are most common in the first year of life with peak incidence between 3 and 6 months.
- DIGs are characteristic in their appearance as large, suprasellar, hemispheric tumors with multiple large centrally located cysts and a solid component that has some desmoplastic dural attachment.
- The cysts usually follow CSF on all images with possible cyst wall enhancement.
- The solid nodule will show intense enhancement with a broad dural attachment, and may have decreased ADC.
- Complete surgical resection is curative, with chemotherapy only for unresectable tumor.

Suggested Readings

Nikas I, Anagnostara A, Theophanopoulou M, Stefanaki K, Michail A, Hadjigeorgi Ch. Desmoplastic infantile ganglioglioma: MRI and histological findings case report. *Neuroradiology*. 2004 Dec;46(12):1039-1043.

Trehan G, Bruge H, Vinchon M, et al. MR imaging in the diagnosis of desmoplastic infantile tumor: retrospective study of six cases. AJNR *Am J Neuroradiol*. 2004 Dec;25(6):1028-1033.

5-year-old female with staring spells

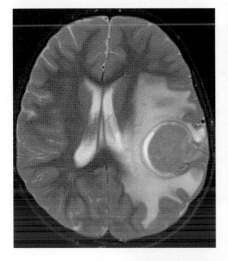
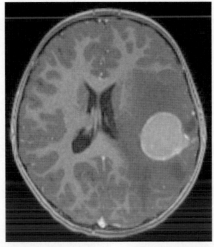
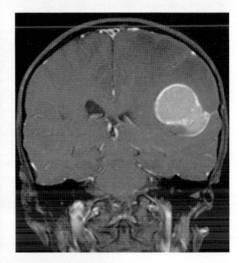
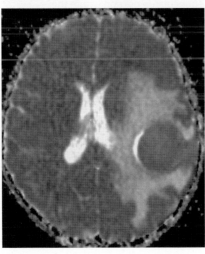
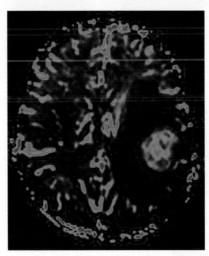

1. What is the differential diagnosis?

2. What imaging finding helps differentiate this lesion from other cortically based tumors?

3. What histologic features can be seen with this tumor?

4. What is the typical WHO grade for this neoplasm?

5. What is the treatment for this disease?

Case ranking/difficulty: **Category:** Intra-axial supratentorial

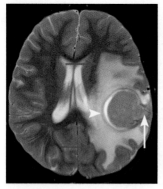

Axial T2 image shows a well-circumscribed mass with uniform low T2 signal, a medial circumferential cyst (*white arrowhead*), extension to the dural surface (*white arrow*), and significant surrounding T2 prolongation, likely edema (*red arrows*).

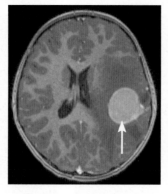

Axial postcontrast image shows intense homogeneous enhancement of the solid mass (*arrow*).

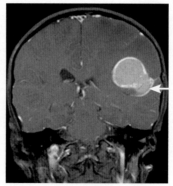

Coronal postcontrast image shows the enhancing mass in the parietal lobe with a pedunculated portion within the sylvian fissure (*arrow*).

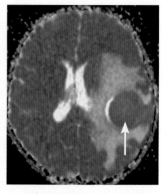

Axial ADC image shows restricted diffusion of the solid mass (*arrow*).

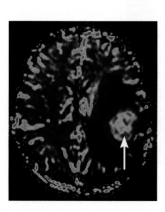

Axial color CBV image from dynamic susceptibility contrast perfusion technique shows increased perfusion of the solid mass (*arrow*). This was an atypical pleomorphic xanthoastrocytoma.

Answers

1. The differential for a well-circumscribed cortically based enhancing mass includes pleomorphic xanthoastrocytoma, ganglioglioma, oligodendroglioma, and pilocytic astrocytoma.

2. Pleomorphic xanthoastrocytomas can characteristically have a dural tail, from dural reaction. While ganglioglioma and oligodendroglioma are cortically based, the enhancing dural tail is not seen in these entities.

3. Pleomorphic xanthoastrocytomas are named for the pleomorphic appearance with different cell types, including large xanthomatous (lipid containing) cells.

4. Pleomorphic xanthoastrocytomas (PXA) are usually WHO grade II tumors. Some classify PXA as WHO grade III when there is atypia, including greater than 5 mitoses per 10 HPF, as in this case.

5. Complete resection is considered curative for pleomorphic xanthoastrocytoma. If there is recurrence, a second resection should be considered prior to chemotherapy or radiation.

Pearls

- Pleomorphic xanthoastrocytoma (PXA) are predominantly WHO grade II tumors, although malignant transformation and atypia can be seen.
- These tumors most commonly occur in the temporal lobe and are usually cortically based.
- Well-circumscribed cyst with mural nodule or simply solid nodule is typical.
- There is T2 hyperintensity of the solid component unless there is atypia.
- There is usually intense enhancement of the solid component, which typically abuts the pial surface with dural reaction, which may appear to be a dural tail.
- Prognosis is generally good with grade II tumors and surgical resection with 70% survival in 10 years.
- Atypia and incomplete resection worsens prognosis.

Suggested Readings

Gallo P, Cecchi PC, Locatelli F, et al. Pleomorphic xanthoastrocytoma: long-term results of surgical treatment and analysis of prognostic factors. *Br J Neurosurg.* 2013 Dec;27(6):759-764.

Mascalchi M, Muscas GC, Galli C, Bartolozzi C. MRI of pleomorphic xanthoastrocytoma: case report. *Neuroradiology.* 1994 Aug;36(6):446-447.

Tien RD, Cardenas CA, Rajagopalan S. Pleomorphic xanthoastrocytoma of the brain: MR findings in six patients. *AJR Am J Roentgenol.* 1992 Dec;159(6):1287-1290.

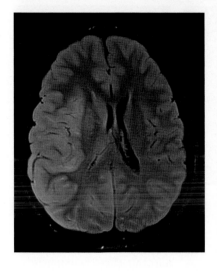
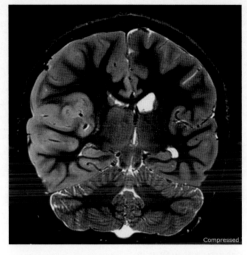
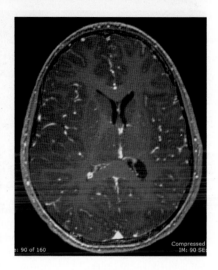

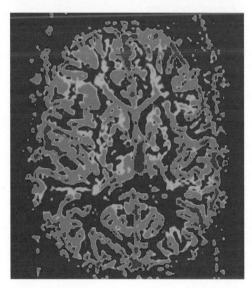

1. What is the differential diagnosis?

2. What is the histopathology of this disease?

3. What are characteristic radiographic findings
   for this disease?

4. What is the best imaging modality for imaging
   the extent of this disease?

5. What is the prognosis?

Case ranking/difficulty:

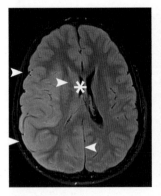

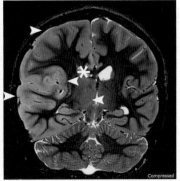

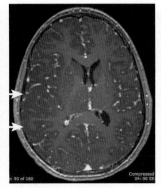

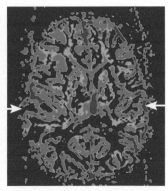

Axial FLAIR image demonstrates diffuse gyral thickening with increased FLAIR signal intensity involving the right insular, frontal, parietal, and temporal lobes as well as in the right basal ganglia, and right thalamus (*white arrowheads*). Also noted is effacement of the cortical sulci and right lateral ventricle (*white asterisk*).

Coronal STIR image demonstrates diffuse gyral thickening with increased STIR signal intensity centered in the right insular and surrounding opercula as well as in the right basal ganglia and right thalamus (*white arrowheads*). Also noted is effacement of the cortical sulci and right lateral ventricle (*white asterisk*). There appears to be relative sparing of the white matter in this case of gliomatosis cerebri.

Postcontrast T1 image demonstrates no abnormal contrast enhancement (*arrows*).

CBV image from dynamic susceptibility contrast perfusion technique demonstrates similar perfusion characteristics with the contralateral hemisphere (*arrows*).

5. Poor prognosis, 50% mortality by 1 year and 75% by 3 years. Surgical resection is not an option due to diffuse disease. Predominantly oligodendrocytic tumors may have a longer mean survival.

Answers

1. The differential for this case of gliomatosis cerebri with predominantly asymmetric mass-like involvement of the gray matter is challenging, but includes encephalitis, metabolic disorder, and lymphoma. Follow-up imaging should show evolution in encephalitis and metabolic disorder while lymphoma and gliomatosis cerebri are likely to show relentless progression.

2. Gliomatosis cerebri can have variable histopathology with astrocytic, oligodendrocytic, or mixed cell lineages with variable proliferation leading to tumor grading from low (II) to high (IV). Typically, elongated glial cells diffusely infiltrate into the parenchyma and myelinated fibers with relative preservation of the brain architecture. The extent of tumor infiltration on imaging is usually disproportionate to the histological features.

3. Typical radiographic features include diffuse, poorly circumscribed, infiltrating, nonenhancing T1 iso- to hypo/T2 hyperintense mass involving predominantly cerebral white matter (76%) and less commonly the cortices (19%). The infiltrating mass typically causes some mass effect, with enlargement but retaining the underlying brain architecture.

4. MRI is the modality of choice due to high-contrast resolution and better characterization of the brain parenchyma. CT may be normal due to isodensity of the infiltrating mass with less appreciable mass effect on the cortical sulci and brain parenchyma.

Pearls

- Rare diffusely infiltrating primary brain tumor.
- Can affect any part of the brain, spinal cord, optic nerves, and any age group, with peak incidence in the fifth to sixth decade.
- Discordance between clinical presentation, imaging, and variable histopathological findings.
- Classic radiographic features include diffuse, poorly circumscribed, infiltrating nonenhancing T1 iso- to hypo/T2 hyperintense lesion, predominantly involving cerebral white matter and at least three contiguous lobes.
- Central gray and white matter structures commonly involved with cortex in a minority of cases.
- Focal neoplastic mass with enhancement and necrosis may develop over time.
- Chemotherapy and radiation may improve neurological function in some patients.

Suggested Readings

Bendszus M, Warmuth-Metz M, Klein R, et al. MR spectroscopy in gliomatosis cerebri. *AJNR Am J Neuroradiol*. 2000 Feb;21(2):375-380.

Shin YM, Chang KH, Han MH, et al. Gliomatosis cerebri: comparison of MR and CT features. *AJR Am J Roentgenol*. 1993 Oct;161(4):859-862.

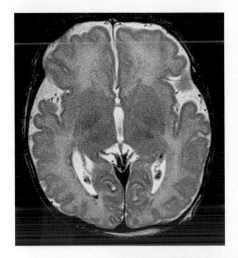
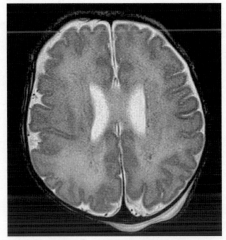
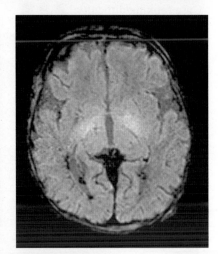

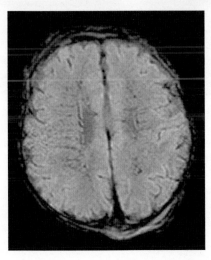
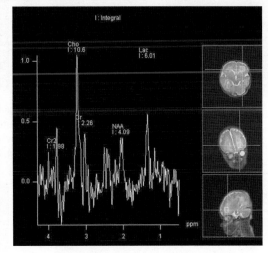

1. What areas of the brain are premature infants most susceptible to injury?

2. What pathophysiologic factors of the premature brain contribute to specific areas being more susceptible to ischemia?

3. When does ADC pseudonormalize in neonates?

4. What is seen on T1, T2, and T2* images in the subacute phase of the disease?

5. What are late-stage imaging sequelae of this disease?

Case ranking/difficulty:

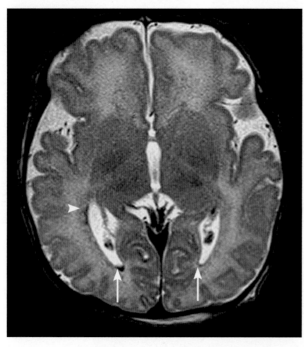

Axial T2 image demonstrates foci of T2 hypointensity along periventricular white matter bilaterally (*white arrowhead*) as well as layering intraventricular blood products (*white arrows*).

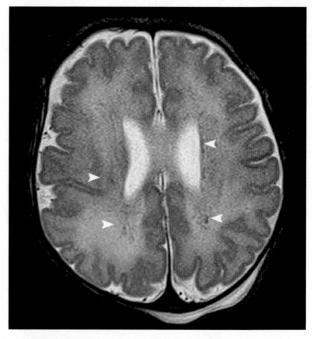

Axial T2 image demonstrates foci of T2 hypointensity along periventricular and deep white matter bilaterally (*white arrowheads*), suggestive of petechial hemorrhage related to reperfusion injury.

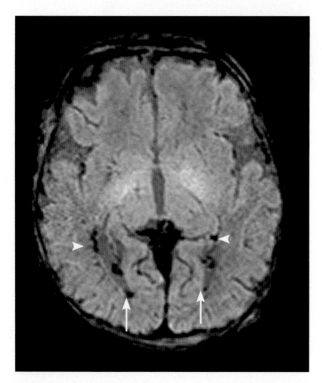

Axial susceptibility-weighted image demonstrates foci of susceptibility artifacts along periventricular white matter bilaterally (*white arrowheads*) and occipital horns of the lateral ventricles (*white arrows*) consistent with blood products.

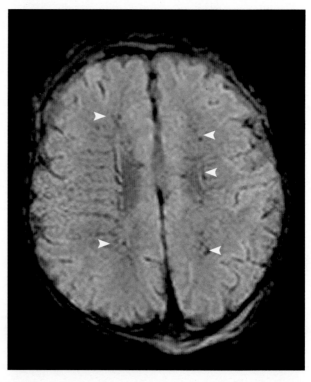

Axial SWI image demonstrates foci of susceptibility artifacts along deep white matter bilaterally (*white arrowheads*), suggestive of petechial hemorrhage related to reperfusion injury.

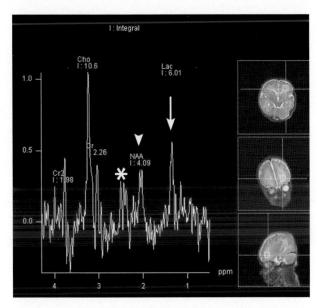

MRI spectroscopy single voxel short echo with voxel placement over the left frontal white matter shows elevated lactate (*arrow*), decreased NAA (*arrowhead*), and elevated glutamate (*asterisk*) consistent with brain injury.

Answers

1. Areas commonly injured in hypoxic ischemic encephalopathy in the premature infant include the periventricular white matter (giving rise to germinal matrix hemorrhages and periventricular leukomalacia), deep white matter, and with severe hypoperfusion, the cerebellum and deep nuclei.

2. Multiple factors of the premature brain contribute to susceptibility to injury in the deep and periventricular white matter, including sensitivity of oligodendrocytic precursors, lack of cerebrovascular autoregulation, increased venous pressure and capillary fragility, with increased susceptibility to reperfusion hemorrhage. Previous theories of ventriculopetal end arteries leading to a water-shed zone have been disputed.

3. ADC pseudonormalization tends to occur faster in neonates (5-7 days compared to adults [7-10 days], with DWI less useful in assessing neonatal hypoxic ischemic injury unless scanned early in the pathologic process.

4. In the subacute phase of hypoxic ischemic injury, T1 hyperintensity and T2 hypointensity can be seen either from hemorrhage or from myelin breakdown products. With hemorrhage, blooming susceptibility artifact can be seen on T2* imaging.

5. Evolution of preterm white matter injury involves cavitation and cystic change that can be incorporated into the lateral ventricle, which, in the chronic stage, can demonstrate large lateral ventricles with angular margins and white matter gliosis.

Pearls

- Very low birth weight (<1500 g) are at greatest risk.
- Typical patterns of premature brain injury involve the periventricular (periventricular leukomalacia, PVL) and deep white matter and the grade I-IV germinal matrix hemorrhages.
- In severe hypoperfusion, the deep gray nuclei, brainstem, and cerebellum are also involved.
- MRI is the most sensitive and specific imaging technique.
- DWI performed between 24 hours and 5 days of life is more sensitive for the detection of cytotoxic edema.
- T1 hyperintensity and T2 hypointensity may be seen in the subacute phase with blooming on T2* with hemorrhage.
- MR spectroscopy with decreasing NAA and increasing lactate correlates with worse prognosis.

Suggested Readings

Chao CP, Zaleski CG, Patton AC. Neonatal hypoxic-ischemic encephalopathy: multimodality imaging findings. *Radiographics*. 2006 Oct;26(suppl 1):S159-S72.

Liauw L, van der Grond J, Slooff V, et al. Differentiation between peritrigonal terminal zones and hypoxic-ischemic white matter injury on MRI. *Eur J Radiol*. 2008 Mar;65(3):395-401.

Liauw L, Palm-Meinders IH, van der Grond J, et al. Differentiating normal myelination from hypoxic-ischemic encephalopathy on T1-weighted MR Images: a new approach. *AJNR Am J Neuroradiol*. 2007 Apr;28(4):660-665.

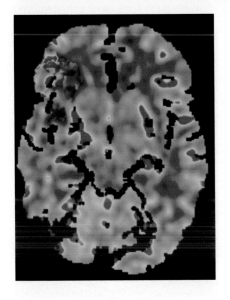 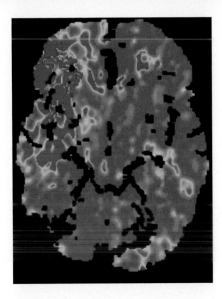 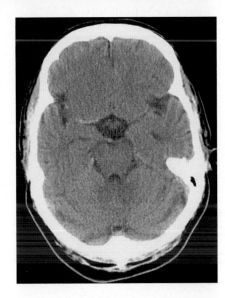

1. What are the findings?

2. What is the diagnosis?

3. What findings indicate a potentially reversible penumbra is present?

4. Is an acetazolamide challenge indicated?

5. What is the most sensitive perfusion map for ischemia?

Case ranking/difficulty:

Category: Intra-axial supratentorial

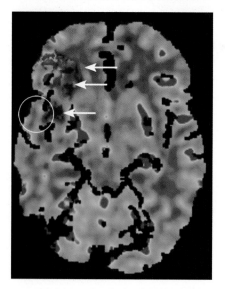

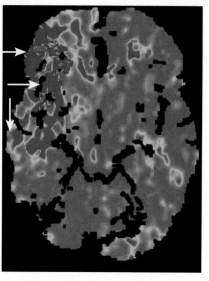

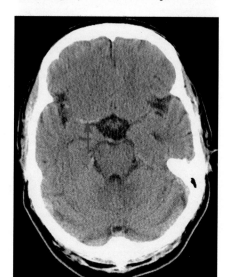

CT perfusion cerebral blood volume (CBV) map shows subtle asymmetry with decrease in the right frontal and temporal lobe cortex (*circle*) and subcortical white matter (*arrows*).

CT perfusion mean transit time (MTT) map demonstrates increase in the right frontal and temporal lobes (*arrows*). Compared to CBV, the mismatched zones in the periphery of the right frontal and temporal lobes indicate reversible ischemic penumbra. Centrally, the areas of matched increased MTT and decreased CBV correspond closely with completed infarct.

CT axial noncontrast image demonstrates no appreciable loss of gray-white differentiation. Asymmetric high density is seen in the right MCA, M1 segment, the "hyperdense MCA" sign (*arrow*).

Answers

1. Elevated mean transit time in the right anterior MCA distribution with only slightly decreased cerebral blood volume.

2. Acute infarct with large penumbra.

3. MTT and CBV mismatch indicates salvageable tissue. Mild decrease in CBV may occur after oxidative stress; however, it is mostly preserved due to autoregulation in potentially salvageable tissue.

4. Acetazolamide challenge is useful to assess vascular reserve after angiography reveals steno-occlusive disease.

5. Most studies in the literature focus on the mean transit time (MTT) as the most sensitive CT perfusion parameter of reversible and irreversible cerebral ischemia.

- Elevated MTT is the most sensitive CT perfusion map for brain ischemia.
- Decrease in CBV is usually seen with irreversible ischemia.
- Matched perfusion defects (elevated MTT with decreased CBV) suggests irreversible ischemia, whereas mismatched perfusion defects (elevated MTT with normal to increased CBV) indicate potentially salvageable tissue (ischemic penumbra).
- Acetazolamide challenge may be helpful to gauge cerebrovascular reserve in patients with vaso-occlusive disease.

Suggested Readings

Allmendinger AM, Tang ER, Lui YW, Spektor V. Imaging of stroke: Part 1, Perfusion CT—overview of imaging technique, interpretation pearls, and common pitfalls. *AJR Am J Roentgenol.* 2012 Jan;198(1):52-62.

Huang AP, Tsai JC, Kuo LT, et al. Clinical application of perfusion computed tomography in neurosurgery. *J Neurosurg.* 2014 Feb;120(2):473-488.

Pearls

- On perfusion imaging, cerebral blood flow (CBF), cerebral blood volume (CBV), and mean transit time (MTT) are physiologic features used to evaluate acute stroke.

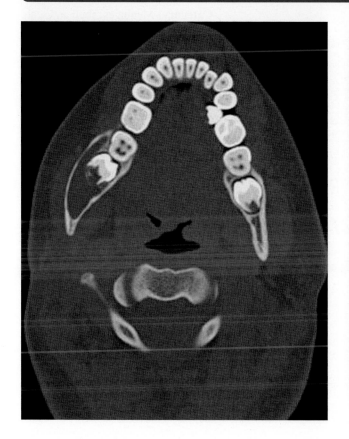
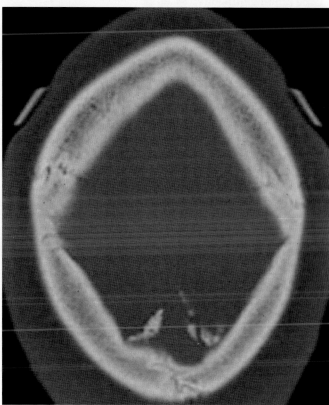

1. What findings are associated in this syndrome?

2. What is the differential diagnosis for the mandibular lesion?

3. What is the best imaging modality in diagnosis?

4. What is the genetic inheritance of this syndrome?

5. Which chromosome is abnormal in this syndrome?

Case ranking/difficulty:

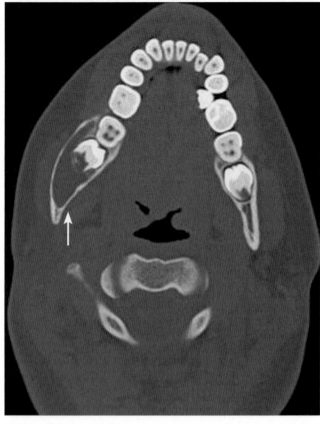

Axial CT image through the mandible shows an expansile lucent lesion (*arrow*) in the right angle of the mandible associated with an unerupted molar without cortical breakthrough.

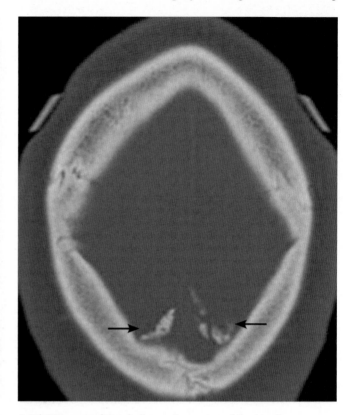

Axial CT image of the skull near the vertex of the head demonstrates prominent dural calcification along a reflection of the superior sagittal sinus (*arrows*).

Answers

1. Basal cell nevi and carcinoma, multiple jaw keratocysts, dural calcification, bifid ribs, and desmoplastic medulloblastoma can be seen in basal cell nevus syndrome (Gorlin syndrome).

2. Periapical (radicular) cyst, dentigerous (follicular) cyst, ameloblastoma, and giant cell granulomas are common differentials for expansile lucent lesions of the jaw. In a child, Langerhans histiocytosis can also be considered.

3. Head and maxillofacial CT is the modality of choice to demonstrate cystic lesions in the jaw and dural calcifications. Head CT is also helpful in assessing for desmoplastic medulloblastomas.

4. Two-thirds of Gorlin syndrome are secondary to autosomal dominant inheritance with complete penetrance and variable expression. One-third of patients are from sporadic mutations.

5. Basal cell nevus syndrome is associated with a mutation of PTCH gene on chromosome 9.

Pearls

- Basal cell nevus syndrome (Gorlin syndrome).
- Autosomal dominant (2/3 of patients) with complete penetrance; sporadic mutation in 1/3 of patients.
- Abnormal gene localized to chromosome 9.
- Characteristic features: multiple odontogenic keratocysts, early dural calcifications, and basal cell nevi and carcinomas.
- Odontogenic keratocysts (keratocystic odontogenic tumor: KOT) in Gorlin syndrome usually develop earlier than nonsyndromic KOT.
- Associated with desmoplastic medulloblastoma.

Suggested Readings

Saulite I, Voykov B, Mehra T, Hoetzenecker W, Guenova E. Incidental finding of lamellar calcification of the falx cerebri leading to the diagnosis of gorlin-goltz syndrome. *Case Rep Dermatol.* 2013 Mar;5(3):301-303.

Stavrou T, Dubovsky EC, Reaman GH, Goldstein AM, Vezina G. Intracranial calcifications in childhood medulloblastoma: relation to nevoid basal cell carcinoma syndrome. *AJNR Am J Neuroradiol.* 2000 Apr;21(4):790-794.

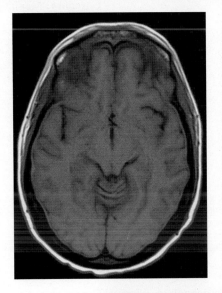
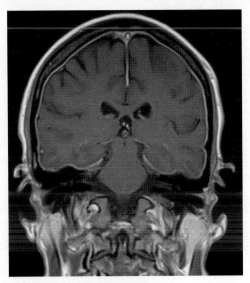

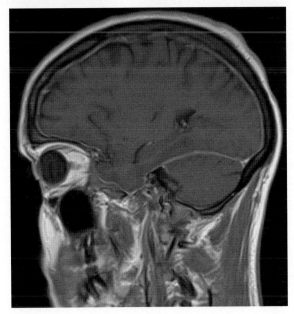

1. Where is the abnormality located?

2. What are the classic imaging findings for this entity?

3. What is the differential diagnosis?

4. What are presenting symptoms for this lesion?

5. What is the treatment for this entity?

Case ranking/difficulty:

Category: Meninges, skull and scalp

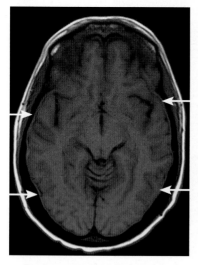

Axial T1 noncontrast image shows thickened appearance to the pachymeninges (*arrows*).

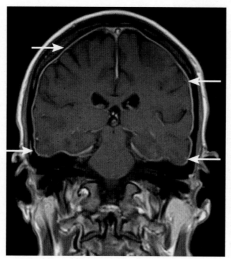

Coronal T1 postcontrast demonstrates diffuse smooth enhancement of the thickened pachymeninges (*arrows*).

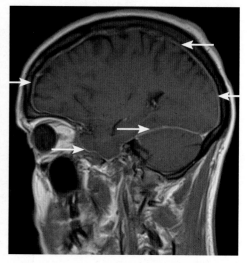

Sagittal T1 postcontrast again shows diffuse pachymeningeal enhancement (*arrows*).

Answers

1. The abnormality involves the dura (which is abnormally thickened).

2. On MRI, the dura is classically isointense to brain on T1- and T2-weighted images. On postcontrast imaging, continuous, smooth linear enhancement is seen, which is usually greater than 2 mm in thickness.

3. The differential diagnosis includes hypertrophic pachymeningitis, dural venous sinus thrombosis, dural metastasis, sarcoid, and meningitis.

4. Patients may presents with ataxia, seizure, cranial nerve dysfunction (commonly optic and vestibular-cochlear), diabetes insipidus, and hoarseness. Of these, headache is the most common symptom.

5. The treatment for this entity includes steroids and immunosuppressants.

Pearls

- Hypertrophic pachymeningitis is the intracranial manifestation of idiopathic inflammatory pseudotumor.
- When the cavernous sinuses are involved = Tolosa-Hunt syndrome.
- Histologically shows a mixed lymphocytic inflammatory infiltrate with fibrosis.

- If brainstem is displaced inferiorly "sagging brainstem" consider intracranial hypotension.
- Diagnoses of neoplasia and infection must be excluded.
- On postcontrast imaging, continuous, smooth, dural enhancement is seen, which is usually greater than 2 mm in thickness.
- The best diagnostic clue is on coronal imaging where continuous enhancement is seen from the vertex extending over the temporal lobes (turn the corner sign).

Suggested Readings

Holodny AI, Kirsch CF, Hameed M, Sclar G. Tumefactive fibroinflammatory lesion of the neck with progressive invasion of the meninges, skull base, orbit, and brain. *AJNR Am J Neuroradiol.* 2001 May;22(5):876-879.

Lee YC, Chueng YC, Hsu SW, Lui CC. Idiopathic hypertrophic cranial pachymeningitis: case report with 7 years of imaging follow-up. *AJNR Am J Neuroradiol.* 2003 Jan;24(1):119-123.

McKinney AM, Short J, Lucato L, SantaCruz K, McKinney Z, Kim Y. Inflammatory myofibroblastic tumor of the orbit with associated enhancement of the meninges and multiple cranial nerves. *AJNR Am J Neuroradiol.* 2007 Mar;27(10):2217-2220.

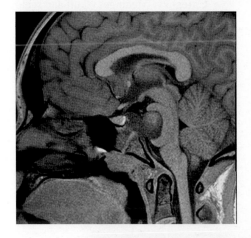
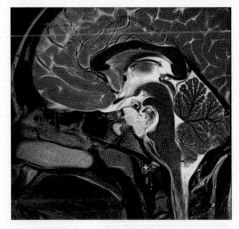
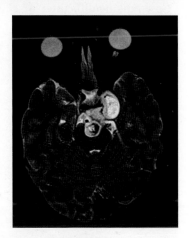

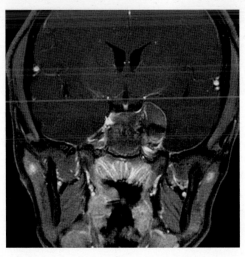
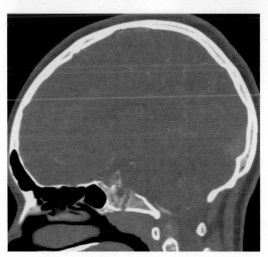

1. What is the differential diagnosis in an adult?

2. What are the characteristic radiographic features?

3. What are possible clinical presentations?

4. What is the best imaging modality?

5. What is the treatment option?

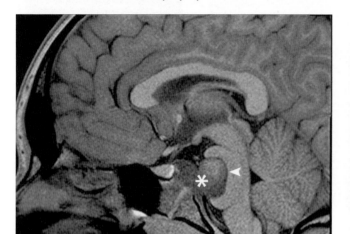

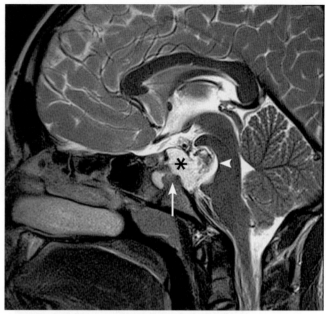

Sagittal T1 image demonstrates a lobulated, destructive mass (*white asterisk*) arising from the posterior basisphenoid clivus with cortical disruption, causing mass effect to the pons (*white arrowhead*) demonstrating the "thumb sign." This mass shows heterogeneous T1 signal intensity, with some foci of T1 shortening, suggestive of hemorrhage or calcification.

Sagittal T2 image demonstrates a lobulated destructive mass (*black asterisk*) arising from the posterior basisphenoid clivus with cortical disruption (*white arrow*), causing mass effect to pons (*white arrowhead*). This mass shows predominantly T2 hyperintensity with focal areas of hypointensity.

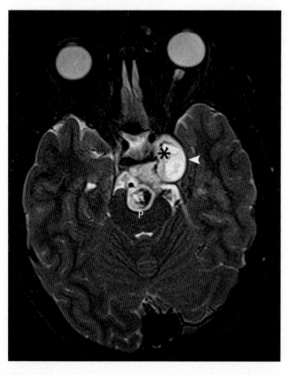

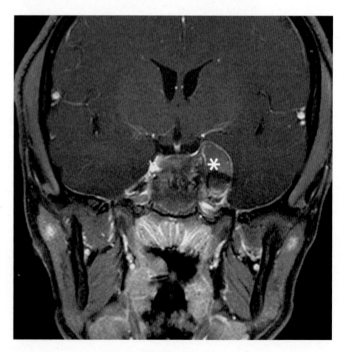

Postcontrast coronal T1 image demonstrates heterogenous contrast enhancement of the skull base mass extending to the left cavernous sinus (*white asterisk*).

Axial T2 image demonstrates an extension of the skull base mass to the left cavernous sinus (*black asterisk*), with mass effect to the left middle cranial fossa (*white arrowhead*) and pons (P).

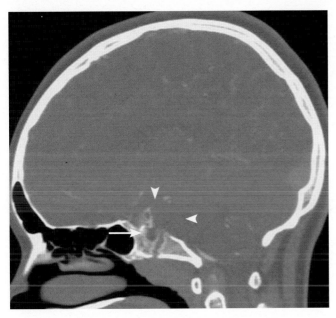

Sagittal CT images demonstrate a soft tissue mass (*white arrowheads*) arising from the posterior basisphenoid with cortical disruption (*white arrow*).

Answers

1. Differential diagnosis of skull base lesions in adults includes chondrosarcoma, chordoma, metastasis, plasmacytoma, and invasive pituitary macroadenoma. This was a typically appearing chordoma in a 10-year-old child, an atypical age presentation.

2. Typical radiographic features include soft tissue mass involving the clivus with destruction of bone, relatively well-circumscribed margins, predominantly T2 hyperintense, with heterogeneous contrast enhancement.

3. Clinical presentations are varied, depending on mass effect of the tumor to adjacent structures and/or cranial nerves. These symptoms include headache, diplopia, ophthalmoplegia, facial pain/palsy, visual loss, and hearing loss.

4. CT and MRI have complementary roles in tumor evaluation; CT is ideal for degree of bone involvement, destruction, and calcification patterns while MRI better characterizes the extent of soft tissue tumor to adjacent structures.

5. Surgery is a mainstay of treatment to obtain tissue for diagnosis and reduce tumor burden. Adjuvant radiation is employed to reduce local recurrence. Prognosis is poor, with 40% 10-year survival.

Pearls

- Rare, slow growing, locally aggressive tumor along the notochord remnant.
- Most common locations are sacrococcygeal (50%), skull base (35%), and vertebral bodies (15%).
- Rarely distant metastasis.
- Divided into three groups: conventional, chondroid chordoma, and dedifferentiation into sarcoma.
- Most common clinical presentations are gradual onset of diplopia and headache.
- CT shows degree of bone involvement, with expansion of the clivus, lytic destruction, and calcified sequestered bone with relatively circumscribed margins.
- MRI features include soft tissue mass with expansile lytic lesion and heterogenous contrast enhancement, predominantly T2 hyperintense with T1 hypointensity and areas of T1 hyperintensity.
- Indentation of the pons in the sagittal plane has been termed the "thumb sign."

Suggested Readings

Meyers SP, Hirsch WL, Curtin HD, Barnes L, Sekhar LN, Sen C. Chordomas of the skull base: MR features. *AJNR Am J Neuroradiol*. 1994 Mar;13(6):1627-1636.

Laine FJ, Nadel L, Braun IF. CT and MR imaging of the central skull base. Part 2. Pathologic spectrum. *Radiographics*. 1990 Sep;10(5):797-821.

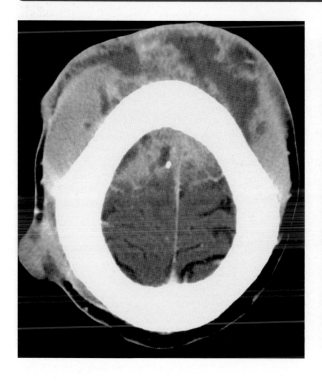 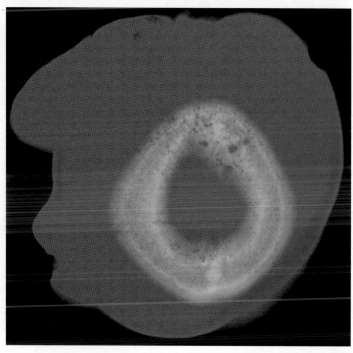

1. Where is the abnormality located?

2. What are the typical imaging findings for this entity?

3. What is the differential diagnosis?

4. What are common presenting symptoms?

5. What is the treatment for this entity?

Case ranking/difficulty:

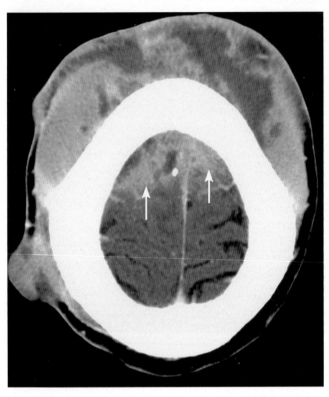

Axial CT with contrast shows heterogeneous enhancing scalp mass extending into the intracranial extraaxial space through the skull (*arrows*).

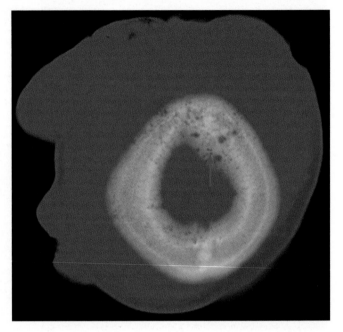

Axial CT without contrast shows lucent permeative lesions of the involved skull (*arrow*).

Answers

1. The abnormality is located within the frontal bone where a permeating pattern is present. Also noted is a large soft tissue scalp mass with extradural extension.

2. Primary non-Hodgkin lymphoma of the skull commonly involves the scalp, bone, and meninges. Typically, there is a permeating pattern within the bone with a large soft tissue component.

3. The differential diagnosis includes metastasis, hemangiopericytoma, and lymphoma.

4. Scalp lymphoma usually presents with a painless scalp lump with headaches due to bone destruction by tumor infiltration.

5. The treatment for this entity is typically a combination of chemotherapy and radiation.

Pearls

- Primary cutaneous B-cell lymphoma of the scalp is rare.
- Primary non-Hodgkin lymphoma of the skull is more likely to have intracranial extradural invasion.
- Scalp lymphoma usually presents with a painless scalp lump with headaches due to bone destruction by tumor infiltration.
- Typically, there is a permeating pattern within the bone with a large soft tissue component.
- The skin is the second most common site of extranodal lymphoma.

Suggested Readings

Kantarci M, Erdem T, Alper F, Gundogdu C, Okur A, Aktas A. Imaging characteristics of diffuse primary cutaneous B-cell lymphoma of the cranial vault with orbital and brain invasion. *AJNR Am J Neuroradiol.* 2003 Aug;24(7):1324-1326.

Kosugi S, Kume M, Sato J, et al. Diffuse large B-cell lymphoma with mass lesions of skull vault and ileocecum. *J Clin Exp Hematop.* 2013;53(3):215-219.

Martin J, Ramesh A, Kamaludeen M, Udhaya M, Ganesh K, Martin JJ. Primary non-Hodgkin's lymphoma of the scalp and cranial vault. *Case Rep Neurol Med.* 2012;616813.

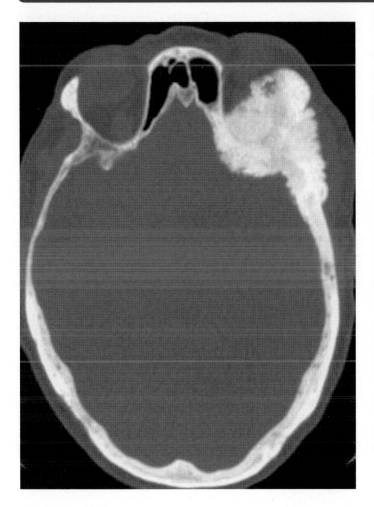
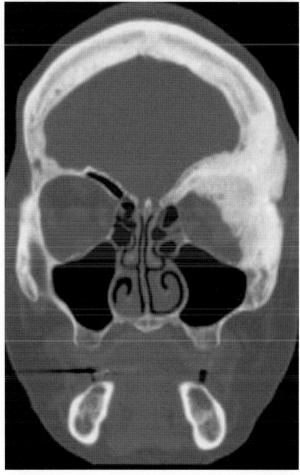

1. What is the differential diagnosis?

2. What are typical imaging findings for this entity?

3. What are common locations for this disease?

4. What is the etiology of this entity?

5. What is the treatment for this disease?

Case ranking/difficulty: **Category:** Meninges, skull and scalp

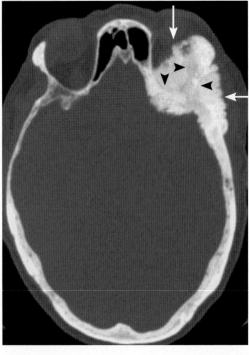

Axial CT bone window image shows an expansile mass centered at the frontal, sphenoid, and zygomatic junctions, which has a "sunburst" appearance without associated soft tissue mass (*arrows*). Note the preservation of underlying internal trabecular architecture (*arrowheads*) consistent with intraosseous meningioma.

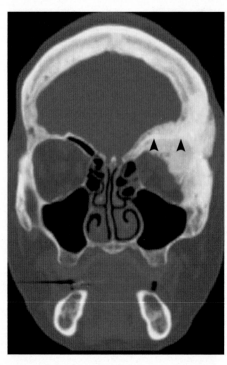

Coronal CT bone window image shows the expansile mass causes mass effect on left orbital structures. There is relative preservation of the internal trabecular architecture (*arrowheads*).

Answers

1. The differential diagnosis for a sclerotic expansile calvarial mass includes intraosseous meningioma (IM), fibrous dysplasia, osteosarcoma, osteoblastic metastasis, and Paget disease.

2. The typical findings for primary IM includes an expansile sclerotic mass with maintenance of the internal trabecular architecture with homogeneous enhancement best seen on MRI.

3. Frontal, parietal, and orbital lesions are the most common sites of calvarial extradural meningiomas. Temporal bone intraosseous meningiomas are also well described in the literature.

4. Primary IM is thought to arise from precursor meningocytes or arachnoid cap cells theoretically trapped in cranial sutures.

5. While primary intraosseous meningiomas are rare, most reported cases only require follow-up with rare findings of cranial neuropathy. While malignant transformation is more common than intradural meningiomas, the reported rate is still low (11%).

Pearls

- Primary intraosseous meningioma is a rare subset of extradural meningiomas.
- Preservation of internal trabecular architecture is a helpful sign for distinguishing from other benign bony tumors.
- 35% can have osteolytic appearance.
- Slightly higher rate of malignant transformation compared to intradural meningiomas.
- Frontal-parietal and orbital lesions most common.
- Has been described in temporal bones and skull base.

Suggested Readings

Hamilton BE, Salzman KL, Patel N, et al. Imaging and clinical characteristics of temporal bone meningioma. *AJNR Am J Neuroradiol.* 2006;27(10): 2204-2209.

Tokgoz N, Oner YA, Kaymaz M, Ucar M, Yilmaz G, Tali TE. Primary intraosseous meningioma: CT and MRI appearance. *AJNR Am J Neuroradiol.* 2005 Sep;26(8):2053-2056.

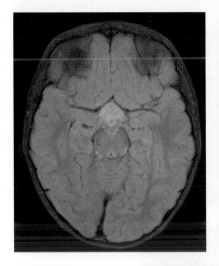
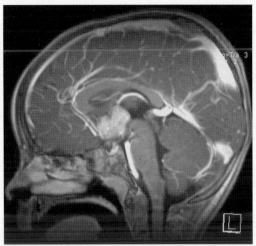
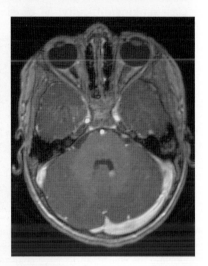
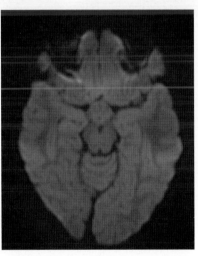
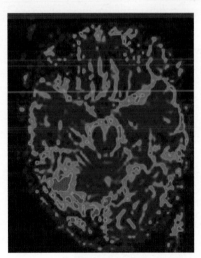

1. What is the differential diagnosis?

2. What are typical MRI findings for this entity?

3. What are clinical differences between pilomyxoid astrocytomas and pilocytic astrocytomas?

4. What are histologic findings in this tumor?

5. What can be seen with perfusion and diffusion imaging?

Case ranking/difficulty:

Category: Sellar/suprasellar

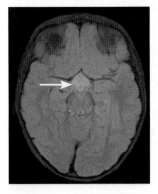

Axial FLAIR image shows a hyperintense mass involving the chiasm and hypothalamus (*arrow*).

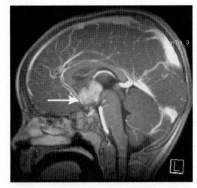

Sagittal T1 postcontrast image shows intense enhancement of the optic chiasmal/hypothalamic mass extending into the third ventricle (*arrow*).

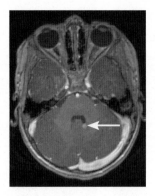

Axial T1 postcontrast image shows a leptomeningeal metastatic deposit in the fourth ventricle (*arrow*).

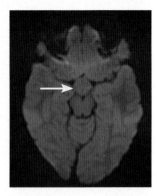

Axial DWI b = 1000 image shows no restricted diffusion of the suprasellar mass (*arrow*).

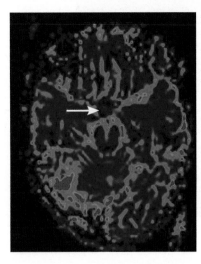

Axial color CBV map from dynamic susceptibility contrast perfusion shows no increased perfusion of the suprasellar mass (*arrow*).

Answers

1. The differential for midline enhancing masses in the suprasellar cistern includes pilomyxoid astrocytoma, pilocytic astrocytoma, and germinomas.

2. Pilomyxoid astrocytomas most commonly involve the hypothalamic/optic chiasm, with T2 hyperintensity, lack of diffusion restriction, and large size at presentation with invasion of adjacent structures.

3. Pilomyxoid astrocytomas tend to occur in younger children and infants, have a greater likelihood to have CSF dissemination, and have a lower overall survival rate than pilocytic astrocytomas. No neuroimaging characteristic is reliable for distinguishing between the two tumors.

4. Pilomyxoid astrocytomas are characterized by neoplastic astrocytes with angiocentric orientation in a myxoid background.

5. Pilomyxoid astrocytoma will usually show increased diffusion and decreased perfusion compared to higher grade tumors.

Pearls

- Pilomyxoid astrocytomas (PMA, WHO grade II) are classified as a more aggressive variant of pilocytic astrocytomas (PA, WHO grade I).
- PMAs are more likely to demonstrate CSF dissemination and are associated with a worse outcome than PAs.
- PMA tend to occur in younger children and infants than PAs.
- The hypothalamic chiasmal region is the most common with extension into the temporal lobes.
- The tumors are typically T2 hyperintense with intense homogeneous enhancement and no restricted diffusion.
- Despite large size and adjacent structure invasion, there is usually little peritumoral edema.

Suggested Readings

Arslanoglu A, Cirak B, Horska A, et al. MR imaging characteristics of pilomyxoid astrocytomas. *AJNR Am J Neuroradiol.* 2003 Oct;24(9):1906-1908.

Linscott LL, Osborn AG, Blaser S, et al. Pilomyxoid astrocytoma: expanding the imaging spectrum. *AJNR Am J Neuroradiol.* 2008 Nov;29(10):1861-1866.

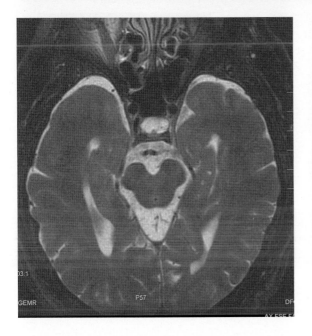
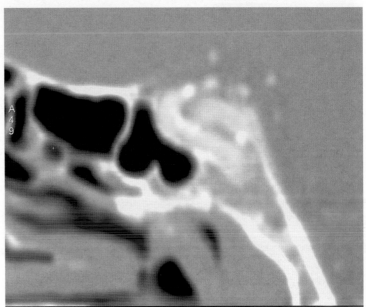

1. Where is the abnormality located?

2. What are the classic imaging findings for this entity?

3. What is the differential diagnosis?

4. What are presenting symptoms for this lesion?

5. What is the treatment for this entity?

Case ranking/difficulty:

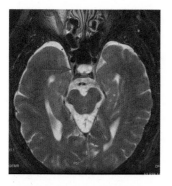

Axial T2 image shows a flow void within the right aspect of the cavernous sinus (*arrow*).

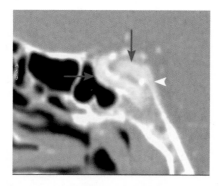

Sagittal CTA image demonstrates a direct connection between the cavernous sinus (*red arrow*) and internal carotid artery (*green arrow*). There is drainage into the basilar venous plexus (*arrowhead*).

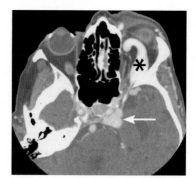

Axial CTA image of an 87-year-old female with left eye proptosis shows a significantly enlarged superior ophthalmic vein (*asterisk*) with associated enlarged vascular structures of the left cavernous sinus (*arrow*).

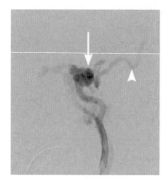

AP view of a left internal carotid artery injection in an 87-year-old female with left eye proptosis shows immediate contrast filling of the left cavernous sinus (*arrow*) in the early arterial injection with filling of the vein of Labbe (*arrowhead*).

Pearls

- Carotid-cavernous fistula (CCF) is a direct connection between the internal carotid artery and the cavernous sinus.
- These fistulas drain via the superior ophthalmic vein or the petrosal sinuses.
- Secondary to trauma or internal carotid artery aneurysm rupture.
- CCF should be considered with unilateral enlargement of the cavernous sinus and superior ophthalmic vein.
- On MRI, CCF is likely present when a flow void is seen in the cavernous sinus.
- On angiogram, contrast is seen filling the cavernous sinus after injection of the ipsilateral carotid artery.

Answers

1. The abnormality is located within the right cavernous sinus.

2. Classic imaging findings for carotid-cavernous fistula (CCF) are an enlarged superior ophthalmic vein, unilateral proptosis, and an enlarged cavernous sinus. On MRI, a flow void may be seen within the cavernous sinus. CTA or MRA may demonstrate the direct connection between the cavernous sinus and internal carotid artery.

3. The differential diagnosis includes aneurysm, carotid-cavernous sinus fistula, and vascular malformation.

4. Patients with this entity may present with cranial nerve deficits (III-VI), visual changes, pulsating exophthalmos, headache, and bruit.

5. The treatment for this entity is typically endovascular, and if this fails, surgery is the final option. Embolization may be performed (with coils, particles, adhesive, and balloons) vs stent deployment.

Suggested Readings

Archondakis E, Pero G, Valvassori L, Boccardi E, Scialfa G. Angiographic follow-up of traumatic carotid cavernous fistulas treated with endovascular stent graft placement. *AJNR Am J Neuroradiol*. 2007 Feb;28(2):342-347.

Horowitz M, Levy E, Bonaroti E. Cavernous carotid origin aneurysm rupture with intracerebral intraparenchymal hemorrhage after treatment of a traumatic Barrow type A cavernous carotid artery fistula. *AJNR Am J Neuroradiol*. 2006 Mar;27(3):524-526.

van Rooij WJ. Endovascular treatment of cavernous sinus aneurysms. *AJNR Am J Neuroradiol*. 2012 Feb;33(2):323-326.

Regional Subject Index

Note: Numbers in parentheses refer to Case IDs.

Subchapter Index

Note: Numbers in parentheses refer to Case IDs.

Alphabetical Subject Index

Note: Numbers in parentheses refer to Case IDs.

Difficulty Level Index

Note: Numbers in parentheses refer to Case IDs.

Author Index

Note: Numbers in parentheses refer to Case IDs.

Acknowledgment Index

Note: Numbers in parentheses refer to Case IDs.